HUMAN NUTRITION

Readings from
**SCIENTIFIC
AMERICAN**

HUMAN NUTRITION

With Introductions by
Norman Kretchmer and William van B. Robertson
Stanford University

W. H. Freeman and Company
San Francisco

Most of the *Scientific American* articles in *Human Nutrition* are available as separate Offprints. For a complete list of more than 950 articles now available as Offprints, write to W. H. Freeman and Company, 660 Market Street, San Francisco, California 94104.

Library of Congress Cataloging in Publication Data

Main entry under title:

Human nutrition.

   Bibliography: p.
   Includes index
   1. Nutrition—Addresses, essays, lectures. I. Kretchmer, Norman, 1923–   II. Robertson, William van B.
III. Scientific American. [DNLM: 1. Nutrition—
Collected works. QU145.3 H9184]
QP141.H79   613.2   78–17367
ISBN 0–7167–0183–9
ISBN 0–7167–0182–0

Printed in the United States of America

9 8 7 6 5 4 3 2 1

PREFACE

Nutrition can be defined as the sum of the processes by which an organism obtains, takes in, and utilizes food substances. Human nutrition is so exceptionally complex that it can only be understood by drawing upon the insights of a large number of scientific disciplines: Agricultural science, anthropology, archeology, the social and behaviorial sciences, economics, and geography, together with classical nutritional science and its allied disciplines of biochemistry, physiology, and medicine. The present collection of articles is designed to introduce the reader to the variety of subjects encompassed within modern nutritional science.

The first section places food in proper perspective as a major component of the biosphere. Two of the most important biological processes that contribute to food supply are photosynthesis and nitrogen fixation. These processes give rise to the molecules that make up the basic building blocks of a number of energy-containing and growth-promoting nutrients utilized by both plants and animals. Ready availability of these nutrients to man was made possible by a series of historical events, a major cultural upheaval known as the Agricultural Revolution, which occurred about 10,000 to 8,000 years ago. The basis of this revolution was the domestication of plants and animals, as a result of which humans learned to live in permanent settlements and thus assure themselves of a year-round supply of food. Thus the Agricultural Revolution not only laid the groundwork for the rise of civilization, it also brought about far-reaching changes in human nutrition.

Section II is concerned with important sources of foods that have been adopted as staples by various human societies. Each of these foods has an extensive history of use and a complicated pattern of geographical dispersion. The history of the selection of specific foodstuffs is described in Section III. Selection is determined by many factors. These factors may be as simple as color, texture, and availability, or they may derive from complex, age-old pressures exerted by religion or culture. A society's choice of foods may in turn influence its culture and its chances of survival.

Section IV surveys the nutrients required by the human body. In a living system nutrients must enter the cells in order to be utilized. Transport of nutrients into the cell is a complicated process that involves expenditure of energy and the participation of specific cellular proteins, carbohydrates, and lipids. Inside the cell, enzymes act upon the incoming molecules of nutrients, catalytically transforming them into a vast array of compounds that enter into the *economy* of the cell and ultimately the whole organism.

Some results of inadequate nutrition are described in Section V. Adequate nutrition is a prerequisite for the proper development of the individual. Poor nutrition plays a major role in the causation of many diseases, and nutrition itself can be manipulated as a factor in the treatment of disease.

The explosive growth of the world's population and the resulting severe competition for food supplies should be of serious concern to any student of nutrition. Section VI touches upon some of the key problems. Present and future nutritional programs will have to incorporate plans for achieving a balance of food supplies, energy sources, and population. The task of achieving this balance is the most urgent problem facing the world today. In the United States, both the Congress and the president have identified nutrition as an area for extreme concern and immediate action by the federal government. In an executive order issued August 25, 1977, President Jimmy Carter stated that the potential benefits from organized federal action in nutrition should be:

More coherent food policy . . . ;

Better integration of food policy and economic policy decisionmaking . . . ;

More consistent and reasonable procedures and standards for food inspection;

More timely decisions on agricultural foreign trade matters;

Improvements in the food supply . . . through more carefully targeted nutrition research; and

A balancing of consumer and economic factors. . . .

Significant progress toward improvement of nutrition for all humankind depends upon increased interest, concern, and action by governments throughout the world.

April 1978   Norman Kretchmer

William van B. Robertson

CONTENTS

V   IMPACT OF DIET ON HUMAN HEALTH AND DISEASE

VI   THE GLOBAL PROBLEM OF HUMAN NUTRITION

Note on cross-references: References to articles included in this book are noted by the title of the article and the page on which it begins; references to articles that are available as Offprints, but are not included here, are noted by the article's title and Offprint number; references to articles published by SCIENTIFIC AMERICAN, but which are not available as Offprints, are noted by the title of the article and the month and year of its publication.

HUMAN NUTRITION

I

NUTRITION
AND THE FLOW OF
ENERGY AND MATTER

NUTRITION AND THE FLOW OF ENERGY AND MATTER

I

INTRODUCTION

All living organisms participate in a *global* flow and transformation of matter and energy. Energy from sunlight is required for transformation of carbon, hydrogen, oxygen, nitrogen, phosphorus, and iron—the inorganic, elemental matter of the earth—into the organic matter of plants, such as carbohydrates, proteins, fats, and nucleotides. The organic material is used by living organisms and returned as inorganic material to the earth and its atmosphere. That portion of the flow of matter that man is able to divert and utilize for his nourishment, and from which he obtains energy, is the proper concern of the study of human nutrition.

In everyday speech the word "energy" has a variety of meanings and is commonly used interchangeably with "power," "strength," "force," and "activity." The scientific concept of energy is more specific, serving as a unifying expression for work or the latent capacity for doing work. Energy can be neither created nor destroyed but only transformed from one form to another. During these transformations a fraction of the energy is converted to heat and is no longer capable of work in that system. For example, when a person metabolizes sugar and fat, some of the chemical energy required to do the work of metabolism is lost to the body in the form of heat. All energy can be converted completely to heat, and all energy eventually ends up as heat. It has thus been common to use a heat unit, the calorie, as the measure of energy. The calorie is the amount of heat necessary to raise a gram of water from 15°C to 16°C. Although the joule, equivalent to 4.18 calories, has been selected as the fundamental energy unit in the Systeme Internationale (SI), it has not yet gained wide acceptance in nutritional work. Energy equivalents of food are still expressed as Calories (kilocalories).

In all living organisms the common medium for energy transformation is a chemical, adenosinetriphosphate, commonly known as ATP. Potentially useful energy absorbed by cells is used to synthesize new molecules of ATP. These molecules are then further metabolized to perform many different types of work within the cell. The processes that have evolved to effect energy transformations by way of ATP are described by A. Lehninger in "How Cells Transform Energy."

Only green plants and some photosynthetic bacteria can transform the radiant energy of the sun into chemical energy by converting inorganic material to organic material having a higher energy content. Animals obtain their energy needs either by eating the organic material of plants (herbivores), eating other animals (carnivores), or by a mixed diet (omnivores). The sequence of transfer of food energy from one organism to another is called a *food chain*. Some chains are simple, as when plants are decomposed by bacteria; others are more complex, as when plants are eaten by herbivorous insects, who are eaten by birds, who in turn are eaten by snakes, who die and are decomposed by bacteria. As material moves along a food chain, about 80 percent of its energy content is converted to heat at each step, a form of energy not utilizable for the nourishment of living organisms. A food chain finally ends when all of the solar energy originally trapped by plants is converted to heat and radiated to outer space, and all of the organic matter converted to inorganic compounds and returned to the earth. (These cycles of energy and matter are discussed in detail in the September 1970 issue of *Scientific American* entitled "The Biosphere.")

Until the present century the input of man and his activities was too small to perturb these grand cycles of nature. Today, however, man's input is significant enough to alter the biosphere. Probably no cycle has felt the impact more than the nitrogen cycle, as a result of the industrial fixation of nitrogen into fertilizer; almost as much nitrogen is fixed industrially as is fixed in nature. Although the use of large quantities of industrially fixed nitrogen has permitted food production to keep pace with food needs in the world, the cost is not negligible. Large quantities of fossil fuel, presently natural gas, are used (30,000 cubic feet of natural gas for each ton of nitrogen fixed). As this resource becomes scarce, the price of synthetic fertilizer will increase to a point where the nations who need it most will not be able to afford it. Considerable research is in progress aimed at developing innovative techniques to make more fixed nitrogen available naturally and thus reestablish the "balance of nature." The present status of our knowledge of this process is discussed by W. J. Brill in "Biological Nitrogen Fixation."

Historically, the world's population has increased only as man has been able to divert more of the cycles of energy and matter to human nutrition. An increased ability to use and control fire has probably been the key factor in developing this increase. Fire was no doubt experienced by the earliest hominids, but only as a phenomenon to be feared. At that time, over a million years ago, man's diet probably consisted of nuts, berries, insects, carrion, and maybe an occasional small animal. Food needs dictated a nomadic existence of small bands in a constant search for food. Although there is some evidence that Peking Man used fire some 600,000 years ago, neither its use nor its production became widespread until toward the latter part of the last glacial period, 50,000 to 75,000 years ago. By that time man had developed a variety of tools (especially the spear). Larger animals could be hunted, killed and utilized. Roasted in the fire, more of this meat became edible than when raw and tough. Hard-shelled seeds that were previously inedible could now be parched, thus cracking the shell and revealing the nutritious endosperm. Caves could be heated and survival thus extended into colder climates. More of the solar energy flow was diverted to man's nutrition. Probably no use of fire had more profound effects on the future than the burning of the land to expose animals to the hunter. Burnt forest lands were replaced by grasses, with their annual yield of seeds. The stage was set for the cultivation of plants and the domestication of animals, the beginnings of the agricultural revolution. (For the epic history of man's association with fire, see "Man the Fire-maker" by Loren Eiseley, *Scientific American*, September 1954.)

This process took place independently in the Near East, in the Americas, and possibly in South East Asia beginning about 6000 to 8000 years ago. No longer was each man's time taken up in the hunt for food. Division of labor was possible, so that some of the group had time to express their creative and inventive abilities. Larger groups of people could be supported by the same land area. Since it was no longer necessary to rove widely in search of food, there was an impetus toward development of settlements; excess food could be accumulated and thus traded for other commodities. An archeological search documenting this transition is presented by Robert J. Braidwood in "From Cave to Village." One chart in this article illustrates the sudden population increase concomitant with man's newfound ability to increase the proportion of solar energy diverted to human nutrition.

Among the accomplishments of agriculture has been its ability to take advantage of the simpler nutritional requirements of other species, such as ruminants, to increase food production for man, even though the overall cost in energy utilization is increased. "The Cycles of Plant and Animal Nutrition" by Jules Janick, Carl H. Noller, and Charles L. Rhykerd looks at food production from the standpoint of the agriculturalist interested in increasing that portion of energy diverted to the use of man.

Beginning about two centuries ago, when man learned to harness energy with the steam engine, significant quantities of fossil fuel have been used in food production. The diversion for human nutrition of solar energy received by the earth eons ago and stored as coal and oil permitted another large increase in population. In the United States in 1974 about seven calories of fossil energy was spent in production, transportation, and preparation of each calorie of food consumed. At no time have so few workers produced so much food as in the United States today. It has been estimated that if the agricultural and food technology available in the United States were applied throughout the world, the world could sustain a population of 6 to 8 billion persons. However, we are beginning to recognize that such massive intervention into the cycles of energy and matter has damaging global consequences, many of which may be unforeseen and irreversible. In a thought-provoking article, "Human Food Production as a Process in the Biosphere," Lester Brown looks at the effects of these interventions and their consequences. Hopefully, we have begun to realize that as part of nature's grand cycles they must be taken into account when we plan long-term activities.

1

How Cells Transform Energy

by Albert L. Lehninger
September 1961

In the chloroplasts of plant cells the energy of sunlight is transformed into chemical fuels. In the mitochondria of animal cells these fuels are oxidized to run the cellular machinery

A living cell is inherently an unstable and improbable organization; it maintains the beautifully complex and specific orderliness of its fragile structure only by the constant use of energy. When the supply of energy is cut off, the complex structure of the cell tends to degrade to a random and disorganized state. In addition to the chemical work required to preserve the integrity of their organization, different kinds of cell transform energy to do the varieties of mechanical, electrical, chemical and osmotic work that constitute the life processes of organisms.

As man has learned in recent times to use energy from inanimate sources to do his work, he has begun to comprehend the virtuosity and efficiency with which the cell manages the transformation of energy. The same laws of thermodynamics that govern the behavior of inanimate substances also govern the energy transactions of the living cell. The first law of thermodynamics says that the sum of mass and energy in any physical change always remains constant. The second law states that there are two forms of energy: "free," or useful, energy; and entropy, or useless or degraded energy. It states furthermore that in any physical change the tendency is for the free energy to decline and the entropy to increase. Living cells must have a supply of free energy.

The engineer gets most of the energy he employs from the chemical bonds in fuel. By burning the fuel he degrades the energy locked in those bonds to heat; he can then use the heat to make steam and drive a turbogenerator to produce electricity. Cells also extract free energy from the chemical bonds in fuels. The energy is stored in those bonds by the cells that manufacture the foodstuffs that serve as fuel. The cell makes use of this energy, however, in a very special way. Since the living cell functions at an essentially constant temperature, it cannot use heat energy to do work. Heat energy can do work only if it passes from one body to another body that has a lower temperature. The cell obviously cannot burn its fuel at the 900-degree-centigrade combustion temperature of coal, nor can it tolerate superheated steam or high voltage. It must therefore obtain energy and use it at a fairly constant and low temperature, in a dilute aqueous environment and within a narrow range of con-

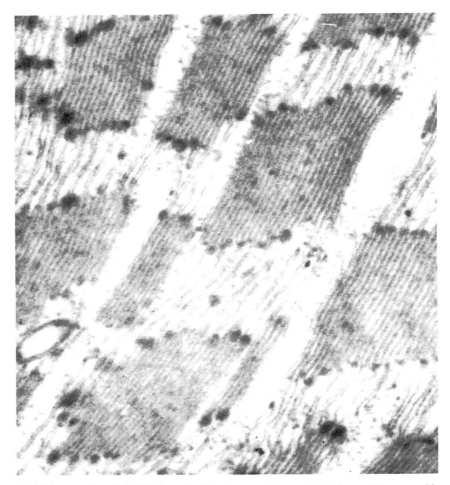

GRANA are enlarged 90,000 times in this electron micrograph by Vatter. They resemble stacks of coins in which chlorophyll is sandwiched between layers of protein and lipid. The lighter material around the grana is the stroma, in which the "dark" reactions take place.

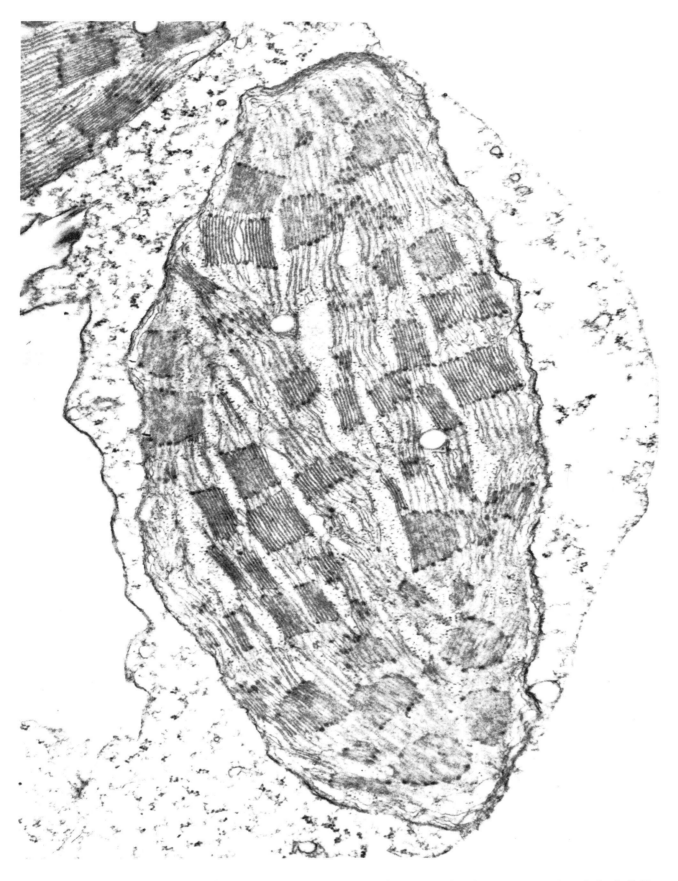

CHLOROPLAST is the site of photosynthesis, whereby light energy is transformed into chemical energy to prime the life cycle of plants and animals. A chloroplast in a maize cell is enlarged 40,000 diameters in this electron micrograph made by A. E. Vatter of Abbott Laboratories. The "light" reactions involving chlorophyll and solar energy take place within the rectangular "grana."

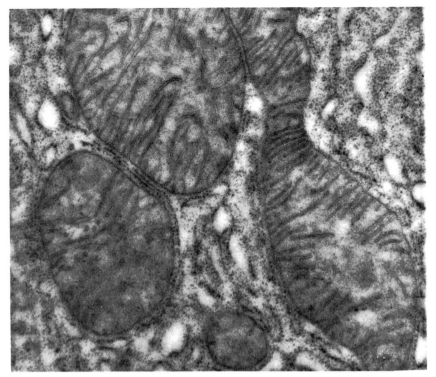

MITOCHONDRION is the site of respiration, the energy-transfer process of animal cells. Four mitochondria of a rat pancreas cell are enlarged 33,000 times in this electron micrograph by George E. Palade of the Rockefeller Institute. The inner membranes of the mitochondria's double wall are involuted to form the characteristic cristae, or folds.

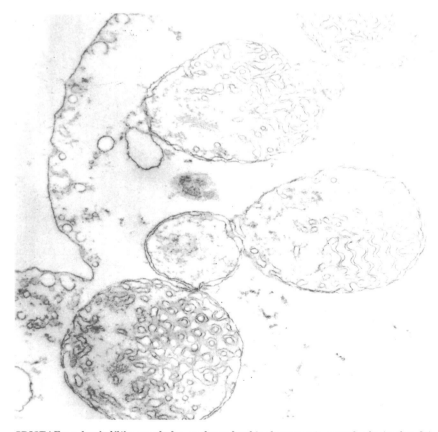

CRISTAE can be shelflike or tubular, as shown by this electron micrograph of mitochondria in a giant amoeba (Chaos chaos) by George D. Pappas and Philip W. Brandt of the Columbia University College of Physicians and Surgeons. Magnification is 27,000 diameters.

centration of hydrogen ions. To secure its primary energy the cell has during the eons of organic evolution perfected extraordinary molecular mechanisms that work with great efficiency under these mild conditions.

The energy-extracting mechanisms of living cells are of two kinds, and they separate all cells into two great classes. The first type of cell, called heterotrophic, includes the cells of the human body and of higher animals in general. This type of cell requires a supply of preformed, ready-made fuel of considerable chemical complexity, such as carbohydrate, protein and fat, which are themselves constituents of cells and tissues. Heterotrophic cells obtain their energy by burning or oxidizing these complex fuels, which are made by other cells, in the process called respiration, using molecular oxygen (O_2) from the atmosphere. They employ the energy so obtained to carry out their biological work, and they give up carbon dioxide to the atmosphere as the end product.

Cells in the other class get their energy from sunlight. Such cells are called autotrophic, or self-reliant. Principal among them are the cells of green plants. By the process of photosynthesis they harness the energy of sunlight for their living needs. They also use solar energy to incorporate carbon from atmospheric carbon dioxide in the elementary organic molecule of glucose. From glucose the cells of green plants and of other organisms build up the more complex molecules of which cells are made. In order to supply energy for this chemical work the cells burn some of the raw material by the mechanism of respiration. From this description of the cellular energy cycle it is clear that living things ultimately derive their energy from sunlight—plant cells directly and animal cells indirectly.

Investigations of the central questions posed here are converging on a complete description of the primary energy-extracting mechanisms of the cell. Most of the steps in the intricate cycles of respiration and photosynthesis have been worked out. Each process has been localized in a specific organ of the cell. Respiration is carried on by mitochondria, large numbers of which are found in almost all cells; photosynthesis is conducted by chloroplasts, the cytoplasmic structures that distinguish the cells of green plants. The molecular devices that make up these structures and perform their functions present the next great frontier to cell research.

From the centers of respiration

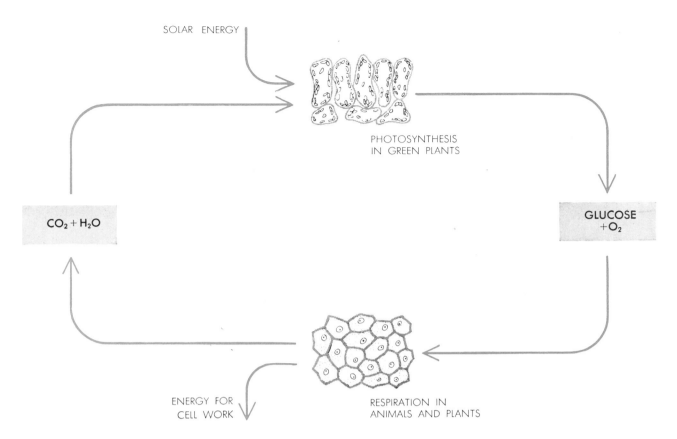

SOLAR ENERGY

PHOTOSYNTHESIS
IN GREEN PLANTS

GLUCOSE
+O_2

CO_2 + H_2O

ENERGY FOR
CELL WORK

RESPIRATION IN
ANIMALS AND PLANTS

CARBON AND ENERGY CYCLE of life is based on the sun as the ultimate source of energy. Solar radiation drives photosynthesis, which builds energy-rich glucose from energy-poor carbon dioxide and water. The glucose and other fuels synthesized from it are then broken down to carbon dioxide and water by animal cells, which use the energy extracted in the process to do their work.

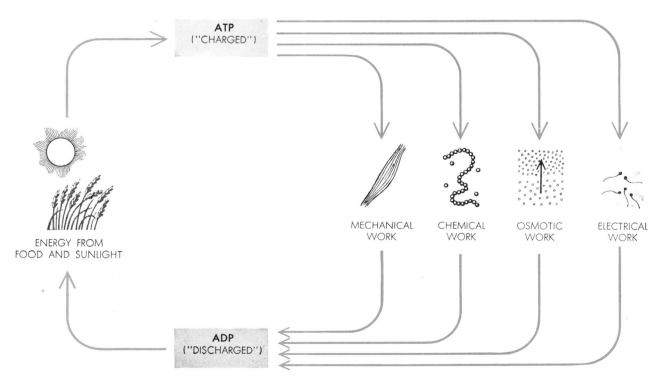

ATP
("CHARGED")

ENERGY FROM
FOOD AND SUNLIGHT

MECHANICAL
WORK

CHEMICAL
WORK

OSMOTIC
WORK

ELECTRICAL
WORK

ADP
("DISCHARGED")

ADENOSINE TRIPHOSPHATE (ATP), the common carrier of energy in animal and plant cells, is formed in the mitochondria and chloroplasts. It supplies energy for muscle contraction, protein synthesis, absorption or secretion against an osmotic gradient and transfer of nerve impulses. "Discharged" adenosine diphosphate (ADP) thus formed is "charged" by solar or food energy.

ADP

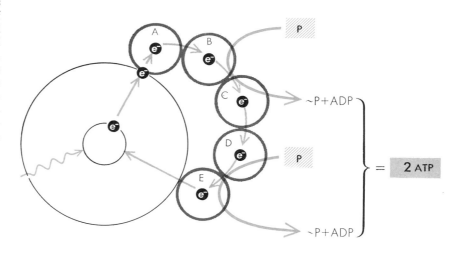

H–N–H

ATP

ATP MOLECULE has one more phosphate group than ADP, attached by a high-energy bond (*wavy line at right of formula*). Solar or food energy is required to make this bond and thus to charge ATP. The chemical energy of the bond is made available again when the ATP is discharged by losing its terminal phosphate, which is transferred to an "acceptor" molecule in the cell. This

and photosynthesis the same well-defined molecule—adenosine triphosphate (ATP)—carries the free energy extracted from foodstuffs or from sunlight to all the energy-expending processes of the cell. ATP, which was first isolated from muscle by K. Lohmann of the University of Heidelberg some 30 years ago, contains three phosphate groups linked together. In the test tube the terminal group can be detached from the molecule by the drastic, one-step reaction of hydrolysis to yield adenosine diphosphate (ADP) and simple phosphate. As this reaction proceeds, the free energy of the ATP molecule appears as heat and entropy, in accordance with the second law of thermodynamics. In the cell, however, the terminal phosphate group is not merely detached by hydrolysis but is transferred to a specific acceptor molecule. The free energy of the ATP molecule is largely conserved by "phosphorylation" of the acceptor molecule, the energy content of which is now raised so that it can participate in an energy-requiring process such as biosynthesis or muscle contraction. Left over from this "coupled reaction" is ADP. In the thermodynamics of the cell ATP may be considered as the energy-rich, or "charged," form of the energy carrier and ADP as the energy-poor, or "discharged," form.

It is, of course, one or the other of the two energy-extracting mechanisms that "recharges" the carrier. In respiration in animal cells the energy of food-

stuffs is released by oxidation and harnessed to regenerate ATP from ADP and phosphate. In photosynthesis in plant cells the energy of sunlight is trapped as chemical energy and harnessed to drive the recharging of ATP. Experiments employing the radioactive isotope phosphorus 32 have shown that the inorganic phosphate passes into the terminal phosphate group of ATP and out again with great rapidity. In a kidney cell the ter-

minal phosphate group turns over so rapidly that its half-life is less than a minute, in consonance with the massive and dynamic flux of energy in the cells of this organ. It should be added that there is really no black magic associated with the action of ATP in the cell. Chemists are familiar with many similar reactions that permit the transfer of chemical energy in inanimate systems. The relatively complex structure of ATP has

CYCLIC PHOTOPHOSPHORYLATION is the process by which an electron in chlorophyll, raised to a high-energy state by a photon of light, provides the energy to make ATP. The excited electron is captured by the first of a chain of "carriers" (*A*) and passed on around a circuit of such molecules (*B through E*), losing energy along the way. Some of the energy couples phosphate to ADP. The cycle ends as the electron returns to chlorophyll.

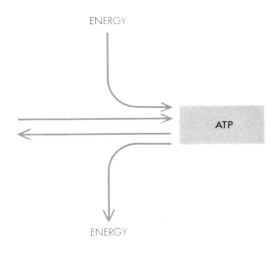

"phosphorylation" raises the energy level of the acceptor molecule. The ADP-ATP reaction is shown in schematic form at the right.

apparently evolved uniquely in the cell to produce maximum control and organization of energy-transferring chemical reactions.

The role of ATP in photosynthesis has only recently been elucidated [see "The Role of Light in Photosynthesis," by Daniel I. Arnon; SCIENTIFIC AMERICAN, November, 1960]. This discovery supplies a major part of the explanation of how photosynthetic cells harness the ultimate energy source of all living things, solar energy, in the synthesis of carbohydrates.

The energy of sunlight comes in packets called photons, or quanta; light of different colors or wavelengths is characterized by different energy content. When light strikes and is absorbed by certain metallic surfaces, the energy of the impinging photons is transferred to electrons of the metal. This "photoelectric" effect can be measured by the resulting flow of electric current. In the green-plant cell, solar energy of a particular range of wavelengths is absorbed by the green pigment chlorophyll. The absorbed energy raises an electron from its normal energy level to a higher level in the bond structure of this complex molecule. Such "excited" electrons tend to fall back to their normal and stable level, and when they do they give up the energy they have absorbed. In a pure preparation of chlorophyll, isolated from the cell, the absorbed energy is re-emitted in the form of visible light, as it is from other phosphorescent or fluorescent organic and inorganic compounds.

Thus chlorophyll itself in the test tube cannot store or usefully harness the energy of light; the energy escapes quickly, as though by short circuit. In the cell, however, chlorophyll is so connected spatially with other specific molecules that when it is excited by the absorption of light, the "hot," or energy-rich, electrons do not simply fall back to their normal positions. Instead these electrons are led away from the chlorophyll molecule by associated "electron carrier" molecules and handed from one to the other around a circular chain of reactions. As they traverse this external path the excited electrons give up their energy bit by bit and return to their original positions in the chlorophyll, which is now ready to absorb another photon. The energy given up by the electrons has meanwhile gone into the formation of ATP from ADP and phosphate; that is, into recharging the ATP system of the photosynthetic cell.

The electron carriers that mediate this process of "photosynthetic phosphorylation" have not yet been fully identified. One of these molecules is believed to contain riboflavin (vitamin B_2) and vitamin K. Others are tentatively identified as cytochromes: proteins containing iron atoms surrounded by porphyrin groups similar in arrangement and structure to the porphyrin of chlorophyll itself. At least two of these electron carriers are able to cause some of the energy they carry to be captured, in order to regenerate ATP from ADP [see illustration at bottom of opposite page]. This appears to be the basic scheme of the conversion of light into the phosphate-bond energy of ATP, as it has been developed by Daniel I. Arnon and his associates at the University of California and by other workers.

The complete photosynthetic process, however, involves the synthesis of carbohydrate as well as the harnessing of

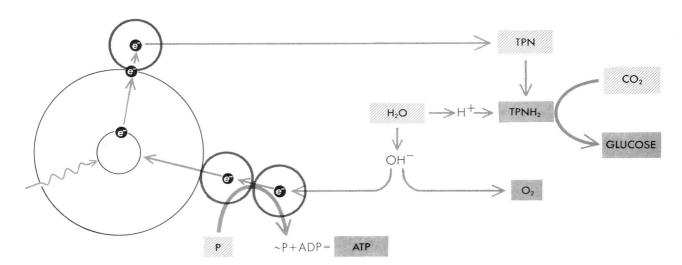

COMPLETE PHOTOSYNTHESIS requires an outside source of electrons and hydrogen ions (protons) to synthesize carbohydrate by "reducing" (adding electrons and hydrogen to) carbon dioxide. The source of electrons is chlorophyll and the source of protons is water. The reducing agent for carbon dioxide is "reduced triphos-phopyridine nucleotide" ($TPNH_2$) formed by the action of protons and electrons on TPN, one of the carrier molecules. The leftover hydroxyl ions (OH^-) of water apparently lose electrons to restore the chlorophyll's supply. In this process oxygen gas, characteristic product of photosynthesis, is evolved and ATP is charged up.

solar energy. It is now believed that some of the "hot" electrons from excited chlorophyll, along with hydrogen ions derived from water, cause the reduction (that is, the addition of electrons or hydrogen atoms) of one of the electron carriers, triphosphopyridine nucleotide (TPN), which in its reduced form becomes $TPNH_2$ [*see illustration at bottom of preceding page*]. In a series of "dark" reactions, so named because they occur in the absence of light, $TPNH_2$ brings about the reduction of carbon dioxide to carbohydrate. Much of the energy necessary for this series of reactions is supplied by ATP [*see illustration at right*]. The pattern of the dark reactions was worked out largely by Melvin Calvin and his associates, also at the University of California. A by-product of the original photoreduction of TPN is the hydroxyl ion (OH⁻). Although the evidence is not yet complete, it is thought that these ions donate their electrons to a cytochrome in the photosynthetic chain, releasing molecular oxygen in the process. The electrons continue down the carrier chain, contributing to the formation of ATP and finally settling—in their energy-depleted state— in the chlorophyll.

As the highly organized and sequential nature of the photosynthetic process suggests, the chlorophyll molecules are not randomly situated or merely suspended in solution inside the chloroplasts. On the contrary, the chlorophyll

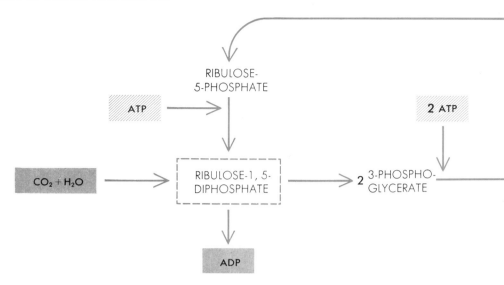

SYNTHESIS OF GLUCOSE from carbon dioxide and water is a dark reaction—that is, it involves a series of reactions that do not directly require light. But it does require two compounds made by light, ATP and $TPNH_2$, as the energy supply and reducing agent respec-

is arranged in orderly structures within the chloroplasts called grana, and the grana in turn are separated from one another by a network of fibers or membranes. Within the grana the flat chlorophyll molecules are stacked in piles. The chlorophyll molecules can therefore be looked on as the single plates of a battery, several plates being organized as in an electric cell, and several cells in a

battery, represented by the chloroplast.

The chloroplasts also contain all the specialized electron-carrier molecules that work together with chlorophyll to extract the energy from the hot electrons and use that energy to synthesize carbohydrate. Separated from the rest of the cell, the chloroplasts can carry out the complete photosynthetic process.

The efficiency of these miniature solar

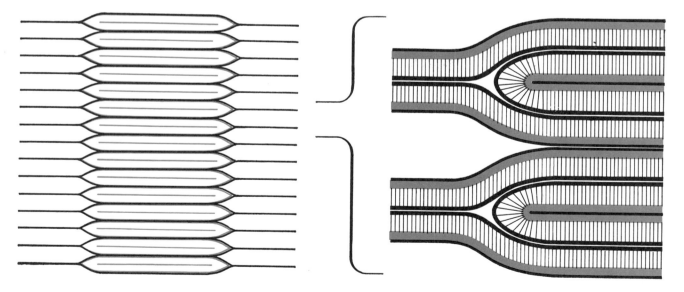

STRUCTURE OF ONE GRANUM in a chloroplast is diagramed in successive magnifications. The chlorophyll (*color*) is concentrated within envelopes stacked to form the granum (*left*), with connecting fibers leading to adjacent grana. In the layers, two of which are magnified (*second from left*), the chlorophyll is sand-

wiched between membranes of protein, according to a hypothetical model proposed by Alan J. Hodge of the California Institute of Technology. In Hodge's model, based on electron microscopy and the "electron carrier" chemistry discussed in the text, the individual chlorophyll molecules are oriented (*third from left*) be-

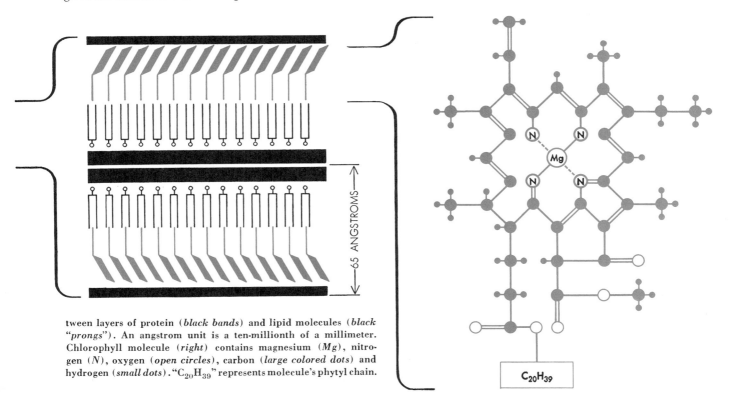

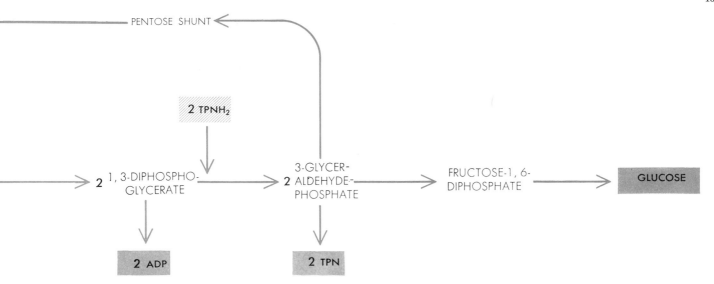

tively. In this complex cycle, shown here only in outline, the key intermediate is ribulose diphosphate, which picks up the carbon dioxide and makes two molecules of phosphoglycerate. This is reduced by TPNH₂ and rearranged in steps, ultimately to become glucose. Meanwhile the ribulose diphosphate is regenerated in a series of reactions abbreviated here as "pentose shunt."

power plants is impressive. Though the exact figures are subject to controversy, it can be demonstrated under special laboratory conditions that the photosynthetic process converts as much as 75 per cent of the light that impinges on the chlorophyll molecule into chemical energy. On the other hand, the efficiency of energy recovery of a field of corn, given the random and uneven exposure of the leaves to sunlight and other conditions of nature, is considerably lower: on the order of only a few per cent.

The molecule of glucose, as the end product of photosynthesis, can therefore be visualized as having a considerable amount of solar energy locked in its molecular configuration. In the process of respiration heterotrophic cells extract this energy by carefully taking apart the glucose molecule step by step, conserving its energy of configuration in the phosphate-bond energy of ATP.

There are different kinds of heterotrophic cell. Some, such as certain marine microorganisms, can live without

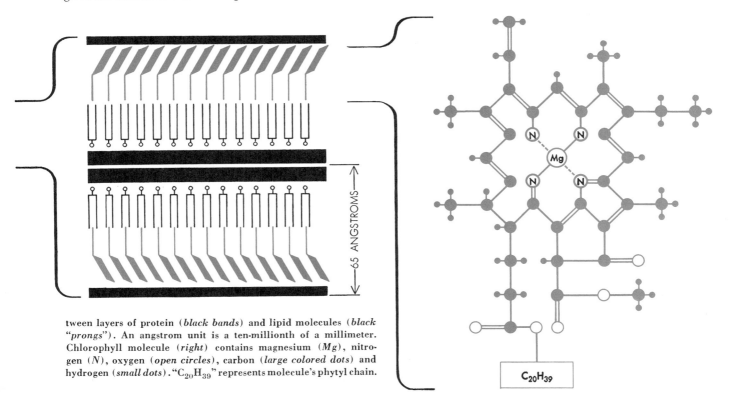

tween layers of protein (*black bands*) and lipid molecules (*black "prongs"*). An angstrom unit is a ten-millionth of a millimeter. Chlorophyll molecule (*right*) contains magnesium (*Mg*), nitrogen (*N*), oxygen (*open circles*), carbon (*large colored dots*) and hydrogen (*small dots*). "C₂₀H₃₉" represents molecule's phytyl chain.

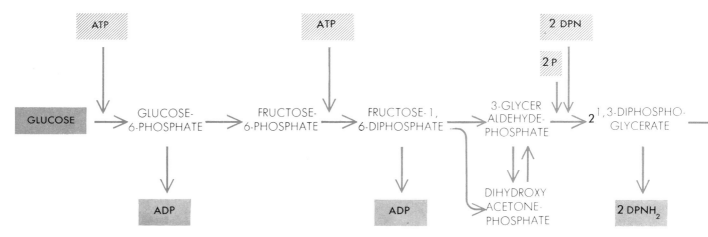

GLYCOLYSIS is the first step in energy recovery from glucose. As comparison of this diagram with the upper one on pages 12 and 13 will show, many of the steps are the reverse of those in the dark synthesis of glucose by plants. Six-carbon glucose is broken down

oxygen; some, such as brain cells, absolutely require oxygen; some, such as muscle cells, are more versatile, being able to function either aerobically or anaerobically. Furthermore, although most cells prefer glucose as the major fuel; some can live exclusively on amino acids or fatty acids synthesized from glucose as the basic raw material. The disassembly of the glucose molecule by the liver cell may be taken, however, as typical of the process by which most known aerobic heterotrophs obtain energy.

The total amount of energy available in a molecule of glucose may be quite simply determined. By burning a sample in the laboratory it can be shown that the oxidation of the glucose yields six molecules of water and six molecules of carbon dioxide, with the evolution of

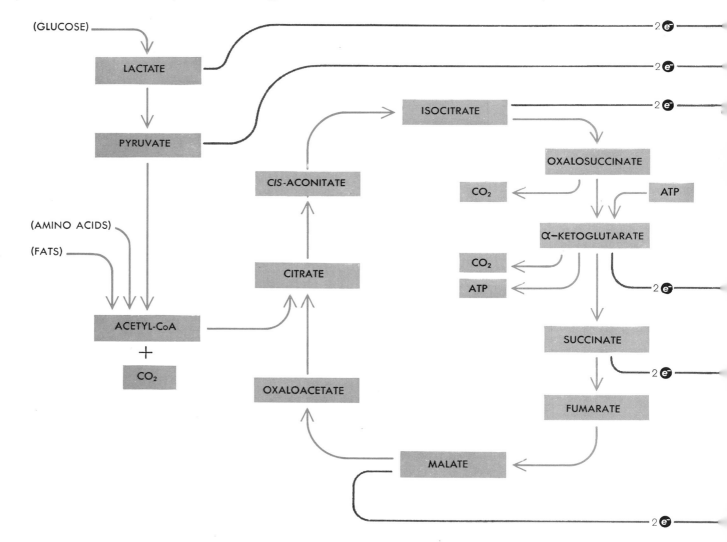

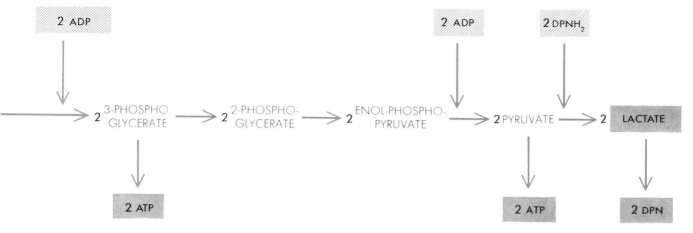

into two molecules of three-carbon lactate (or lactic acid; the ionic rather than the acid form of the intermediate compounds is shown in the diagrams). Two molecules of ATP are used up in glycolysis but four are formed, for a net gain of two molecules of ATP.

some 690,000 calories of energy per gram molecular weight (that is, per 180 grams of glucose) in the form of heat. Energy in the form of heat is, of course, useless to the cell, which functions under essentially constant temperature conditions. The step-by-step oxidation of glucose achieved by the mechanism of respiration occurs in such a way, however, that much of the free energy of the glucose molecule is conserved in a form that is useful to the cell. In the end more than 50 per cent of the available energy is recovered in the form of phosphate-bond energy. This recovery compares most favorably with the standard of the engineer, who rarely converts more than a third of the heat of combustion into useful mechanical or electrical energy.

The oxidation of glucose in the cell proceeds in two major phases. The first, or preparatory, phase, called glycolysis, brings about the splitting of the six-carbon glucose molecule into two three-carbon molecules of lactic acid. This seemingly simple process occurs not in one step but at least 11 steps, each catalyzed by a specific enzyme. If the complexity of this operation seems to contradict the Newtonian maxim *Natura enim simplex est*, then it must be borne in mind that the function of the reaction is to extract chemical energy from the glucose molecule and not merely to split it in two. Each of the intermediate products contains phosphate groups, and a net of two molecules of ADP and two phosphates are used up in the reaction.

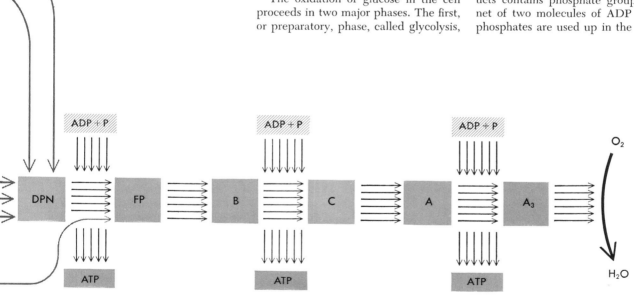

KREBS "CITRIC ACID" CYCLE finally oxidizes the products of glycolysis to carbon dioxide and water. Lactate is first converted to pyruvate, which in turns goes to acetyl coenzyme A. (Here fat and protein join carbohydrate in the metabolic process.) There follows a cycle of reactions, involving the regeneration of oxaloacetate, in which carbon compounds are broken down to carbon dioxide. Electrons removed at various stages are passed down a "respiratory chain" of electron carriers: diphosphopyridine nucleotide (DPN), a flavoprotein enzyme (FP) and a series of iron-containing enzymes: cytochromes B, C, A and A₃. As the electrons pass down the chain, ultimately to reduce oxygen to water, they drive the phosphorylations in which ATP is formed. Each molecule of lactate contributes six pairs of electrons; five of these charge up three ATP molecules each and the sixth makes two ATP's. One more ATP is formed in the citric acid "mill" itself, so a total of 36 molecules of ATP is produced by the two molecules of lactate that were formed from the original glucose molecule.

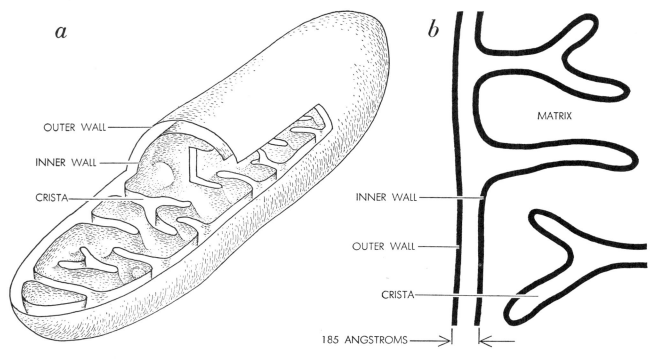

STRUCTURE OF MITOCHONDRION is basically that of a fluid-filled vessel with an involuted wall (*a*). The wall consists of a double membrane (*b*), with infoldings of the inner one forming cristae. Each membrane is apparently constructed of a layer of pro-

Ultimately the splitting of glucose not only yields two molecules of lactic acid but also generates two new molecules of ATP [*see illustration at top of preceding two pages*].

What does this mean in terms of energy? Thermodynamic equations show that the splitting of a gram molecule of glucose to lactic acid makes a total of 56,000 calories available. Since the charging of each gram molecule of ATP captures about 10,000 calories of energy, the yield at this stage is about 36 per cent, a respectable figure by engineering standards. The conversion of 20,000 calories represents, however, a small fraction—only 3 per cent—of the total of 690,000 calories bound in the glucose. Yet many cells, such as anaerobic cells or muscle cells in exercise (which are unable to conduct the process of respiration), function on this small yield.

With glucose now broken down to lactic acid, aerobic cells proceed to extract a major portion of the remaining energy by the process of respiration, in which the three-carbon lactic acid molecule is broken down to single-carbon molecules of carbon dioxide. The lactic acid, or rather its oxidized form pyruvic acid, undergoes an even more complex series of reactions, each step again being catalyzed by a specific enzyme system [*see illustration at bottom of preceding two pages*]. First the three-carbon compound is broken down to an activated form of acetic acid—acetyl coenzyme A —and carbon dioxide. The two-carbon acetic acid compound then combines with a four-carbon compound, oxaloacetic acid, to make the six-carbon citric acid. This is degraded again to oxaloacetic acid by a series of reactions, and the three-carbon atoms of pyruvic acid that were fed into this cyclic mechanism at last appear as carbon dioxide. This "mill," which oxidizes not only glucose but also fat and amino acid molecules previously broken down to acetic acid, is known as the Krebs citric acid cycle. It was first postulated by Sir Hans Krebs in 1937 in one of the great landmarks of modern biochemistry and honored by a Nobel prize in 1953.

Although the Krebs cycle accounts for the oxidation of lactic acid to carbon dioxide, it alone does not explain how the large amount of energy remaining in these molecules is extracted in useful form. The process of energy recovery that accompanies the action of the Krebs cycle has been an intensely active field of investigation in recent years. While the over-all picture can be described with some assurance, there are many details yet to be solved. In the course of the cycle, it appears, electrons are extracted from the intermediates by enzymes and fed into a series of electron-carrier molecules, collectively called the respiratory chain. This chain of enzyme molecules is the final common pathway of all electrons removed from foodstuff molecules during biological oxidation. At the last link in the chain, the electrons combine with oxygen to form water. The breakdown of foodstuffs by respiration therefore in essence reverses the process of photosynthesis in which electrons are removed from water to form oxygen. Moreover, it is striking that the electron carriers in the respiratory chain bear many chemical similarities to those of the corresponding chain in photosynthesis. They contain, for example, riboflavin and cytochrome structures similar to those in the chloroplast. The Newtonian simplicity of nature is thereby affirmed.

As in photosynthesis, the energy of the electrons passing along the chain to oxygen is tapped off and used to drive the coupled synthesis of ATP from ADP and phosphate. Actually this respiratory-chain phosphorylation, or oxidative phosphorylation, is better understood than the more recently discovered photosynthetic phosphorylation. One thing known with certainty is that there are three points along the chain at which ATP is recharged. For each pair of elec-

c

d

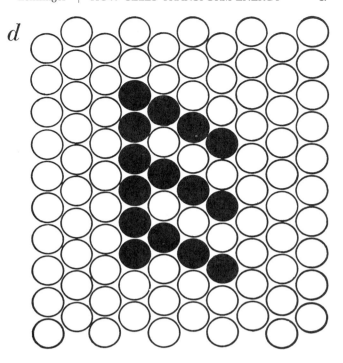

|←————— 185 ANGSTROMS —————→|

tein molecules (*spheres at "c"*) lined by a double layer of lipid molecules (*black-tailed spheres*). The respiratory-chain electron

carriers and enzymes appear to be regularly spaced elements (*black spheres at "d"*) of the protein monolayers. The "matrix" is fluid.

trons split from lactic acid in the course of its oxidation in the Krebs cycle, therefore, an average of three molecules of ATP are formed.

From the total yield of ATP molecules it' is now possible to calculate the thermodynamic efficiency with which the cell extracts the energy made available by the oxidation of glucose. The preliminary splitting of glucose to two molecules of lactic acid yields two molecules of ATP. Each molecule of lactic acid in turn delivers ultimately six pairs of electrons to the respiratory chain. Since three molecules of ADP are "charged up" to ATP for each pair of electrons traversing the chain, 36 molecules of ATP are formed in the respiratory process proper. On the rough estimate of 10,000 calories each, the 38 molecules of ATP incorporate in their phosphate bonds some 380,000 of the 690,000 calories contained in the original gram molecule of glucose. The efficiency of the combined processes of glycolysis and respiration can therefore be estimated as a minimum of 55 per cent.

The intricacy of the respiratory process in particular suggests again that the enzymatic machinery involved could not do its work if its component parts were randomly mixed together in solution. Just as the molecular devices of photosynthesis appear to be spatially

oriented to one another in the chloroplast, so the organ of respiration in the cell, the mitochondrion, presents the same picture of structured order. There may be anywhere from 50 to 5,000 mitochondria in a cell, depending on its type and function. A single liver cell of the rat contains about 1,000 mitochondria. They are large enough (three to four microns long) to be seen in the cytoplasm with a light microscope. But their ultrastructure requires the electron microscope in order to be seen.

In electron micrographs it can be seen that the mitochondrion has two membranes, the inner one occurring in folds in the body of the structure. Recent research on mitochondria isolated from cells of the liver has shown that the Krebs-cycle enzyme molecules are located in the matrix, or soluble portion of the inner contents, but the respiratory-chain enzymes, in the form of molecular "assemblies," are located in the membranes [see "Energy Transformation in the Cell," by Albert L. Lehninger; SCIENTIFIC AMERICAN Offprint 69]. The membranes consist of alternating layers of protein and lipid (fatty) molecules, just as do the membranes of the grana of the chloroplasts. Indeed, there is a remarkable similarity in the structure of these two fundamental power plants of

all cellular life, one capable of capturing solar energy in ATP and the other of transforming the energy of foodstuffs to ATP energy.

Modern chemistry and physics have recently been able to specify the three-dimensional structure of certain large molecules, such as those of proteins and of DNA, the molecules that carry genetic information. The next great step in cell research is to find out how the large enzyme molecules, themselves proteins, are arranged together in the mitochondrial membranes, together with the lipids, so that each catalyst molecule is properly oriented and therefore able to react with the next one in the working assembly. The "wiring diagram" of the mitochondrion is already clear!

If the classical engineering science of energy transformation is humbled by what is now known about the power plants of the cell, so are the newer and more glamorous branches of engineering. The technology of electronics has achieved amazing success in packaging and miniaturizing the components of a computer. But these advances still fall far short of accomplishing the unbelievable miniaturization of complex energy-transducing components that has been perfected by organic evolution in each living cell.

2

Biological Nitrogen Fixation

by Winston J. Brill
March 1977

Only a few bacteria and simple algae have the cellular equipment needed to "fix" the nitrogen of the atmosphere into ammonia. They are the major suppliers of this limited agricultural resource

Antoine Laurent Lavoisier gave nitrogen the name "azote," meaning "without life," because it differed from the other main component of air (oxygen) in being unable to sustain the metabolism of living organisms. The name has turned out to be an ironic one. Nitrogen is an essential constituent of proteins, and we now know that large amounts of it are required by all forms of life. Indeed, for both plants and animals nitrogen is probably the commonest limitation to growth, and an inadequate supply of nitrogen for agriculture is an important factor contributing to human hunger.

Nitrogen is at once an abundant element, making up almost 80 percent of the earth's atmosphere, and a scarce nutritional resource. The paradox is easily

explained: the form of nitrogen in air is so inert that it is useless to the vast majority of organisms. Nitrogen can enter biological systems only when it has been "fixed," or combined with certain other elements, such as hydrogen or oxygen. Today the fixation can be accomplished industrially, through the manufacture of ammonia from hydrogen and atmospheric nitrogen. The making of ammonia and of other chemical fertilizers derived from it is now a major industry, but the bulk of all fixed nitrogen is of biological origin.

In nature, nitrogen fixation is a faculty reserved to a few genera of bacteria. (Included among these bacteria are several blue-green algae, a group of organisms that today are generally classified with the bacteria under the name cyano-

bacteria.) No higher organisms have developed the capability, although several participate indirectly by forming symbiotic associations with nitrogen-fixing bacteria. The best-known of these relations is the one between the plants called legumes and various bacteria of the genus *Rhizobium*. Other nitrogen-fixing bacteria associate with other host plants, and many live freely in the soil or in water. A few are photosynthetic; some require oxygen; others can grow only when oxygen is excluded from their environment. All these organisms apparently share a common mechanism for nitrogen fixation; as in the industrial process, the initial product is ammonia. They also share a unique enzyme: nitrogenase. We are just beginning to unravel the structure of nitrogenase, to learn how it functions and how it is regulated and to understand what characteristics distinguish the organisms that possess it. The potential benefits of this knowledge can be reckoned in a higher worldwide standard of living. The cost of fertilizer has increased dramatically in the past few years, affecting the cost of food in the more affluent countries and restricting the supply of food in the less affluent ones. If the nitrogen-fixing activities of bacteria can be understood, they might also be improved, and ultimately they might be conferred on other organisms, perhaps including cereal crops. The result would be reduced dependence on nitrogenous fertilizer.

Nitrogen Chemistry

The nitrogen in the atmosphere is a diatomic gas, that is, it consists of molecules made up of two atoms each, denoted N_2. Molecular nitrogen is nearly inert because the chemical bond joining the atoms is exceptionally strong and stable; it is a triple bond and a large quantity of energy must be supplied in order to break it.

In industrial fixation the required energy is provided by fossil fuels. In a process developed in the early years of the 20th century by Fritz Haber and Karl Bosch atmospheric nitrogen is

SUBSTANCE	FORMULA	STRUCTURE
MOLECULAR NITROGEN	N_2	
NITRATE ION	NO_3	
AMMONIA	NH_3	
PEPTIDE (SUBSTRUCTURE OF PROTEINS)	$-NH-CH-C-$ (R, O)	

FIXATION OF NITROGEN is the conversion of the abundant but nearly inert molecular gas N_2 into compounds useful to living organisms. In biological fixation and in the industrial Haber process the immediate product is ammonia. Nitrates are another source of fixed nitrogen common in soil and in chemical fertilizers. Most of the nitrogen that enters biological systems is made into proteins, molecules made up of amino acids linked by a carbon-nitrogen bond.

combined with hydrogen at high temperature and pressure in the presence of a catalyst containing iron. The product is ammonia (NH_3), which is itself an effective fertilizer and which can be converted into other useful nitrogen compounds, such as urea and nitrates.

The energy cost of the Haber process becomes apparent when the source of the required hydrogen is considered: it is extracted from natural gas or petroleum. For this reason the cost of nitrogenous fertilizers is closely correlated with the cost of fossil fuels.

In the soil fixed nitrogen from industrial fertilizer or from natural sources is taken up by plant roots and is ultimately employed in the synthesis of biological molecules. By far the largest share is incorporated in the structure of proteins, the versatile molecules that are responsible for metabolism in living cells. Proteins are made up of amino acids, all of which contain at least one atom of nitrogen. A typical protein might be composed of a few hundred amino acid units. A crucial structural element is the peptide bond, which links one amino acid to the next; the bond connects a nitrogen atom in one amino acid to a carbon atom in another.

Through plant and animal wastes and dead tissues fixed nitrogen is returned to the soil, where much of it can be recycled. Proteins are dismantled to yield amino acids, and these are often broken down further to ammonia or nitrate; these substances can then be absorbed anew by living roots. Competing with plant roots, however, are a class of decay bacteria, the denitrifiers, that break down fixed nitrogen and return it to the form of a diatomic gas. The denitrifying bacteria thus complete the nitrogen cycle by returning the element to the atmosphere. As a result of their activities the reservoir of fixed nitrogen in the soil must be continually replenished. In agriculture there is an even greater drain on the supply of fixed nitrogen: each time a crop is harvested for market, the nitrogen it contains is lost to the soil.

Small quantities of fixed nitrogen are

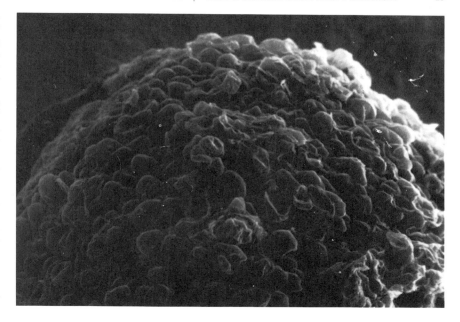

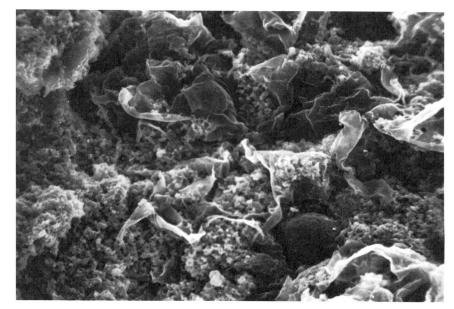

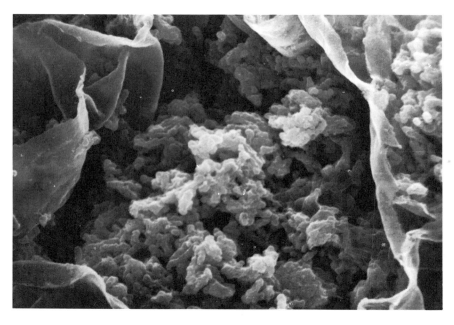

SOYBEAN ROOT NODULE consists of plant cells crammed full of nitrogen-fixing bacteria. A single nodule is seen at progressively greater magnification in this sequence of scanning electron micrographs made in the author's laboratory at the University of Wisconsin. At the top is the pebbly surface of a small root nodule. In the middle photograph the nodule has been sliced open to expose the interior. At the bottom one region of the interior surface is enlarged, showing a dense mass of bacteria spilling out of a ruptured plant cell. The bacteria are of the species *Rhizobium japonicum*, which associates exclusively with soybeans; other plants of the family Leguminosae harbor other *Rhizobium* species. Associations of legumes and *Rhizobium* account for 40 percent of all nitrogen fixed by biological means, and for virtually all that fixed by crop plants.

added to the biosphere each year by inorganic processes, such as the formation of nitrates in automobile engines, in lightning discharges and in volcanic emissions. A somewhat larger amount—about a fourth of the total world production of fixed nitrogen—is ammonia made by the Haber process. The remainder is the bacterial product. It is estimated to amount to 150 million metric tons per year.

Legumes

The activities of nitrogen-fixing bacteria were harnessed for human benefit centuries before either the bacteria or the nitrogen-fixing process was discovered. Farmers have long experience in the growing of legumes, such as soybeans, peanuts, alfalfa, beans, peas and clover. These crops can revitalize the soil, an effect that is now understood to result from nitrogen fixation by species of *Rhizobium* that form nodules in the roots of the legumes. Commercial *Rhizobium* inoculants are employed in planting legumes to ensure that the soil contains the appropriate bacteria. Legume crops are often grown in rotation with nonlegumes, such as corn. In this way nitrogenous substances from one season's legume crop help to fertilize the next season's grain crop. For a maximum yield of grain industrial fertilizer must still be applied, but the amount needed is reduced.

The *Rhizobium* enters the legume root through a root hair, a cell on the surface of the root that is specialized for absorption. The cell wall of the root hair invaginates to form an infection thread, which contains many proliferating *Rhizobium* cells. Most of these infections are abortive, but a few grow back to the base of the root hair and, by repeating the invagination process, enter the cortical cells of the root. Eventually the tip of the infection thread ruptures, releasing the bacteria into the cortical cells, which then develop into a bulbous enlargement: a root nodule. The nodule consists of enlarged plant cells, most of which are packed with bacteria. Ammonia produced by the bacteria is combined with carbon compounds derived from plant photosynthesis to yield amino acids, which are then incorporated into plant proteins.

As the term "infection thread" implies, the introduction of *Rhizobium* into legumes resembles a disease process, but it is one in which the plant cooperates. The welfare of the plant is served best if it encourages infection by *Rhizobium* but excludes all other bacteria, some of which might be pathogens or parasites. This discrimination is accomplished through a system of chemical markers by which the plant and the bacterium recognize each other.

Each legume is associated with a distinct species of *Rhizobium*. The bacteria that form nodules in soybeans, for example, will not infect alfalfa. In 1974 the first element of the recognition mechanism responsible for this specificity was discovered by Benjamin B. Bohlool and Edwin L. Schmidt of the University of Minnesota. They identified a protein from soybean that binds to cells of *Rhizobium japonicum,* the bacterial species that infects soybeans, but not to any other *Rhizobium* species. Frank B. Dazzo and David H. Hubbell of the University of Florida subsequently found another protein that seems to bear the same relation to clover and to *Rhizobium trifolii,* the bacterium that infects clover roots. They named the protein trifoliin.

Dazzo has continued his work at the Center for Studies of Nitrogen Fixation at the University of Wisconsin. He has recently shown that trifoliin is found on the surface of clover root hairs, the initial site of infection. Furthermore, he has shown that trifoliin binds to a polysaccharide on the surface of the infecting *Rhizobium trifolii* but not to surface polysaccharides from other *Rhizobium* species.

A plausible hypothesis derived from these experiments is that trifoliin acts as a link between bacterium and plant. Further studies, employing labeled antibody molecules, have provided preliminary information on the sites where trifoliin binds to the plant root and to the bacterial surface. Remarkably, the two binding sites are antigenically similar, that is, they have an affinity for the same antibody molecules. The significance of this similarity is not yet understood, but analogies are known. For example, the surfaces of some pathogenic bacteria are structurally similar to the surfaces of mammalian cells. As a result of this mimicry host responses that would normally eliminate an invading microorganism can sometimes be deceived.

Nonrhizobial Fixation

The symbiotic association between legumes and *Rhizobium* is the most highly developed and most sophisticated system for biological nitrogen fixation, but it is not the only one. For exam-

	FREE-LIVING BACTERIA				
NITROGEN-FIXING ORGANISM	AZOTOBACTER VINELANDII	CLOSTRIDIUM PASTEURIANUM	KLEBSIELLA PNEUMONIAE	RHODOSPIRILLUM RUBRUM	CITROBACTER FREUNDII
ASSOCIATED ORGANISM	NONE	NONE	VARIOUS	NONE	TERMITE
NATURAL HABITAT	AEROBIC SOILS	ANAEROBIC SOILS	AEROBIC AND ANAEROBIC SOILS; WATER; ALSO IN ASSOCIATION WITH PLANTS, MAN	SURFACE OF POLLUTED PONDS (A PHOTOSYNTHETIC BACTERIUM)	TERMITE GUT

NITROGEN-FIXING ORGANISMS include several genera of bacteria and cyanobacteria, or blue-green algae. These are among the simplest and presumably the most primitive organisms, being distinguished by the absence of cell nuclei. Among the nitrogen-fixing or-

ple, the alder tree, a hardwood species common in the northwestern U.S., encapsulates nitrogen-fixing bacteria in root nodules not unlike those of the legumes. Another symbiosis involves a small aquatic fern, *Azolla,* and a cyanobacterium that is capable of both photosynthesis and nitrogen fixation. Occupying cavities in the fern leaves, the cyanobacterium supplies nutrients that enable the fern to propagate in waters deficient in fixed nitrogen. Farmers in Vietnam have made use of the alga's capabilities by allowing *Azolla* to grow in flooded rice paddies; the fern might also be grown in ponds and harvested as a nitrogen-rich mulch.

Another apparent symbiosis, although it is probably a rather loose one, was discovered by Johanna Döbereiner of the Agricultural Research Institute in Brazil. She found nitrogen-fixing bacteria growing in association with the roots of certain tropical grasses. For example, the grass *Digitaria* was found to support populations of the bacterium *Spirillum lipoferum,* which is known to fix nitrogen. The bacteria do not form specialized structures such as nodules but simply grow on the surface of the roots. It is notable that most important grain crops, including wheat and corn, are genetically derived from tropical grasses.

A further intriguing discovery was made when a colleague of Döbereiner's noticed that among corn plants growing in nitrogen-deficient fields a few were taller than the rest. When the exceptional plants were dug up, Döbereiner found *Spirillum lipoferum* associated with the roots. It was a finding of great potential importance, since it implied that corn might be grown without fertilizer if the bacterium-root association could be reliably established. In subsequent experiments in several other laboratories, however, attempts to increase the yield of corn by inoculation with *Spirillum lipoferum* have had variable results. The nature of the association is still under investigation.

Among the more unusual symbioses are those involving nitrogen-fixing bacteria that colonize termites and shipworms. These pest species, which survive on a diet of wood, have long been known to harbor microorganisms that secrete enzymes for the digestion of cellulose. It has now been established that they also receive dietary assistance from another population of microorganisms. Wood is a poor source of biological nitrogen; bacteria living in the intestines of the termites and shipworms provide a supplement derived from atmospheric nitrogen.

In addition to obligatory symbionts, there are a number of organisms that fix nitrogen while living independently. Many cyanobacteria, for example, fix atmospheric nitrogen while growing freely at the surface of ponds. In many cases these blue-green algae constitute a nuisance: the organic nitrogen, released from the dead algal cells, promotes the growth of aquatic weeds and contributes to the process called eutrophication. On the other hand, the same algae might be cultivated and harvested as fertilizer or animal feed.

There are also free-living bacteria with the capacity to fix nitrogen. They include members of the genus *Clostridium,* which are anaerobic bacteria; they cannot grow in the presence of oxygen. Others, members of the genus *Klebsiella,* can grow either with or without oxygen and are found both free-living and in association with plants and animals. Finally, there is the genus *Azotobacter,* a group of aerobic bacteria whose name derives from Lavoisier's term for nitrogen. The contribution of these free-living bacteria to global supplies of fixed nitrogen is probably modest, but their contribution to the study of nitrogen fixation has been quite large. Because the complications of symbiosis are avoided, free-living bacteria are favored organisms for investigations of the biochemistry of fixation.

Nitrogenase

The overall chemical reaction of nitrogen fixation is the same whether it is achieved by the Haber process or takes place in the living cell. First the triple bond of the N_2 molecule must be broken; then three hydrogen atoms must be bound to each nitrogen atom. In the Haber process the hydrogen is supplied as a molecular gas; in most nitrogen-fixing bacteria it is extracted from organic molecules such as glucose, the principal carbohydrate product of photosynthesis. Hydrogen atoms are transferred from glucose to nitrogen through a network of intermediate molecules. Actually it is only the electrons that are actively transported; the aqueous medium of the cell is a sea of protons, or hydrogen nuclei, and these are readily supplied to complement free electrons. A transfer of electrons between two substances is called an oxidation-reduction reaction; the donor of electrons is said to be oxidized by the reaction and the acceptor to be reduced. Thus in nitrogen

SYMBIOTIC BACTERIA					
NONLEGUMES			LEGUMES		
FRANKIA ALNI	*NOSTOC MUSCORUM*	*ANABAENA AZOLLAE*	*RHIZOBIUM JAPONICUM*	*RHIZOBIUM TRIFOLII*	*RHIZOBIUM MELILOTI*
ALDER	*GUNNERA MACROPHYLLA* (TROPICAL HERB)	*AZOLLA* (AQUATIC FERN)	SOYBEAN	CLOVER	ALFALFA
ROOT NODULES OF THE ALDER TREE	IN STEMS; A CYANOBACTERIUM	IN LEAF PORES; A CYANOBACTERIUM	ROOT NODULES OF THE SOYBEAN	ROOT NODULES OF CLOVER	ROOT NODULES OF ALFALFA

ganisms are free-living forms and those that thrive only in symbiotic association with higher plants and animals; a few can adopt either mode of life. The bacteria that live in an anaerobic habitat cannot survive exposure to oxygen; aerobic bacteria need oxygen for growth.

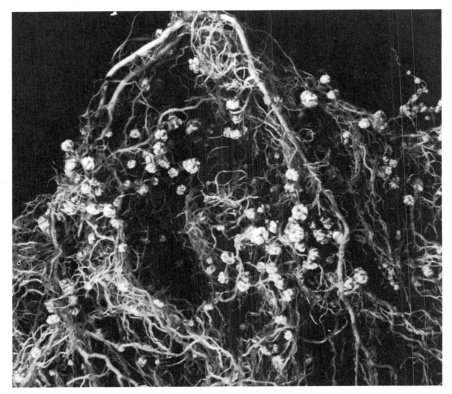

SOYBEAN ROOTS have many bulbous nodules that result from infection with *Rhizobium*. In this symbiotic association the plant supplies carbohydrate to the bacterium, which in turn supplies plant with fixed nitrogen. In legumes the plant also protects the bacteria from exposure to oxygen, which permanently denatures nitrogenase, the crucial enzyme in nitrogen fixation.

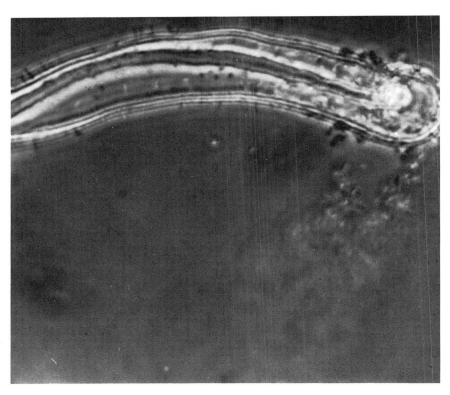

INFECTION WITH RHIZOBIUM takes place through the root hairs, cells at the periphery of roots. In this photomicrograph, made by Frank B. Dazzo of the University of Wisconsin, many bacteria (*fuzzy black objects*) adhere to a root hair. In addition the bacteria have already entered the cell through an infection thread, the long tube extending through the root hair. The infection thread is formed by the invagination of the cell wall; the eventual release of the bacteria from the thread into the cortical cells of the root leads to the development of a nodule.

fixation glucose is oxidized and nitrogen is reduced. Of course the two molecules do not interact directly; the pathway that connects them is a complex one, and some segments of it have not yet been thoroughly explored.

One of the mystifying features of the nitrogen-fixing reaction is the amount of energy consumed. The energy, which is derived from the breakdown of glucose or other carbohydrates, is supplied in the form of adenosine triphosphate (ATP), the universal energy currency of the cell. The conversion of one molecule of N_2 into two molecules of ammonia requires from 12 to 24 molecules of ATP. Part of this energy must be applied to breaking the stable bond between the nitrogen atoms, but far more is required than a naïve analysis would suggest. The likely explanation for the inefficiency is that not all the ATP goes toward reducing nitrogen; some of it may be diverted to competing reactions. In any case it appears that nitrogen fixation has a high cost in energy for the cell, just as it does for the industrial chemist.

The key molecule in the nitrogen-fixation pathway is the enzyme nitrogenase. All nitrogen-fixing organisms contain nitrogenase, which does not seem to vary significantly in structure from one species to another. No organisms that lack nitrogenase are able to fix nitrogen.

The enzyme consists of two proteins, labeled Component I and Component II. Component I has a molecular weight of 220,000 and is made up of four subunits, each of which is a single strand of amino acids; in addition Component I contains 24 iron atoms and two molybdenum atoms. Component II has a molecular weight of 55,000, consists of two protein subunits and includes four iron atoms.

Rather little is known of how this array of proteins and metal atoms is assembled to make an enzyme. The structure of the entire molecule may eventually be mapped through X-ray-diffraction analysis. In the meantime less direct methods have provided some information on the chemical environments of the various metal atoms. It is probably not a coincidence that the most effective catalysts in the Haber process are transition metals such as iron and molybdenum. In nitrogenase the role of the two molybdenum atoms is particularly fascinating because they seem to be part of the active site of the enzyme. The molybdenum is bound not to the large proteins of Component I but to a small cofactor, which Vinod K. Shah, working in my laboratory at the University of Wisconsin, has purified. A surprising recent finding is that the cofactor also contains some of the iron atoms associated with Component I. The molecule Shah isolated is capable of reactivating nitrogen fixation in a mutant strain of bacteria that lacks the cofactor. Edward I. Stiefel of the Charles F. Kettering Research

Laboratory has pointed out that among all the metals found in enzymes molybdenum is uniquely capable at both higher and lower oxidation states of transferring two electrons and two protons, and that may be its role in nitrogenase. Only a few other enzymes contain molybdenum; one of them, interestingly, is nitrate reductase, an enzyme required by plants for the conversion of nitrates into amino acids.

Much of the progress made in the past 15 years toward understanding the biochemistry of nitrogen fixation can be ascribed to two experimental techniques of uncommon importance. One of these techniques is the acetylene-reduction assay. In 1965 Robert Schöllhorn and Robert H. Burris of the University of Wisconsin and Michael J. Dilworth of Murdoch University in Australia discovered that the gas acetylene inhibits nitrogenase activity. Subsequent experiments showed that the enzyme reduces acetylene (C_2H_2) to another gas, ethylene (C_2H_4). Nitrogenase activity can therefore be evaluated simply by incubating an organism with acetylene and then measuring the production of ethylene by gas chromatography. Earlier methods for estimating nitrogen fixation involved tracing heavy isotopes of nitrogen or measuring an increase in the nitrogen content of an organism, a time-consuming procedure. The acetylene-reduction assay is both quick and comparatively accurate.

The other improvement in experimental methods was the development of a system for observing nitrogen fixation in vitro, that is, in the absence of living cells. Extracts of bacterial cells can be prepared in which the nitrogenase is not destroyed, but ordinarily the enzyme cannot function without its associated cellular machinery. In the early 1960's it was discovered that cell-free extracts could be made to fix nitrogen if small amounts of ATP were added along with a strong reducing agent, such as sodium dithionite. With such an in vitro system nitrogen fixation becomes a laboratory process that can be manipulated and measured with comparative ease.

What is the progress that has been made in understanding nitrogenase biochemistry? The present state of knowledge is summarized in recent findings of William H. Orme-Johnson of the University of Wisconsin, Leonard E. Mortenson of Purdue University and Barry E. Smith and his colleagues at the University of Sussex. They have shown that the first event in the sequence that leads to fixation is the reduction of enzyme Component II by an electron-transport protein external to the nitrogenase. The reduced Component II reacts with ATP and then reduces Component I. Finally Component I reduces molecular nitrogen, eventually forming ammonia. The same sequence of events can be described in another way. Component II

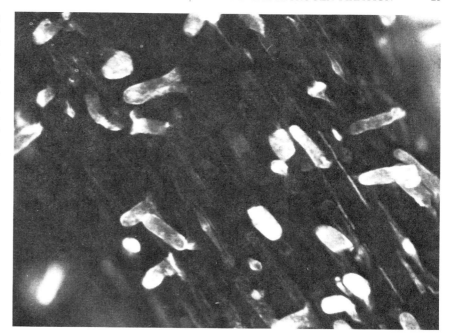

EXCLUSIVE RELATION between a legume and a nitrogen-fixing bacterium is demonstrated by the binding of *Rhizobium trifolii* to the root hairs of clover. A fluorescent dye was first linked to a polysaccharide in the bacterial capsule, an amorphous sheath that surrounds the cell wall. The labeled polysaccharide was then incubated with clover roots. Fluorescence of the clover root hairs indicates that capsule polysaccharide has preferentially bound to them. Similar experiments show that polysaccharide molecules from other *Rhizobium* species do not bind to the clover roots and that *Rhizobium trifolii* does not bind to the roots of other legumes.

first accepts an electron from a transport protein; the electron is then transferred to Component I and finally to nitrogen. No substances intermediate between nitrogen and ammonia have been discovered, so that all the intermediate states must remain bound to the nitrogenase. There is evidence corroborating the intuitive supposition that the electrons are transferred by iron and molybdenum atoms, but the actual mechanism of transfer remains a mystery.

It is the final event in this sequence—the actual reduction of nitrogen—that is at once the most interesting and the most baffling. The process probably will

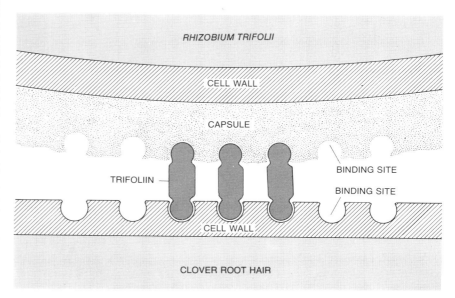

RECOGNITION OF RHIZOBIUM by a legume seems to be mediated by a protein that links the bacterium to the root hair. In the case of clover the protein has been given the name trifoliin. The binding sites for trifoliin in the cell wall of the plant and in the bacterial capsule are antigenically related; presumably they are also similar in structure. One interpretation of this surprising discovery is that bacterial binding site developed through imitation of plant; such mimicry may have helped to defeat the plant's defenses against invasion by foreign organisms.

not be understood in detail until the structure of the active site of nitrogenase has been determined. One hypothesis is that one of the bound intermediate states is a diimide, a molecule with the structure HN = NH. It is supposed, in other words, that at least one hydrogen atom is bound to each nitrogen before the bond between the nitrogen atoms is completely dissolved. There is an appealing symmetry between this process and the presumed mechanism by which nitrogenase reduces acetylene to ethylene, but there is little evidence either proving it or disproving it.

Competing Reactions

One discovery made possible by the development of in vitro nitrogenase systems was the peculiar behavior of the enzyme in the absence of its substrate. When nitrogenase is supplied with ATP but is isolated from nitrogen, hydrogen gas is evolved. Apparently the transport of electrons to the enzyme proceeds normally in the absence of nitrogen; when the electrons reach the active site of the enzyme, they merely recombine with protons. In fact, even in a normal atmosphere some electrons and ATP seem to be wasted in forming hydrogen. Karel Shubert and Harold J. Evans of Oregon State University have determined that most *Rhizobium*-legume associations waste about half of the electrons reaching the nitrogenase. They estimate that the annual U.S. soybean crop produces a volume of hydrogen gas with an energy equivalent to that of 300 billion cubic feet of natural gas. Plainly the efficiency of fixation could be improved if the parasitic production of hydrogen could be eliminated. An encouraging finding is that at least two symbioses—those involving the cowpea and the alder tree—do not lose electrons by forming hydrogen gas. In all likelihood the hydrogen is created at the nitrogenase active site as it is in other organisms but is recycled before it can escape the cell.

An alternative to suppressing hydrogen production is to exploit it. For example, ponds of cultivated blue-green algae might convert solar energy into both fixed nitrogen and free hydrogen. The principal difficulty would be in collecting the hydrogen.

A peculiarity of all nitrogenase systems is that both protein components of the enzyme are denatured by contact with oxygen. The oxygen poisoning is irreversible; the activity of the enzyme cannot be restored, even by removing the oxygen or by adding strong reducing agents. This sensitivity to oxygen is vexing to the biologist studying nitrogenase, since all his experimental apparatus must be designed to exclude oxygen; it would seem to present as great a challenge to the nitrogen-fixing organism. Indeed, those organisms have adopted a variety of strategies for protecting their enzymes.

The problem of oxygen-labile enzymes is a trivial one for the anaerobic nitrogen-fixing bacteria. For these organisms oxygen is a toxic gas in any case, and they live only in those environments, such as the deeper strata of soil, from which oxygen is naturally excluded. The bacterium *Klebsiella pneumoniae* is able to grow with or without oxygen as long as ammonia or nitrate is present. It is able to grow on atmospheric nitrogen, however, only in the absence of oxygen; apparently the bacteri-

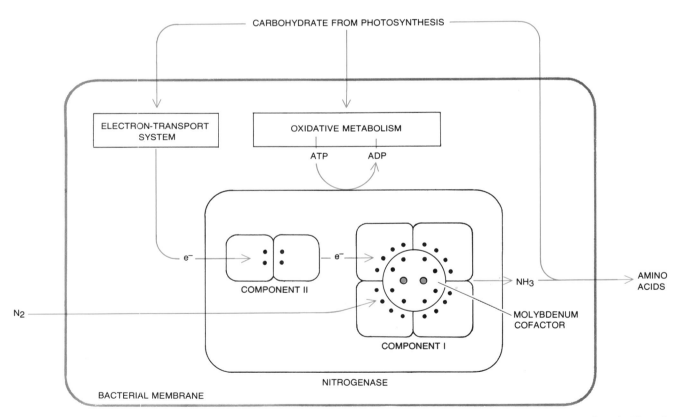

BIOCHEMISTRY OF FIXATION involves the transfer of hydrogen atoms from carbohydrates, such as glucose, to nitrogen. The site of transfer is the enzyme nitrogenase, a complex protein with two main components. The smaller component, Component II, has two subunits and contains a total of four iron atoms. The larger component, Component I, consists of four protein molecules together with 24 iron atoms; it also has a small cofactor containing two molybdenum atoms. Vinod K. Shah in the author's laboratory has recently shown that the cofactor also contains some of the Component I iron atoms. In order to transfer hydrogen atoms active transport is required only for the electrons; protons, or hydrogen nuclei, can be freely deposited in and withdrawn from the aqueous medium of the cell. Electrons derived from carbohydrate are donated first to Component II, then to Component I, where the actual reduction of nitrogen to ammonia takes place. The functioning of both components requires energy, which is supplied in the form of adenosine triphosphate (ATP). Mechanism of ammonia synthesis is apparently the same in all nitrogen-fixing species, although in photosynthetic bacteria the electrons and the ATP are transferred directly from the photosynthetic apparatus to the enzyme nitrogenase without the intermediate stage of carbohydrates.

um has no means of protecting its nitrogenase from deactivation.

Many of the blue-green algae that fix nitrogen have specialized, thick-walled cells, called heterocysts, that contain the nitrogenase. Presumably the heterocysts isolate the enzyme from atmospheric oxygen. Bacteria that fix nitrogen in an aerobic habitat have developed still another means of defense. They possess enzymes that reduce oxygen to water as soon as it enters the cell.

The most sophisticated oxygen barrier is the one found in *Rhizobium*-legume symbioses. Oxygen is trapped before it can reach the bacteria by an oxygen-binding protein, leghemoglobin, that is synthesized by plant tissue in the root nodules. It is the only form of hemoglobin found in the plant kingdom, and like the more familiar animal hemoglobins it has the ability to bind oxygen tightly and to give it up on demand. As a result the *Rhizobium* can adopt an efficient, aerobic metabolism while still protecting the nitrogenase from oxygen. This arrangement may be one of the principal benefits to the bacterium of the symbiotic way of life. In a larger context the oxygen lability of nitrogenase, along with the large amount of energy required for its activity, may be responsible for confining nitrogen fixation to a relatively few species.

The large energy requirement of the biological fixation process argues that a parsimonious organism should not fix nitrogen unless it is necessary for growth. That is indeed the behavior observed: if fixed nitrogen is present in the bacterial environment, ammonia production is suppressed. Fertilizer applied to a legume crop reduces the number of root nodules and hence the amount of nitrogen fixed by *Rhizobium*.

Regulation of Nitrogenase

The responsiveness of bacteria to fixed nitrogen in the environment implies that the fixation system is under metabolic control. The basic mechanism of control has been determined: fixed nitrogen suppresses further fixation by halting the synthesis of nitrogenase. As in many other biological systems, control is exercised by the repression of gene expression. The regulation of nitrogenase has been studied in greatest detail in *Klebsiella pneumoniae;* in that bacterium the crucial molecule in the regulatory pathway is an enzyme, glutamine synthetase.

In several species of bacteria glutamine synthetase participates in important aspects of nitrogen metabolism. Its primary role is to catalyze the first step in the synthesis of amino acids. Ammonia, whether it is derived from nitrogen fixation or from some other source, first enters the biochemical pathway by reacting with glutamate, an amino acid, to form another amino acid, glutamine; it is this reaction that is mediated by glutamine synthetase. Most of the other amino acids are then made by transferring the nitrogen from glutamine to other compounds. Boris Magasanik and his colleagues at the Massachusetts Institute of Technology have shown, in bacteria that do not fix nitrogen, that glutamine synthetase also regulates the synthesis of enzymes that degrade certain nitrogenous substrates.

Glutamine synthetase is itself regulated by feedback inhibition from several of the ultimate products of amino acid synthesis. High concentrations of glutamine or of some other amino acids diminish the activity of the enzyme and hence suppress the production of additional amino acids. A plausible interlocking mechanism for the regulation of nitrogen fixation is easily imagined: fixation might be encouraged by the presence of active glutamine synthetase, since that would imply a relative deficiency in the ultimate nitrogen-containing products, the amino acids. The inactivation of glutamine synthetase, on the other hand, would suppress fixation, since the enzyme would be inactivated only when amino acids were abundant.

This hypothesis seemed to be confirmed by studies of mutant strains of *Klebsiella pneumoniae* with defective genes coding for glutamine synthetase. These strains do not synthesize nitrogenase, indicating that glutamine synthetase must play a key role in the regulation of nitrogenase synthesis in this organism. It is not yet understood, however, exactly how the one enzyme controls the synthesis of the other. Moreover, the regulatory mechanism in *Klebsiella pneumoniae* is now known to be even more complex, in that both molybdenum and oxygen have an influence on the synthesis of nitrogenase.

The regulation of nitrogenase synthe-

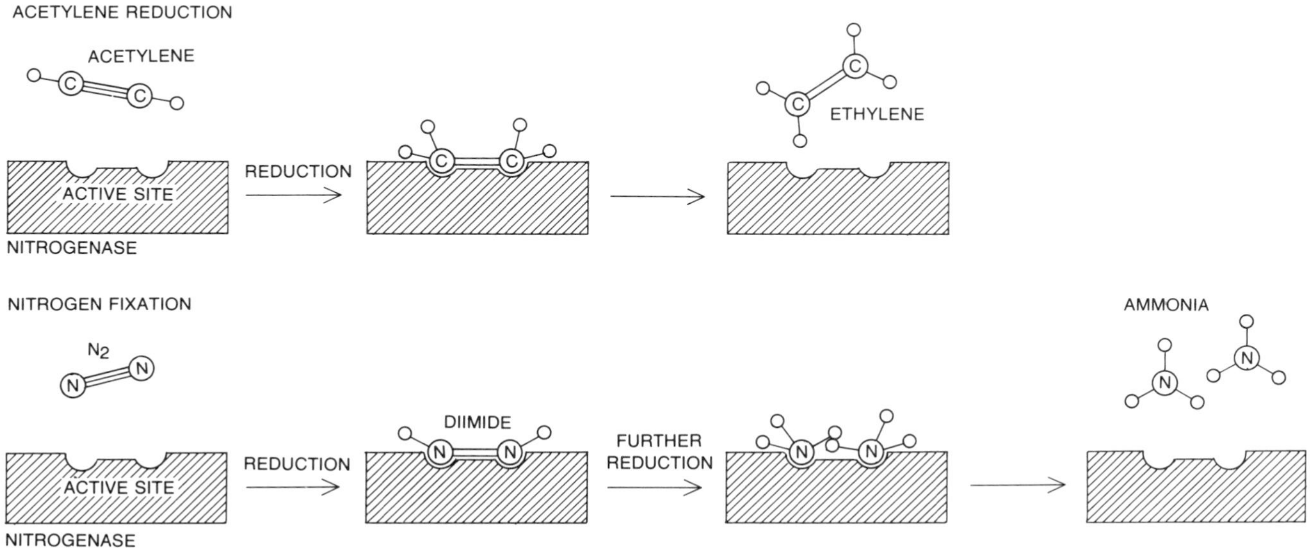

HYPOTHETICAL SEQUENCE of events in nitrogen fixation assumes that all intermediate states remain bound to nitrogenase. The sequence is based in part on the presumed mechanism of the acetylene-reduction assay, a test of nitrogenase activity. In the absence of nitrogen, nitrogenase converts acetylene to ethylene; a triple bond is reduced to a double bond and two atoms of hydrogen are added. In shape and in the presence of a triple bond molecular nitrogen resembles acetylene, and it is plausible to suppose nitrogenase acts on the two molecules approximately the same way. If that is the case, an intermediate compound in nitrogen fixation would be a molecule called a diimide. When acetylene is the substrate of nitrogenase, the reduction halts after a single step and the product is released as ethylene. The action of the enzyme on nitrogen is obviously different: each nitrogen atom is reduced three times, acquiring three electrons and becoming a molecule of ammonia. Just as this proposed mechanism is hypothetical, so the nitrogenase active site that is shown here is an arbitrary one; little is known about the actual structure of the active site. Neither the diimides nor other intermediates have been detected.

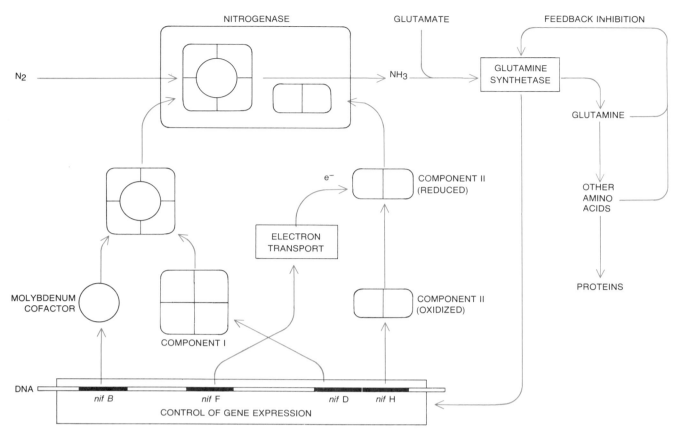

CONTROL OF NITROGEN FIXATION is apparently achieved by regulating the genes, labeled *nif*, that code for nitrogenase. The regulatory molecule is an enzyme, glutamine synthetase. Ammonia made by nitrogen fixation is combined with glutamate, in a reaction catalyzed by glutamine synthetase, to form the amino acid glutamine. Other amino acids are made by modifying glutamine, and high concentrations of several of these have been shown to inhibit glutamine synthetase. It follows that the activity of that enzyme is a measure of the cell's need for fixed nitrogen. In logical confirmation of this finding the enzyme glutamine synthetase seems to regulate the rate of fixation, if only indirectly, by turning the *nif* genes on and off. The mechanism of fixation control, however, is still not fully understood.

sis in other free-living bacteria has been studied through experiments with a substance that is structurally similar to glutamate. This glutamate analogue, methionine sulfoximine, is a powerful inhibitor of enzymes involved in the metabolism of ammonia. A bacterial growth medium that contains ammonia will ordinarily inhibit the synthesis of nitrogenase. Joyce K. Gordon in my laboratory has shown that ammonia does not prevent nitrogen fixation in the presence of methionine sulfoximine. When bacteria are grown with this analogue of glutamate, they accumulate high concentrations of nitrogenase and even excrete ammonia. A similar response has been observed in many kinds of bacteria, including cyanobacteria and other photosynthetic bacteria. This consistent result is evidence that all the cells regulate nitrogenase synthesis through some enzyme involved in the assimilation of ammonia or through the amino acid products of such an enzyme.

Improved Efficiency

Although our understanding of biological nitrogen fixation is still far from perfect, it is not presumptuous to consider improving on nature. Several methods of enhancing fixation might be practical now, and for some of the more radical approaches it is at least apparent what must be learned and achieved.

One of the most obvious methods of increasing the production of biological nitrogen is by improving the efficiency of the *Rhizobium*-legume association. Perhaps the simplest way to achieve that is by genetic screening of both plants and bacteria to determine the combinations best suited for a particular environment. The development of the acetylene-reduction assay makes possible rapid screening of plants for nitrogen-fixing capacity.

Through such a technique Robert Maier, a graduate student in my laboratory, isolated a mutant strain of *Rhizobium japonicum,* the soybean-nodulating bacterium, that fixed more nitrogen in a laboratory assay than did its parent strain. We wondered if the mutant bacteria would also give superior performance in the field. It is often difficult to introduce a new *Rhizobium* strain to a cultivated field because of competition from bacteria already present, and so the bacteria were tested on a plot of land at the University of Hawaii that was free of soybean-nodulating *Rhizobium* species. The soybeans were inoculated with the mutant and with the parent strain; preliminary experiments have achieved greater yields with the mutant. The problem of competition from indigenous bacteria remains, however, if such "superstrains" are to be adopted on a large scale. One possible solution would be to introduce the genes responsible for superior fixation into the strains that are already successful in the field.

The vigor and efficiency of the host plant in legumes also has a strong influence on the amount of nitrogen fixed. Ralph W. F. Hardy and his colleagues at E. I. du Pont de Nemours and Company have found that adding carbon dioxide gas to small plots of soybeans greatly improves the yield of beans, presumably because of greater production of carbohydrate by photosynthesis. Moreover, nitrogen fixation was found to proceed at a higher rate and to continue longer into the life cycle of the plant. It is not practical to flood farmers' fields with carbon dioxide, but the same effect might be achieved by breeding plants with a higher photosynthetic efficiency.

Another improvement in efficiency would result from the selection of *Rhi-*

zobium-legume associations that do not dissipate photosynthetic energy by evolving hydrogen gas. As I have mentioned, two such plants are known: the cowpea and the alder. Perhaps it would be possible to transfer whatever mechanism suppresses hydrogen production in these species to some of the more desirable crop plants.

Rhizobium-legume associations are responsible for about 40 percent of the nitrogen fixed by biological means, and for virtually all the nitrogen fixed by cultivated plants. The best prospects for an immediate improvement in the supply of biological nitrogen are almost certainly to be found among these organisms. There are more than 10,000 species of Leguminosae, of which only about 10 percent have even been examined for nodulation. Fewer than 50 species are cultivated. There may well be other plants in the family that could be exploited for agriculture.

Another approach to increasing the nitrogen supply is through manipulating the biochemical mechanisms that regulate fixation in bacteria. For example, Gordon has isolated mutant strains of *Azotobacter* that continue to fix nitrogen and even excrete ammonia in the presence of nitrogenous fertilizer. Such bacteria could be cultured in ponds on a substrate of cheap organic carbon, such as paper-mill wastes. If ammonia-excreting strains of blue-green algae were available, even the organic carbon could be eliminated, since photosynthesis would supply carbohydrate. The contents of the pond would be harvested as fertilizer.

Ammonia-excreting bacteria might also be adapted to living in the soil near the roots of plants such as wheat or corn. Perhaps an artificial symbiosis could be contrived by selecting plant varieties whose roots exude carbon-rich substances that would nourish the bacteria. The bacteria in turn would enrich the soil in fixed nitrogen.

Altering the bacterial regulatory mechanism could even benefit legumes. If *Rhizobium* species could be made insensitive to the concentration of ammonia, legume crops might supply more fixed nitrogen to the soil, rather than depleting what is already present.

Genetic Manipulation

Certainly the most ambitious program for raising nitrogen output is one based on genetic modification, and in particular on the transfer of genes from one organism to another. In at least one bacterium, *Klebsiella pneumoniae*, a substantial number of the genes involved in fixation (the *nif* genes) have already been mapped in the laboratory of Raymond C. Valentine of the University of California at Davis and in my laboratory. They are clustered in a small region of the bacterial chromosome.

Ray A. Dixon and John R. Postgate of the University of Sussex have transferred the cluster of *nif* genes in *Klebsiella pneumoniae* to another bacterium, *Escherichia coli,* a favored pet of biologists and a common inhabitant of the human gut. The transfer was accomplished by first incorporating the *nif* genes in a plasmid, a bit of extrachromosomal DNA, and then introducing the plasmid into *E. coli* cells. *E. coli* is not a nitrogen-fixing bacterium. The new strain created by addition of the plasmid was found to synthesize nitrogenase, and was able to fix nitrogen provided that it was protected from oxygen.

The success of this experiment has justifiably aroused excitement. It suggests the possibility, by a further genetic transfer, of creating a corn or wheat plant capable of independently fixing atmospheric nitrogen. That is indeed a possibility, but it should be emphasized that it is still a remote one. A few simple genes have been transposed from *E. coli* into cells of higher plants grown in culture, but no one has yet grown a mature plant containing bacterial genes. The difficulties of creating a nitrogen-fixing corn plant seem formidable.

Even if *nif* genes could be incorporated into the cells of a plant such as corn, that would probably not be enough to create a self-fertilizing crop. One problem that would remain to be solved, for example, is the protection of the nitrogenase from oxygen. It appears that creating a higher plant capable of efficient nitrogen fixation would require an extensive modification of the plant's structure and metabolism. The technology for accomplishing that remains far in the future.

Until this century deposits of sodium nitrate, principally the nitrate deposits of Chile, were the major source of fixed nitrogen for agriculture and incidentally for munitions. In 1893 Sir William Crookes warned the British Association for the Advancement of Science that the Chilean deposits were approaching depletion. It was the knowledge of impending scarcity that provided the incentive for the development of industrial ammonia manufacture. It now appears that the oil and natural gas required for fertilizer production are also being depleted, and yet another source for agricultural nitrogen must be found. Biological processes, which are already the major contributors to the world nitrogen cycle, are obvious candidates.

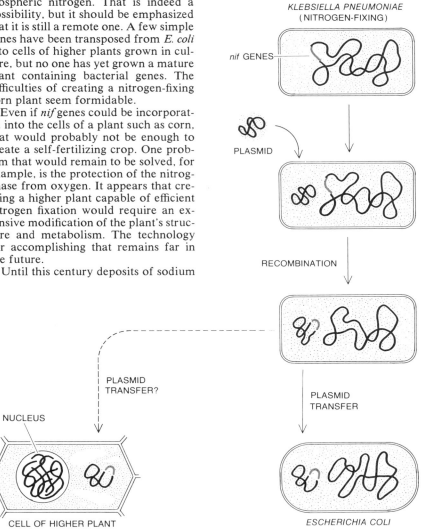

TRANSFER OF GENES from a nitrogen-fixing bacterium to some other organism, such as a crop plant, offers the most spectacular means of increasing the world supply of fixed nitrogen. A first stage in such a transfer has already been accomplished: *nif* genes from *Klebsiella pneumoniae* were incorporated into a plasmid, a bit of extrachromosomal DNA, and implanted in *Escherichia coli,* a bacterium that has no nitrogenase. A similar transfer into the cells of higher plants, however, would be far more difficult. Moreover, the possession of *nif* genes would not by itself ensure that a plant would fix nitrogen. The *nif*-containing *E. coli,* for example, are able to manufacture the enzyme nitrogenase but do not fix nitrogen because the enzyme cannot be protected from oxygen. A nitrogen-fixing cereal plant thus seems a remote possibility.

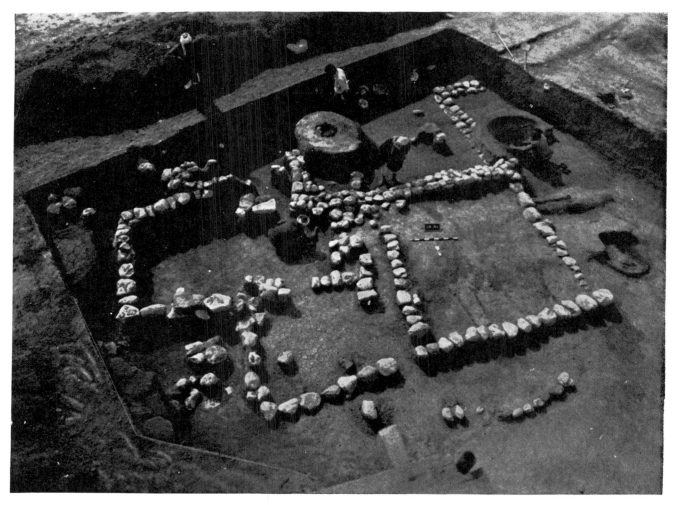

MASONRY excavated at Jarmo had provided the foundation for houses made of *touf*, or pressed mud. These remains are in one of Jarmo's upper architectural levels. Earlier houses had been built without foundations.

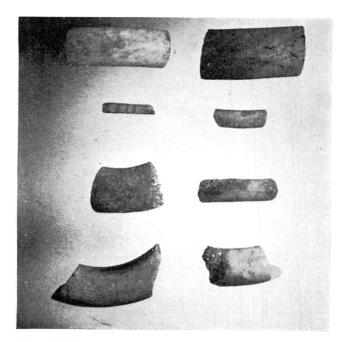

BRACELETS worn by the people of Jarmo were made of stone. Numerous fragments of these have been found.

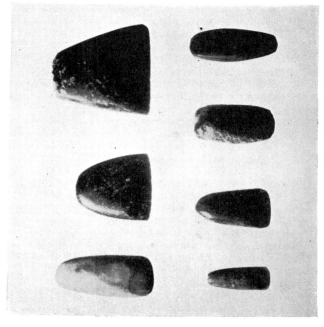

TOOLS were also made of stone. Shown here are several stone axes and adzes found at the site of the village.

From Cave to Village

by Robert J. Braidwood
October 1952

*An account of a recent expedition to Iraq which
sought the remains of a prehistoric revolution in the
life of man: the Birth of agriculture and animal
husbandry*

THUS FAR in human history there have been two principal economic revolutions. One is the Industrial Revolution, which began 175 years ago and which, to judge by the stresses of our period, is still far from complete. The other is the food-producing revolution—the invention of agriculture and animal husbandry—which began in prehistoric times. Although there is no contemporary written record of this earlier revolution, its material remains may be read by the prehistoric archaeologist. This article is concerned with some meaningful remains of the food-producing revolution uncovered by a recent expedition of the Oriental Institute of the University of Chicago to the Near East.

For 500,000 years before the food-producing revolution small groups of men lived mostly in caves. They were obliged to spend almost all of their time in the quest for food; they hunted, fished and gathered a few edible wild plants. After the revolution larger groups of men lived in villages. Tilling the soil and tending the animals gave them enough food, and thus enough leisure, to develop specialized skills. It is easiest for the archaeologist to comprehend the economic and technological features of such a profound development, but it must have embraced all the other aspects of culture: social, political, religious, moral and esthetic. To say that the economic and technological aspects came before the others would be rather like asking the conundrum: "Which came first, the chicken or the egg?"

WHERE did the food-producing revolution occur? There is overwhelming evidence that the first experiments in food production and village life were made in the Near East. Similar experiments in China and India surely came later, and quite possibly were due to Near Eastern influence. The beginnings of food production in the New World were independent, but still later.

The Near East also appears to have been the natural habitat of the plants and animals that were later domesticated to provide the basis for the agriculture and animal husbandry of the western Old World. One might assume that these species grew, as did the earliest civilizations, on the classic plains of the Tigris and the Euphrates and the Nile—the region that the great historian James H. Breasted called "The Fertile Crescent." Actually it now seems that they and the first villages were native to the hills that flank this region. These hilly grasslands were independent of irrigation; in them the winter rains of any normal year assure a spring crop even today. Thus it would appear that as the revolution progressed the basic food plants and animals were brought to the Fertile Crescent from the hills.

But exactly when and how did the food-producing revolution come about? In 1947, when we began to organize our expedition at the Oriental Institute, we held the following view of Near Eastern prehistory. The remains of preagricultural cave dwellers had been found in Palestine and Egypt, and to a lesser extent in Syria, Lebanon and Iraq. The latest of these cultures, the Natufian of Palestine, differed from the others only in that its people had domesticated the dog and devised a flint sickle, apparently for the collection of a wild food plant. Then there was an abrupt break in the historical sequence. The next remains are those of villages in full flower: established settlements with architecture, pottery and weaving—a vastly larger Sears, Roebuck catalogue than that of the cave dwellers.

In Iraq, for example, the latest remnants of the preagricultural people had been found in the cave of Zarzi; they were represented by tools of chipped flint. Next came the village materials of Hassuna, whose people first camped around hearths in the open and later built mud houses, made several different kinds of pottery and altogether lived a full peasant existence. After Hassuna followed an uninterrupted succession of excavated cultural materials, in which

were presently seen the settlement of the Mesopotamian plain, the building of towns and temples, the invention of writing and the founding of city-states. Between the cave of Zarzi and the village of Hassuna there was clearly a large gap in culture and time. In this gap occurred the food-producing revolution.

We chose to seek evidence of the revolution in Iraq, where the sequence of villages after the gap had been thoroughly worked out, where the world's earliest civilization later developed and where the Government Directorate-General of Antiquities was cordial and cooperative. Early in 1947 Dr. Naji-al-Asil, the Director-General, had sent us a list of promising sites, and in the fall of that year three of us departed for Iraq. From March to May of 1948 we excavated the remains of a village south of the great modern oil-producing town of Kirkuk. These remains resembled those of Hassuna, but we were unable to find anything more primitive. In May and June we spent a month digging at another site that had been listed by the Director-General. This was Qalat Jarmo, 30 miles east of Kirkuk in the Kurdish hills. Our test soundings showed that Jarmo was surely part of what we were after.

A large-scale prehistoric excavation is expensive, and its financing is not easy. It took us two years to get back to Iraq. We reopened our excavation at Jarmo in the fall of 1950, and, with the exception of time lost to winter rains, continued to dig until the spring of 1951.

THE village of Jarmo lay on the crest of a hill overlooking a deep *wadi,* or gully. It covered an area of at least three acres. It was inhabited for a moderately long time; the debris of its life is 25 feet deep. When we dug into the debris, we discovered that it was made up of perhaps 12 different levels, each represented by a change in architecture.

The people of Jarmo lived in houses made of what the modern Iraqi calls *touf:* pressed mud. At any one time there

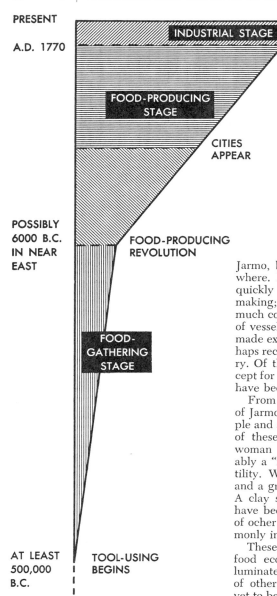

PRESENT

A.D. 1770

INDUSTRIAL STAGE

STEAM ENGINE INVENTED

FOOD-PRODUCING STAGE

CITIES APPEAR

POSSIBLY 6000 B.C. IN NEAR EAST

FOOD-PRODUCING REVOLUTION

FOOD-GATHERING STAGE

AT LEAST 500,000 B.C.

TOOL-USING BEGINS

CHART shows place of the food-producing revolution in human history.

were about 30 of these structures, sheltering perhaps 200 people. In the uppermost levels of the debris the touf walls rested on foundations of stone. The houses had mud floors, often packed over a layer of reeds. Each house was equipped with an oven; in one case we found a fairly intact oven vault, with its fire door opening into an adjoining room. Another feature of the houses, especially those in the lower levels of the debris, was a basin that was baked into the floor; this was apparently used as a permanent receptacle.

In the five uppermost levels of Jarmo we found portable pottery vessels. The earliest fragments of pottery are few in number, but have painted and burnished exteriors. Their advanced workmanship suggests that they were not made at

Jarmo, but were brought in from elsewhere. However, the people of Jarmo quickly adopted the notion of pottery making; the resulting product was a much coarser and very poorly fired type of vessel. Throughout their history they made excellent vessels of stone, and perhaps receptacles of skin, wood or basketry. Of the latter we found no trace except for impressions in the mud that may have been made by mats or baskets.

From the beginning the inhabitants of Jarmo made little clay figures of people and animals. The most characteristic of these represents a seated pregnant woman with rather fat buttocks—probably a "mother goddess" symbol of fertility. We also found beads, pendants and a great variety of marble bracelets. A clay stamp with a spiral motif may have been used to apply a tattoo mark of ocher paint—red ocher occurred commonly in the debris.

These things give us little clue to the food economy of Jarmo. This was illuminated, however, by a vast number of other remains, most of which have yet to be analyzed in the laboratory. We found weights for digging sticks, hoelike celts, flint sickle-blades and a wide variety of milling stones. Bone was abundantly employed in the manufacture of hafts, awls, needles, blades and spoons. We also discovered several pits that were probably used for the storage of grain. Perhaps the most important evidence of all was animal bones and the impressions left in the mud by cereal grains.

One of our collaborators, Hans Helbaek of the Danish National Museum, has already shown that the people of Jarmo grew at least two varieties of wheat and a legume. Fredrik Barth of the University of Oslo, who was with us in the field, classified the bones of pigs, cattle, dogs, sheeplike goats and a relative of the horse, as well as those of wild animals. Barth found that the proportion of sheep-goat bones was very high, and that the teeth of these animals indicated that almost all of them had

been yearlings—a selection that does not suggest hunting.

All of these things indicate that Jarmo is the earliest village site yet uncovered in the Near East. One of our keenest hopes was to determine its actual age by means of the radiocarbon method, in which organic substances such as charcoal, shell or burnt bone can be dated by their radioactivity. Even in 1948 we had brought snail shells from Jarmo to the Institute of Nuclear Studies at the University of Chicago, where Willard Libby and his associates developed the radiocarbon method. To these shells Libby's laboratory assigned an age of 4757 B.C. ± 320 years. Libby was reluctant to accept this as a firm date because shell is less reliable than charcoal for radiocarbon purposes. During the past summer, however, he has run tests on two samples of charcoal from Jarmo, one taken from exactly the same site as the shell. The ages of these charcoal samples are 4654 B.C. ± 330 years and 4743 B.C. ± 360 years. In other words, the shell and charcoal dates corroborate one another with a surprising degree of accuracy. This not only suggests the validity of shell dates, but also leaves little doubt that Jarmo began to flourish around 4750 B.C.

Our own date for Jarmo, reckoned by fitting its remains into the accepted "relative" chronology of Near Eastern archaeology, had been 6000 B.C. We suspect that as the possibility for errors is reduced in the still experimental radiocarbon instrumental procedure, and as more samples from the Near East are tested, it will be necessary to bring the whole sequence of Near Eastern prehistoric dates forward in time.

ON BEHALF of the American Schools of Oriental Research we began in March of 1951 to explore the region around Jarmo for even earlier settlements. We first selected Karim Shahir, a two-acre site on a hill two miles up the wadi that runs past Jarmo. Karim Shahir has only one archaeological level; architecturally it consists only of an incomprehensible scatter of stones, each about the size of a human fist. These had been definitely carried to the site, but we could make no architectural sense of them. There was no trace of either stone or pottery vessels. We did find a storage pit, fragments of stone mills and a fair number of chipped and ground stone-hoes—all of which suggest an incipient agriculture.

At Karim Shahir we gathered a great many of the tiny stone blades that the archaeologist calls microliths. We had also found microliths at Jarmo, but there was an important distinction between those of the two sites. All of the Karim Shahir microliths were made of flint; some of those at Jarmo were of the volcanic glass obsidian. The lack of obsid-

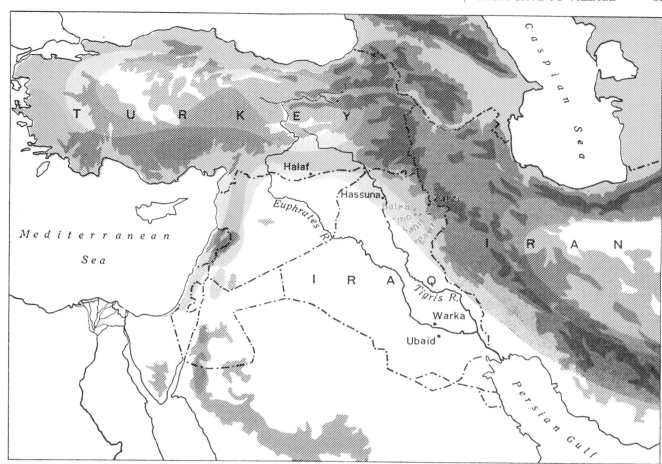

MAP of the Near East shows the location of the sites described in this article. Lighter gray shading denotes land higher than 3,000 feet; darker gray shading, land higher than 6,000 feet. Blue shading indicates rainfall.

ECONOMY	HISTORICAL CHARACTERISTICS	PERIOD IN IRAQ
		— 2000 B.C.
FOOD-PRODUCING ↑	*Civilization:* Fully efficient food production, cities, formal political state, formal laws, formal projects and works, classes and hierarchies, writing, monumentality in art.	AKKADIAN
		EARLY DYNASTIC
		— 3000 B.C.
	Era of Incipient Urbanization: New social and political aspects of culture crystallize.	PROTO-LITERATE
	Era of Established Peasant Efficiency: Market towns, temples, expansion into river valleys.	WARKA
		UBAID
	Era of Primary Peasant Efficiency: Permanent villages, pottery, metal, weaving.	HALAF
		HASSUNA
	Incipient Agriculture and Animal Domestication.	
		JARMO
	Incipient Agriculture and Animal Domestication.	KARIM SHAHIR
FOOD-GATHERING ↓	*Era of Cave-dwelling Hunters, Fishermen and Food-collectors:* Cultural unit probably small mobile band.	ZARZI
		PALEGAWRA

DIAGRAM locates the sites shown on the map at the top of this page in time and in cultural development. The names of the sites excavated by the expedition, and the historical gap that is filled by them, are in blue.

ian at Karim Shahir is an example of the difference between the two settlements. The closest known sources of obsidian are several hundred miles away in Turkey; it must have been imported to Jarmo. Thus Jarmo represents a new era in which trade has begun. Karim Shahir is only on the verge of that era.

In every way Karim Shahir seems to represent the cultural stage just before Jarmo: a time when men were probably making their first experiments with agriculture and animal domestication—as well as with that most significant consequence of deliberate food production, village life. We purposely do not call Karim Shahir a village; the deposit there was very thin and it is possible that its population was only seasonal.

From Karim Shahir we extended our exploration in time by investigating the cave of Palegawra, some 15 miles east of Jarmo. Judging by the bones we found in the cave, its occupants were successful hunters of wild horses, deer, goats, gazelles, sheep and pigs. They made long stone blades and minute microlithic tools which must have been mounted, perhaps as harpoons or arrow points. But we found no evidence of agriculture or animal husbandry.

Finally we inspected one still earlier site called Barda Balka. Here the remains indicated men who made flint and limestone hand-axes, pebble-tools and scrapers. They lived a catch-as-catch-can existence, along with extinct elephants and rhinoceroses, in a landscape that must have been very different from the now almost treeless countryside. Although Barda Balka shed no light on our central problem, it provided an archaeological and geological check point for the early cave materials of Iraq.

As of now the account cannot be any more complete than this. It is clear, however, that we have bracketed the gap in knowledge between the terminal cave-stage and the established village stage in Iraq. Our work adds four new phases to the known sequence of prehistory in a "nuclear" area of cultural activity, but I do not suspect that we have completely closed the gap. Nevertheless, when the reports are all in and the full story can be written, there will be a new understanding of a range of time and of cultural activities which were of vast consequence to human history. The people of Jarmo were adjusting themselves to a completely new way of life, just as we are adjusting ourselves to the consequences of such things as the steam engine. What they learned about living in a revolution may be of more than academic interest to us in our troubled times.

The Cycles of Plant and Animal Nutrition

4

by Jules Janick, Carl H. Noller and Charles L. Rhykerd
September 1976

Energy and inorganic nutrients are processed for human consumption by plants, animals and microorganisms. Modern agriculture ensures man's food supply by subsidizing the growth of these other species

The nutrition of all forms of life is necessarily in equilibrium. The solar energy absorbed by photosynthetic plants is passed along to a variety of other organisms, and it may take a long and complicated path through the biosphere. Ultimately, however, all of it is radiated back into space; if it were not, the temperature of the earth would rise. Similarly, inorganic substances in soil, water and air are absorbed by photosynthetic plants and incorporated into organic molecules that become the nutrients for animals, for certain other plants and for microorganisms. Some of these substances may be sequestered for long periods in an inaccessible form, but if the biological system is stable, all of them must eventually be returned to the pool of plant nutrients.

Because of the requirement of equilibrium the global biological system can be considered as being a continuous flow of energy and nutrients through a network of interlocking cycles. The function of agriculture is to divert this flow to the benefit of a single species. Natural forms of vegetation are replaced by cultivated varieties that have been selected for their efficiency in manufacturing foodstuff for man. Domesticated animals are introduced for a similar purpose. A third essential link in the food chain—the microorganisms—still consists mainly of wild species, but agricultural technology may eventually intervene in this part of the cycle as well.

The diversion of the flow of nutrients through the food cycle is the aim of all agricultural technologies. The distinction of modern agriculture is that it has augmented the food supply by increasing the rate at which nutrients flow through the cycle. This has been accomplished by several methods, but by far the most common and one of the most important consists in speeding the return of nutrients to the soil, where they can be reabsorbed. Hence in order to feed the human population we must ensure the nutrition of an assortment of plants, animals and microorganisms.

The earth intercepts a vast amount of solar energy, but only a little of it is available for biological purposes. About 60 percent is reflected without interacting further and most of the remainder is absorbed by the atmosphere or by oceans and landmasses and is promptly reradiated as heat. On the scale of the planetary energy budget the amount of sunlight absorbed by green plants and stored in chemical form is almost insignificant. It is less than 1 percent of the total incident energy, and it is well within the range of computational error.

In the plant, sunlight is absorbed by pigments: molecules whose bright colors signify that they strongly absorb some part of the optical spectrum. The most important pigment is chlorophyll,

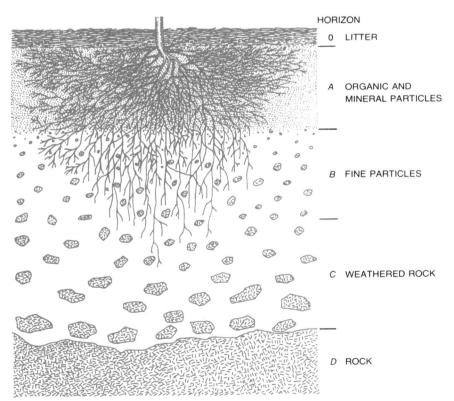

SOIL is the principal source of nutrients for plants and the site of a number of important transformations in the food cycle. The inorganic constituents of soil, produced by the weathering of rock and by the crystallization of minerals, are classified by texture as clay, silt, sand and gravel. An additional component of great importance is the organic material called humus. Clay and humus are colloids whose particles have a large surface area; they readily adsorb nutrients and retain them for later absorption by roots. A cross section of soil generally reveals a sequence of layers, or horizons; the *A* horizon corresponds to what is commonly called topsoil.

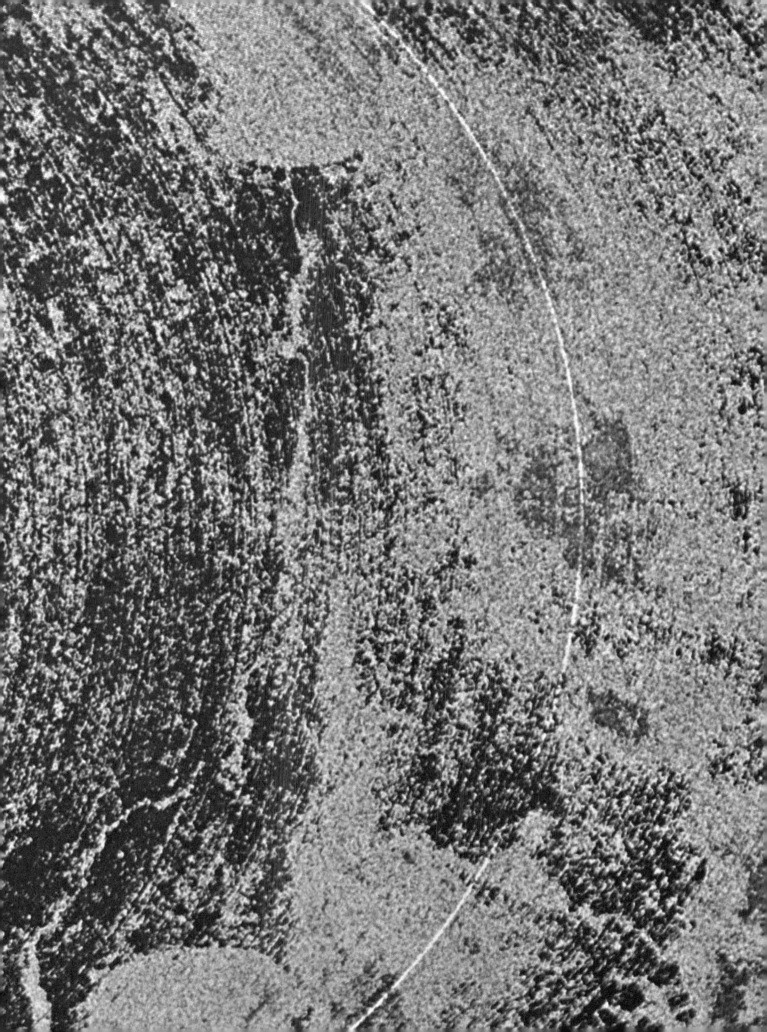

which absorbs both red and blue light, but several others are also found in almost all plants; together they can make use of almost all wavelengths in the visible part of the spectrum.

The solar energy absorbed is employed by the plant to drive a complicated sequence of chemical reactions that has the net effect of transferring two atoms of hydrogen from a molecule of water to a molecule of carbon dioxide. The products of the reaction are free oxygen, which is released to the atmosphere, and carbohydrates, compounds made up of carbon, hydrogen and oxygen. The energy of these products is greater than that of the carbon dioxide and the water; the added energy can be recovered and put to work. It can be recovered most simply by recombining the oxygen and the carbohydrates; that process, respiration, is the principal mechanism from which the vast majority of organisms derive their energy.

Carbon that has been converted to organic form through photosynthesis is called fixed carbon. Some of it is utilized immediately to meet the metabolic needs of the plant, including the synthesis of other essential molecules, such as the amino acids that make up proteins. The rest of the fixed carbon is stored, usually in the form of polysaccharides: large molecules made of many simple sugar units linked together. By far the commonest polysaccharide in plants is cellulose, the fibrous material responsible for the rigidity and structural integri-

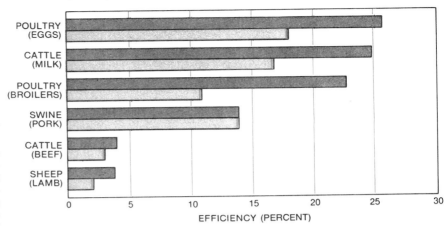

EFFICIENCY OF LIVESTOCK measures the percentage of dietary crude protein and energy converted to products edible by man. The highest efficiencies in the conversion of both protein (*gray bars*) and energy (*color*) are found in the production of eggs and milk. Cattle and sheep raised for slaughter have a low efficiency, but because their diets can be composed largely of material that is inedible to man their production can result in a net gain for human nutrition.

ty of leaves and stems. Energy reserves for the plant and its progeny are often provided by another polysaccharide, starch, stored in seeds and in specialized organs such as tubers, rhizomes, bulbs and corms. Animals derive almost all their energy directly or indirectly from the decomposition of these two polysaccharides. Cellulose and starch are closely related: both consist of long chains of the sugar glucose. They differ only in the geometry of the bonds between the glu-

cose units. This small difference in structure, however, brings vast differences in the physical properties of the two molecules and in their suitability as a constituent of animal diets.

Green plants capture solar energy with an efficiency of from 15 to 22 percent, which exceeds the efficiency of energy conversion in many industrial technologies. The energy represented by the fixed carbon is passed along the food chain when plant materials are consumed by other organisms. With each transition a portion of the energy is lost, in some cases the major portion. A hundred thousand pounds of marine algae must be transferred through the food chain to produce a pound of codfish. All the remaining energy of the algae is dissipated, mainly as heat. The codfish itself is soon reduced to heat and a few low-energy substances: carbon dioxide, water and minerals.

This enormous loss of energy may seem improvident, but it is not germane to the problem of feeding the human population. The annual production of fixed carbon by green plants on land and in the seas is about 150 billion tons; human consumption is about 260 pounds per person. Thus the energy captured by plants far exceeds human needs; if it could all be directed to human nutrition, it could support a population of 1.15 trillion, more than 280 times the present population. The food supply is not limited by a scarcity of sunshine.

The quantity of energy that is important in calculations of agricultural efficiency is the energy that must be supplied by man in order to concentrate and extract nutrients. Under natural conditions plant life is often sparsely distributed and little of the available organic matter is in a form directly useful to man. The intermediary use of a grazing steer is an inefficient step in the conver-

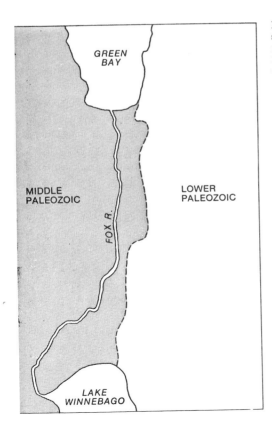

ENERGY EQUILIBRIUM of the earth's surface is suggested by the image on the opposite page, made with radiation in the thermal infrared portion of the electromagnetic spectrum. The photograph was made in August, 1973, from an altitude of 275 miles by an instrument on *Skylab 3*. It covers the region in the vicinity of Green Bay, Wis., shown in the map at the left. The intensity of the thermal infrared radiation emitted by a surface is determined mainly by its temperature. Here the relative level of emissions is indicated by color; in order of increasing intensity the colors are white, cyan, red, green, blue, yellow, magenta and black. The broad belt of land that appears mainly yellow and magenta borders on Lake Michigan, which is just beyond the frame of the image to the right. Yellow and magenta also predominate in Lake Winnebago and Green Bay. The most distinctive feature of the landscape is an abrupt transition to stronger thermal emissions, which appear black. The transition corresponds to a boundary between regions of different underlying geology and different topography. The yellow-and-magenta area is mainly wet lowlands; the black area is more hilly and somewhat drier. The entire region is one of intense agricultural development, being given over mainly to dairy farms. All the solar energy absorbed by the earth is eventually reradiated into space, much of it at thermal infrared wavelengths. The small part employed by plants for photosynthesis passes through food chain before being reradiated.

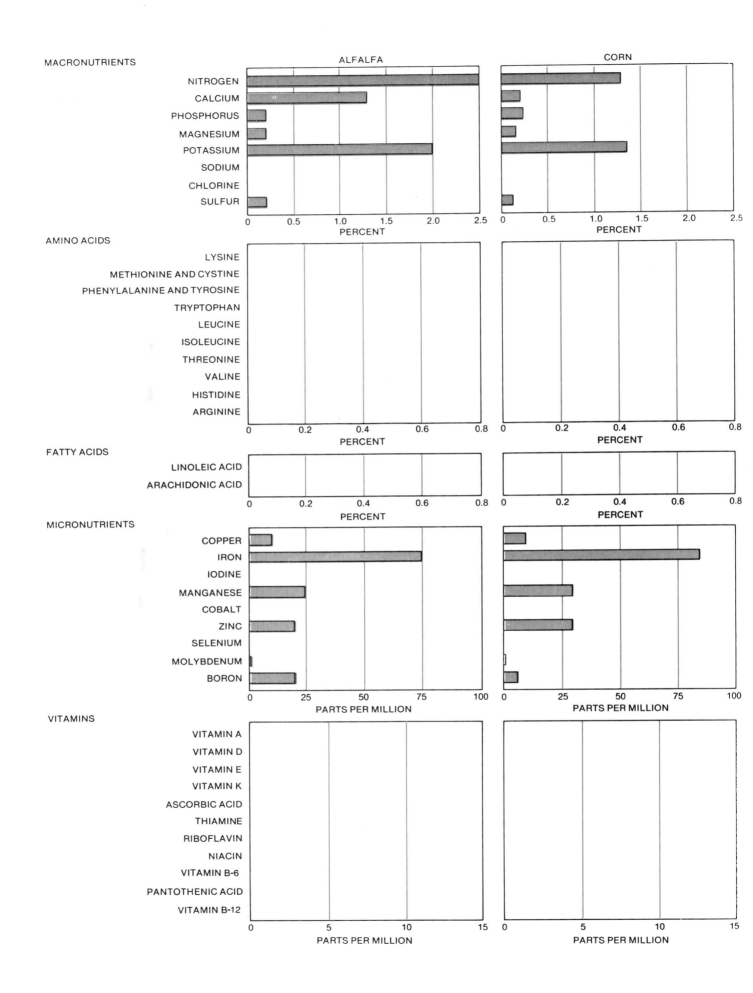

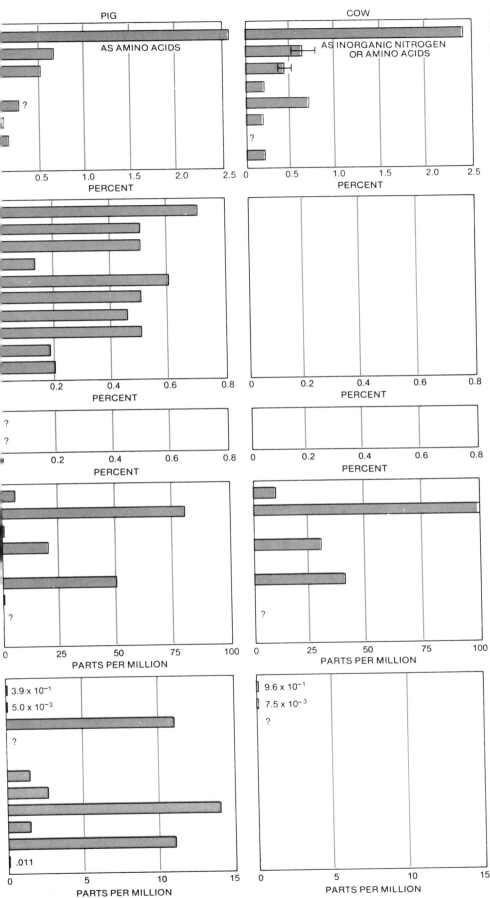

PIG

AS AMINO ACIDS

COW

AS INORGANIC NITROGEN
OR AMINO ACIDS

sion of sunlight to human food. On rangeland, however, where the available plant life is scattered and consists mainly of grasses and other species with a high fiber content, the steer harvests the nutrients under its own power, with only a small energy subsidy from man. Most of the final product—beefsteak—represents a net gain.

Few habitats are so harsh that nothing will grow: the arctic and alpine regions have their tiny wildflowers, and even the urban sidewalk is pierced by crabgrass. Under such circumstances plants make effective use of very scarce nutrients. Agriculture is profitable, however, only where a plant species of some value to man can be grown with a high yield. If a worthwhile yield is to be achieved, all the nutrients needed by the plant must be supplied in virtually optimum amounts.

Compared with the complex nutritional requirements of man and of other animals the needs of plants are quite simple. Plants subsist entirely on inorganic materials, and even they make up only a short list. The major nutrients are carbon dioxide, oxygen and water, and these substances are required in quantities so large that they are often considered in a category apart from the other nutrients. Carbon dioxide and oxygen are of course universally available (at least to land plants), and under field conditions they probably never fall to levels low enough to impair growth. Water is also an abundant resource, although it is less uniformly distributed. The relation of water supply to plant growth has surely been understood since before the beginnings of agriculture. Water is often a factor limiting growth, and the correction of water deficiency by irrigation can yield spectacular benefits.

In all, 16 elements are known to be necessary for the growth of plants. Air and water supply carbon, hydrogen and oxygen. In addition to these three elements, nitrogen, potassium and calcium are required in relatively large quantities. The remaining nutrients are needed in lesser amounts, and for some only a trace is needed. They are phosphorus,

NUTRITIONAL NEEDS of plants and animals are fundamentally different. The nutritional needs of plants can be expressed as a list of elements, whereas animals require more complex, organic molecules, such as amino acids (the constituents of proteins), fatty acids and vitamins in addition to minerals. Among animals the ruminants are exceptional in that many of their nutritional requirements can be met through the synthetic activities of microorganisms in the rumen. In addition to the nutrients shown, all organisms require carbon, hydrogen and oxygen.

magnesium, sulfur, manganese, boron, iron, zinc, copper, molybdenum and chlorine.

Except for carbon, hydrogen and oxygen, all the nutrients must be absorbed from the soil. The nutrition of plants is thus dependent on the ability of the soil to store essential elements and to make them available in a biologically active form. Many of the most important events in the growth of a crop take place below the surface of the soil; as a result soil occupies a central position in several biological cycles.

Soil is formed by the weathering and disintegration of rock and by the synthesis of both crystalline and amorphous minerals. In addition, the character and composition of the soil are altered by biological activity. The process of soil formation is a continuous, evolutionary one. Vertical sections of most soils re-veal a sequence of horizons, or layers: at the surface there may be a layer of loose litter, below that a layer rich in organic material and often called "topsoil," be-low that the "subsoil" and finally the parent rock in various stages of weather-ing. The soil profile is a historical docu-ment, recording the sequence of proc-esses that contributed to the develop-ment of the soil.

The mineral components of soil are classified according to the size of their particles as clay, silt, sand and gravel. In addition there is an important organic constituent, humus, that is made up of decay-resistant residues such as lignins, waxes, fats and some proteinaceous ma-terials. Humus has a profound influence on the physical and chemical properties of the soil. The coarser particles of silt, sand and gravel have properties essen-tially like those of the rock from which they are derived. Clay and humus, how-ever, are colloids, or suspensions of mi-croscopically fine particles, and they are the most active components of the soil. They are particularly well adapted to the retention of mineral nutrients.

The texture and structure of a soil are important in determining its suitabil-ity for agriculture. Texture is mainly a function of particle size, which in turn determines the size of the voids between particles. Sandy soils have large pores, with the result that water tends to drain through them quickly; the water itself is thereby lost to roots, and it also carries away soluble nutrients. The very small pores of clay soils retain water by capil-lary action, providing the aqueous me-dium that is essential for the transport of nutrients. On the other hand, soils with too much clay can become permanently waterlogged, blocking the aeration of the roots.

The most productive soils have a crumbly structure developed when small colloidal particles are cemented together by organic materials, particu-larly the exudates of microorganisms. Such soils are well aerated and have a large capacity for retaining water.

The great importance of the colloidal particles of clay and humus is their capacity for adsorbing ions. The col-loids have an enormous surface area with respect to their volume: in clay the surface area may reach 800 square me-ters per gram. Moreover, the particles bear a negative electric charge and therefore attract cations, or positively charged ions, to their surface. In this way nutrients that otherwise would be lost by leaching are held in reserve for later use by plants.

The cations are not rigidly bound to the colloidal particles, and they can be displaced by other ions. If all the ions are present in equal concentration, sodi-um ions are replaced by potassium ions, and they in turn are replaced by magne-sium. Calcium ions replace the magnesi-um, and finally hydrogen ions replace the calcium. Hydrogen ions are evolved continuously as carbon dioxide dis-solves in the groundwater and forms carbonic acid; the carbon dioxide is re-leased by the respiration of living roots and by the biological decay of carbohy-drates. The steady release of hydrogen ions promotes the exchange of cations, making them available for plant growth. The supply of the other cations is re-plenished by the decomposition of rock and the degradation of organic materi-als. In an agricultural context, of course, the concentrations of all the cations can be altered at will by the application of fertilizers, but the importance of clay and humus in storing the nutrients and making them available to roots remains.

The cation-exchange capacity of a soil depends on the amount of humus

ENERGY CYCLE in the biosphere is driven by the photosynthetic activities of green plants. The plants employ solar energy to convert inorganic nutrients into energy-rich organic com-pounds, particularly carbohydrates and proteins. Almost all other organisms sustain life by breaking down the products of photosynthesis into their simpler constituents. All animals, for example, depend for their nutrition entirely on plant life, directly in the case of herbivores, in-directly in the case of primary and secondary predators. Finally, the waste products and dead tissues of both plants and animals make up the diet of decay organisms, which extract the re-maining available energy from these materials and return them to inorganic form. The relative quantities of radiant energy received by the earth and radiated back into space and the bio-mass of the various organisms in the food chain are represented by the volume of the cubes.

and clay present and on the composition of the clay. Sand is relatively inert, and sandy soils low in organic matter are unreactive and infertile, although they can be made productive by fertilization and irrigation. Silt is slightly more reactive than sand but is generally much less reactive than clay. Clays differ in their ability to exchange cations by a factor of 10; humus may be twice as reactive as the most reactive clays. For this reason humus plays a role in plant nutrition out of proportion to the modest amounts of it found in most soils.

In the humid Tropics soils tend to be of low productivity: their clays have a low capacity for cation exchange and humus does not accumulate because the high temperatures of equatorial climates promote the rapid decomposition of organic matter. The problem is exacerbated by copious precipitation, which leaches nutrients from the soil. The lush vegetation of the humid Tropics seems to suggest great agricultural potential; actually the fertility of the soil is low. The plants of the rain forest are able to achieve their luxuriant growth only because they are adapted to their habitat and rapidly absorb the nutrients released by decaying organic matter before they can be leached away. This equilibrium is fragile. The direct extension of the agricultural practices of the Temperate Zone to tropical climates is seldom successful because the nutrient cycle is broken and productivity steadily declines.

The pH of the soil has a profound effect on plant growth. Abnormally alkaline soils (those with a pH of 9 or above) and very acid soils (with a pH of 4 or below) are in themselves toxic to roots. Between these extremes the direct effect of soil pH on most plants is minor, but the indirect effect on the availability of nutrients can be tremendous. Phosphorus, for example, becomes insoluble and therefore unavailable if the soil is either very acid or very alkaline. The pH also affects soil organisms, particularly bacteria. High acidity, which is typical of humid areas, inhibits both nitrogen fixation and the decay process. Acid soils can be neutralized by applying limestone (ground calcium carbonate and magnesium carbonate rock); excessive alkalinity, which is typical of arid areas, can be corrected by the addition of acid-forming fertilizers or by leaching to remove excess salts.

A final component of soil that must not be neglected is the indigenous population of living organisms. An acre-foot of fertile soil may contain more than three tons of living matter, including bacteria, fungi, protozoa, algae, nematodes, worms and insects. These organisms are entirely responsible for the breakdown of organic matter into simple nutrients that can be absorbed by plant roots. The microorganisms feed on plant and animal refuse and the

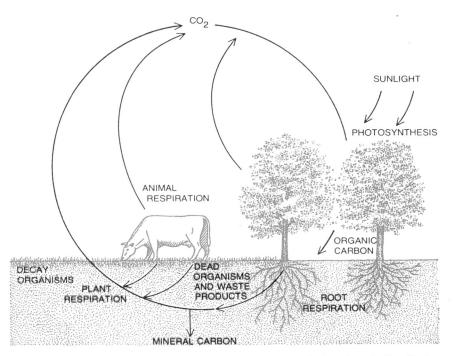

CARBON CYCLE involves two competing processes: photosynthesis and respiration. During photosynthesis plants convert carbon dioxide and water into carbohydrates and free oxygen. The latter combination of substances represents a rich store of energy, which is utilized in respiration as the carbohydrates and oxygen are recombined to yield carbon dioxide and water again. Respiration is common to all organisms that can live in the presence of oxygen, and thus all contribute to the return of carbon dioxide to the atmosphere. Some carbon is sequestered in minerals such as coal and petroleum, but that too is returned to the cycle when it is burned.

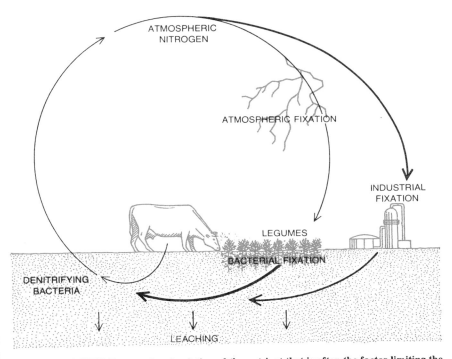

NITROGEN CYCLE traces the circulation of the nutrient that is often the factor limiting the growth of plants. Atmospheric nitrogen is useless to plants; the element must be supplied in "fixed," or combined, form, as in ammonium ions (NH_4^+) or nitrate ions (NO_3^-). A little nitrogen is fixed by lightning and other processes in the atmosphere, and a more important contribution is made by bacteria, notably those that live symbiotically in the root nodules of legumes. Nevertheless, the pool of available nitrogen in most soils remains small. The element is removed by leaching and by bacteria that return it to the atmosphere, and it is lost through the harvesting of crops. To compensate for these losses nitrogen fixed industrially is applied to the soil as fertilizer; industrial fixation has become a major component of the nitrogen cycle.

plants feed on the excretions and decay products of the microorganisms. Soil fauna and microorganisms also help to maintain soil structure and aeration.

In the mid-19th century Justus von Liebig formulated his law of the minimum, which states that plant growth is limited by the availability of whatever nutrient is scarcest. Thus it is of little benefit to irrigate a crop that is stunted for lack of nitrogen, and if the nitrogen deficiency is corrected, some other nutrient will become the limiting factor. The strategy of agriculture must be to provide all nutrients in adequate amounts and in optimum proportions.

Nitrogen is commonly the limiting element. Because it is a constituent of all proteins and of many other biological molecules it is required in relatively large amounts. Furthermore, much nitrogen is removed from the soil by leaching and erosion, by the action of microorganisms and by the plants themselves. The amount readily available in most soils is small.

Nitrogen, of course, is the major constituent of the atmosphere, and the column of air above an acre of land contains 75 million pounds of it. This form of nitrogen, however, is useless to most plants; to be biologically active the nitrogen must be "fixed" by being combined with other elements. In nature nitrogen fixation is accomplished in the soil, primarily by bacteria. The most efficient of these bacteria are symbiotic: they fix nitrogen only in association with the roots of legumes and of some tropical grasses.

Nitrogen in the soil is found largely in organic matter in various stages of decomposition, but the nitrogen remains unavailable to plants until it is converted to ammonium ions (NH_4^+) or nitrate (NO_3^-) ions. The circuitous route of nitrogen from element to amino acid to protein and back to the elemental form is the most intensely studied of the nutrient cycles. Much of plant and animal nutrition pivots on the availability of nitrogen-containing compounds.

The breakdown of proteins into amino acids in the soil is carried out by bacteria, which utilize the energy released by this process for their own growth. Only after the death and disintegration of the bacteria is the nitrogen available to roots.

The further breakdown of amino acids into inorganic nitrogen compounds is accomplished in several steps, each mediated by a specific group of bacteria. First, ammonium ions are liberated from the amino acids; then the ammonium ions are converted to nitrite ions (NO_2^-) and finally to nitrate ions (NO_3^-). The bacteria that produce nitrites and nitrates are autotrophic and aerobic, that is, they do not require organic nutrition but do require oxygen. They are greatly affected by soil aera-

tion and by temperature and moisture.

Like the conversion of nitrogen to a form in which it can be assimilated, the removal of nitrogen from the soil is largely a biological process. Much of it is lost to plants, and when a crop is harvested, the loss is permanent. Fixed nitrogen is also removed from the pool of nutrients by certain soil bacteria, which convert nitrates back to atmospheric nitrogen. This process is an anaerobic one: it can proceed only in the absence of oxygen. Thus a lack of proper aeration results in the loss of available nitrogen. Furthermore, nitrates are readily soluble in water, and if they are not utilized by microorganisms or higher plants, they can be lost by leaching. The level of available nitrogen is therefore dependent on the amount of organic matter in the soil, on the population of microorganisms and on the extent of leaching.

Under natural, nonagricultural conditions an equilibrium is reached between the rate of plant growth and the forces that affect the supply of nitrogen in the soil. In many agricultural systems, however, this equilibrium is disturbed. The harvesting of a crop tends to deplete nitrogen not only through the direct effects of removing the plant life but also through increased erosion and a reduction in soil organic matter. For this reason intensive agriculture depends on the addition of nitrogen as fertilizer.

Traditionally nitrogen fertilizers were derived from organic sources, particularly animal manures such as guano: the accumulated droppings of birds. Later supplies included sodium nitrate, mined in Chile, and ammonium sulfate, a byproduct of coke ovens. Today most nitrogen fertilizer is synthesized by the Haber process, in which atmospheric nitrogen is reacted with hydrogen to form ammonia. The ammonia can be applied directly or it can be employed as a raw material for the manufacture of urea, nitrates or other nitrogen compounds.

The hydrogen required by the Haber process is generally extracted from natural gas, and the cost of that fuel makes up most of the cost of the manufactured nitrogen fertilizer. The synthesis of a ton of anhydrous ammonia requires 30,000 cubic feet of natural gas. Hence through industrial nitrogen fixation fossil fuels enter directly into the nutrient cycle; their cost is recouped through the value added to the crop by fertilization.

The remaining nutrient elements are somewhat less likely to present a limitation to growth, but that is not to say they are less important. In some cases the amount required is small, but it is an absolute requirement. Phosphorus is a constituent of nucleic acids and of several molecules involved in the transport of energy, but it is required only in small amounts. Dry plant materials contain about 2 percent nitrogen but only .2 percent phosphorus. Nevertheless, most soils are unable to supply enough phos-

phorus for maximum growth. Phosphorus, unlike nitrogen, is relatively stable in the soil and leaching is negligible; on the other hand, the availability of phosphorus is dependent on soil pH. Phosphate fertilizer is widely applied, most

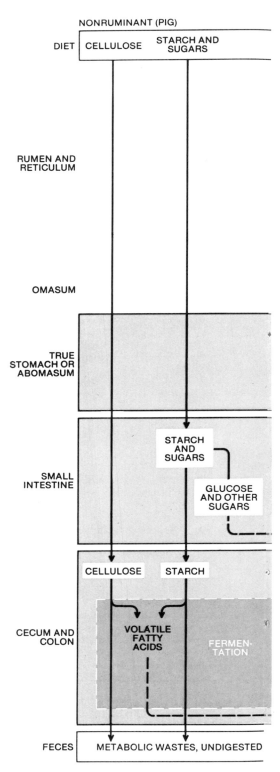

DIETARY STRATEGY of ruminants and nonruminants differs markedly. Nonruminants simply assimilate that portion of their

often in the form of "superphosphates" obtained by treating rock phosphate with sulfuric acid or phosphoric acid.

Potassium is required in relatively large amounts, although its precise role in plant physiology is not well understood. It is available as an exchangeable ion adsorbed on the soil colloid. Soils that contain relatively little humus are often rich in potassium, but it is in an insoluble form and therefore unavailable. Organic soils are usually deficient in potassium. Hence fertilization is often required; the major fertilizer is potassium chloride.

The calcium content of plants varies by species (it is low in grasses and high in legumes), but calcium is seldom defi-

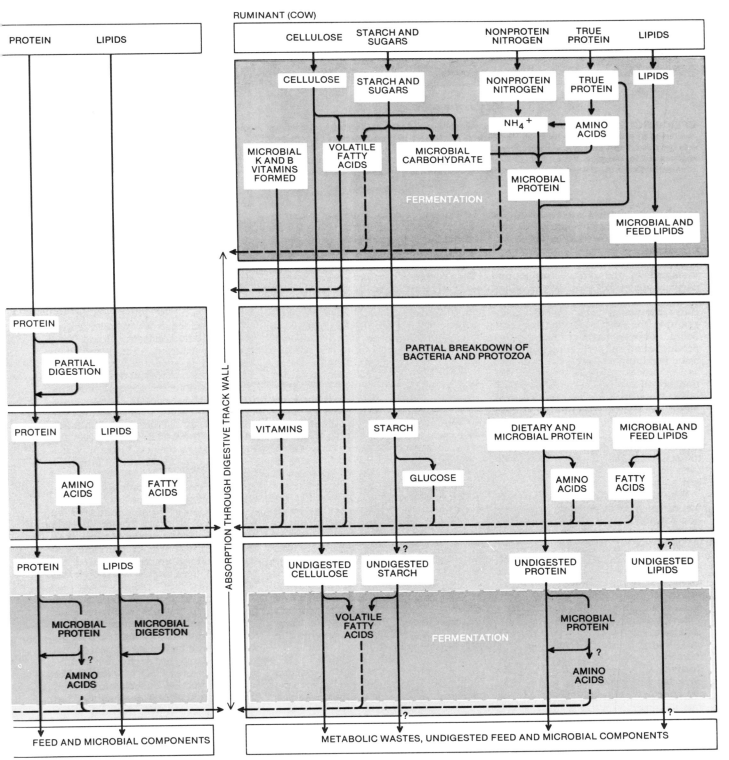

diet which is digestible and excrete the rest. Ruminants divert a portion of their food in order to raise an internal crop of bacteria. Both the waste products and the breakdown products of the bacteria can then be absorbed as nutrients. The ruminant digestion is not more efficient than that of the nonruminant, but by breaking down cellulose it makes use of a food that otherwise would not be available at all.

cient as a nutrient. The collateral effects of calcium on the soil, however, are numerous, with the result that the calcium content is frequently amended. The element has an influence on the activities of microorganisms, on pH and on the absorption of other ions. Calcium is present in the soil as a water-soluble, exchangeable cation, in combination with organic compounds and in insoluble minerals such as the feldspars hornblende and calcite.

Magnesium, a constituent of the chlorophyll molecule, is absorbed by roots as an ion. It is found in the soil solution as an exchangeable cation, and deficiencies are rare.

Sulfur, a constituent of two amino acids, cystine and methionine, and of the vitamins biotin and thiamine, is not available in large amounts in the soil. It is continually leached, but new supplies are also continuously added by the breakdown of sulfur-containing minerals, such as pyrite. In industrial regions sulfur is also added by rainfall, since rain absorbs sulfur dioxide from industrial pollution.

Manganese, boron, iron, zinc, copper, molybdenum and chlorine are required by plants only in minute amounts. Deficiencies, although not widespread, can severely limit productivity. Molybdenum deficiency has been implicated as a factor causing low levels of nitrogen fixation in some areas.

Apart from light, air and water, the most conspicuous demand a plant makes on its environment is for minerals. Animals too require minerals, but they also have more complex dietary needs, which cannot be expressed by a simple list of chemical elements. The nourishment of animals is dependent on organic substances: carbohydrates, fats, vitamins and proteins or the amino acids of which proteins are made. All these substances must be derived directly or indirectly from green plants, and animals are therefore effectively parasites on the plant community. They obtain energy by breaking down the energy-rich products of photosynthesis into simpler, less energetic molecules. For example, an animal can ingest glucose and combine it with oxygen to release energy, carbon dioxide and water; this process, respiration, is the exact opposite of photosynthesis.

Virtually all animals feed in essentially the same way: organic substances are ingested and partially decomposed by digestive enzymes so that the nutrients can be absorbed. The partial decomposition is the function of the digestive tract. The species differ, however, in the kinds of food that are acceptable to them. Among the vertebrates the most significant distinction is between those animals that gain sustenance from cellulose and those that require other forms of carbohydrate.

The importance of this distinction reflects the extraordinary importance of cellulose in the global nutrient cycle. A major share of the energy budget of most green plants is dedicated to the manufacture of cellulose, and cellulose is the most abundant material in the structure of plants. It represents an enormous energy resource.

Mammals do not make enzymes that are capable of breaking the bonds between the glucose units in cellulose, and it therefore has no direct nutritive value

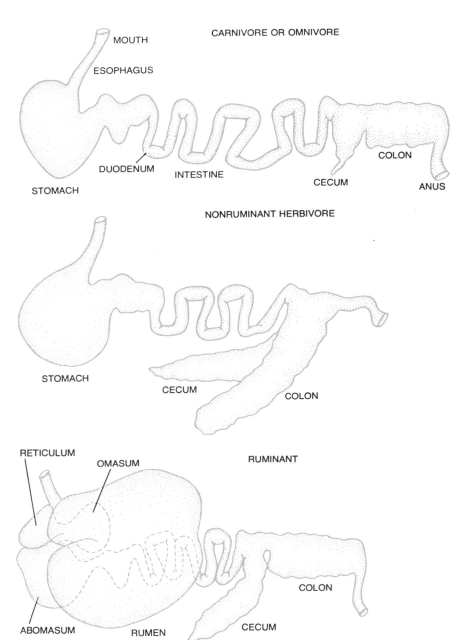

ANATOMY OF THE DIGESTIVE TRACT is the principal determinant of animal diet; in particular it determines whether or not an animal can derive sustenance from cellulose, the most abundant plant product. The digestion of cellulose is dependent on enzymes secreted by bacteria. In animals with simple stomachs, including carnivores such as the dog and omnivores such as man and the pig, the appropriate bacteria are found only in the cecum and colon, and the food passes through these structures too quickly for digestion to be effective. In nonruminant herbivores such as the horse the cecum and colon are more highly developed, but residence time is still limited and some nutrients required by the bacteria are removed earlier in the tract, so that cellulose digestion is inefficient. In ruminants, such as the cow, the bacterial degradation of cellulose is accomplished at the start of the alimentary tract, in the rumen. The full length of the intestine, cecum and colon is available for the absorption of the nutrients.

for them. A number of bacteria do secrete the appropriate enzymes. Mammals that sustain themselves on a diet rich in cellulose are able to do so by virtue of the fact that these bacteria grow in their digestive tract. Through fermentation the bacteria partially decompose the cellulose, skimming off some of the energy to support their own life cycle. The decomposition is completed by the host animal, which by reducing the molecules to carbon dioxide and water extracts the remaining energy. Moreover, the dead bacteria can also be digested. The dietary strategy amounts to a kind of internal agriculture.

Animals can be classified in three groups based on their abilities to assimilate cellulose, a classification that is reflected in the structure of their digestive apparatus. Carnivores, such as the dog, and omnivores, such as man and the pig, have simple stomachs and have difficulty digesting cellulose. Nonruminant herbivores, such as the horse, the rabbit and the guinea pig, can derive sustenance from cellulose, but they assimilate it less efficiently than the ruminants. Ruminant herbivores, such as cattle,

sheep, goats, deer, buffalo and many others, can efficiently break down cellulose and extract a large proportion of their dietary calories from it.

In animals with simple stomachs digestion is carried out mainly by indigenous enzymes: those secreted by the animal itself. Most of the enzymes are manufactured in the pancreas and by mucosal cells in the wall of the stomach and the small intestine. The main site of nutrient absorption is the small intestine. Bacteria are found in the cecum and colon, but food residues pass through these parts of the digestive tract quickly, with little bacterial digestion.

In nonruminant herbivores the bacterial populations of the cecum and colon are more important. Dietary cellulose is digested there by the bacteria, producing acetic acid, propionic acid and butyric acid; these organic acids are waste products of the microorganisms but energy-rich foods for the host animal. Some of the amino acids and vitamins synthesized by the bacteria can also be absorbed.

The efficiency of this process may be limited because some nutrients required

by the bacteria are absorbed in the small intestine, before they reach the microorganisms. Moreover, some of the nutritionally valuable products of the bacteria may be lost in the feces because of inefficient absorption in the cecum and colon.

The superlative adaptation to the challenge of a diet rich in cellulose is found in the ruminants. Bacterial fermentation of fibrous foods is concentrated in an extensive fermentation vat, the rumen, at the beginning of the digestive tract. There cellulose is broken down into smaller molecules, and the capabilities of the bacteria for synthesizing amino acids and certain vitamins are exploited. The bacterial transformation is accomplished before the food enters the small intestine, so that the full length of the intestine is available for the absorption of nutrients extracted from the food and synthesized by the microorganisms.

Farm animals have traditionally been sustained by the direct consumption of plant materials, such as grains and grasses, but many other nutritive materials are potential dietary resources. For example, the meal produced from soy-

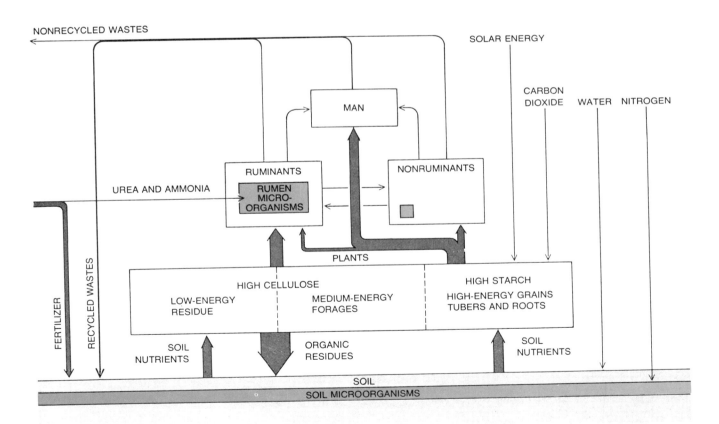

OVERALL NUTRIENT CYCLE includes man as the ultimate consumer and as the architect of the agricultural system. High-energy plant products, such as grains, are consumed by man directly or processed through animals. Lower-energy plant materials that are high in cellulose are processed through ruminants, thereby drawing on the capabilities of the rumen bacteria. The growth of the crops that support both the livestock and the human population is enhanced by returning wastes to the soil and by the application of fertilizers.

beans, cottonseed and peanuts as a by-product of oil extraction, and the wheat bran, beet pulp and molasses produced as a by-product of carbohydrate extraction, are all suitable feeds for many animals. Slaughterhouse wastes, such as blood, bone meal and offal, and even animal wastes, such as the manures of cattle and poultry, can be fed to cattle. Because of the ability of rumen bacteria to synthesize amino acids cattle can even be fed sources of inorganic nitrogen, such as ammonia or urea.

With the variety of feedstuffs available, the number of potential animal-ration formulations is almost unlimited. In poor countries livestock and man are in competition for the available grain. As a result grain is fed only to animals that are efficient converters of calories to tissue, such as the chicken and the pig, and to animals needed for work. Ruminants either graze or consume wastes.

In rich and agriculturally productive countries, on the other hand, there is only limited competition for food. It is therefore possible to increase the productivity of animals by supplementing their diet with grain. Swine and poultry can consume essentially all their nutrients in concentrated form. In the U.S. beef breeding cows spend almost their entire life on pasture with little or no grain, but their offspring destined for slaughter generally receive a generous portion of grain in a feedlot to increase their rate of weight gain and to improve their carcass characteristics.

Productive dairy cows are generally fed rations containing from 20 to 50 percent grain. Dairy cattle can grow, maintain themselves, reproduce and remain healthy when fed entirely on forages. On a forage of average quality, however, cows have difficulty obtaining sufficient nutrients to produce more than 10 to 20 pounds of milk per day. High-quality forages can support from 30 to 40 pounds of milk per day. With liberal grain feeding, dairy cows can produce more than 100 pounds of milk per day.

Nonruminant animals require a diet that in many respects does not differ much from the human diet. In the event of a food shortage it would theoretically be more efficient to bypass the animal and reserve the available food for human consumption. Animals, however, offer a way of refining unpalatable or inedible products and storing them in useful forms. Of the solar energy transformed into chemical energy by the plant only about 20 percent can be directly utilized by man. Animals convert plant products into human food with an efficiency that varies between 2 and 18 percent. That inefficient conversion, however, is not a loss but a gain if the photosynthetic energy consumed by the animals could not have been recovered otherwise. The justification for animals in agriculture is their ability to trans-

form products of little or no value into nutritious human food.

In an undisturbed ecological system a balance is soon achieved between the resources of the soil, the plant life and all the organisms that feed on the plants. The biomass, or total amount of biological material that can be supported, is determined by a combination of environmental factors, of which climate is the most important. In primitive agricultural systems the natural flora and fauna are merely replaced by crops and domesticated animals. The interaction of plants and animals may be altered only slightly; any change in the total biomass is probably small and could be either a gain or a loss. The economic impact, however, is enormous, because a much larger proportion of the biomass is of use to man.

Primitive agriculture is characterized by a small energy subsidy, low output and high overall efficiency. Animals consume excess feed, roughage and waste products; wastes from plant decay, and from animals and people, are utilized or recycled back to the soil. Power requirements are met through the labor of men, women and animals. Little is added to the system in fuel, machinery, fertilizer or pesticide, but little is removed in food in spite of unrelenting toil. Properly managed, the system is at best self-sustaining; mismanagement, either by overgrazing or by cultivation practices that lead to excessive erosion, destroys the system.

Modern agricultural systems emphasize high production and labor efficiency. The natural plant and animal cycles, the mainstay of primitive agriculture, are modified to fit a technology in which a large energy subsidy is possible. This subsidy often takes the form of manufactured goods: machinery, gasoline, fertilizer, pesticide. For maximum efficiency, production of particular crops is geographically concentrated and farms become specialized. Animals and plants are raised in widely separated places. These changes represent the response of farmers to a combination of economic forces involving climate, the concentration of population, land values, the low cost of energy and the high cost of labor. The preferences of consumers have also had a strong influence. In the U.S. it is the demand for tender cuts of beef combined with the relatively low cost of grain that makes the feeding of high-energy grains to cattle feasible.

Liebig's law of the minimum need not be confined in its application to plant nutrients; it can be extended to cover all the factors that bear on the success of the agricultural enterprise. Indeed, the history of agricultural technology has been a search for economic ways of overcoming factors that limit production. Some of the most productive lands

were once worthless because they were too dry; similarly, in many parts of the world today a lack of investment capital has proved to be just as effective in limiting production as a lack of water. On the whole the success of technology in increasing agricultural productivity has been remarkable. The alarming graph of world population increase is also the reassuring graph of increasing world food production.

For additional improvements in yield many of the most promising opportunities involve intervention in the cycles that connect plants, soil, animals and microorganisms. For example, there is the potential for a large increase in the biological fixation of nitrogen. The legume alfalfa has been grown with annual yields of 16 tons per acre without the application of nitrogen fertilizers. In alfalfa containing 3 percent nitrogen the bacteria associated with the plant roots must fix at least 1,000 pounds of nitrogen per acre per year, which is five times the amount generally accepted as being typical. Nitrogen fixation in the soil might be further improved by artificially selecting efficient strains of symbiotic bacteria, coupled with more widespread adoption of improved legumes, particularly in the Tropics. It was recently discovered that bacteria capable of nitrogen fixation live in a partial symbiotic association with certain tropical grasses, including maize. The genetic manipulation of bacteria offers hope that the capacity to fix nitrogen may eventually be conferred on all crops. A development with a more immediate prospect of application is the discovery of an inexpensive substance (nitropyrin) that retards the bacterial conversion of ammonia to nitrite in the soil. Since ammonia is a cation and is retained by soil colloids, whereas nitrite and nitrate are readily leached away, nitropyrin could retard the loss of nitrogen from the soil. Finally, the absorptive capacity of some plant roots is increased by an intimate association, called mycorrhiza, between the roots and a fungus. The encouragement of mycorrhizal associations might benefit certain crop plants, particularly in infertile soils and where specific nutrients are low in availability.

A number of potential improvements in the agricultural efficiency of industrial societies are merely a matter of thrift. Many residues that are now burned or discarded could be returned to the soil to improve fertility; better still, they could be processed through animals to produce food. Organic wastes such as sewage sludge, cannery by-products and animal manures are rich sources of plant nutrients. About 44 percent of the live weight of cattle slaughtered for meat is inedible to man but is of high nutritional value as a protein concentrate for animal feeding. Nutrients are also wasted in the discarded by-products of grain milling, oil extraction, fish processing and fermentation. Billions of tons of crop residues, including straw, sugarcane refuse and sawdust, are potential feed for ruminants. In the U.S. alone 60 million acres of corn are grown for grain, which contains only half of the plant's potential energy; the other half, contained in the stalks and cobs, could be fed to animals. So could poultry and cattle manures; in fact, they are already being included in ruminant diets. The greater use of such bulky residues and by-products is limited mainly by the high cost of transportation. One possible strategy for avoiding those costs would be to decentralize animal agriculture in the U.S.

Competition for protein suitable for human consumption could be reduced and perhaps eliminated in ruminants by replacing protein in the ruminant diet with other sources of nitrogen. A lactating cow on a diet of waste roughage and urea produces more protein than it consumes. Rumen efficiency might be enhanced by rumen stimulants and digestive aids. Even nitrogen fixation has been demonstrated in the bacteria of the ruminant digestive tract and might someday be exploited.

Although man has become a manipulator of the food cycle, he is made of flesh and must still remain a participant in the cycle. A viable system of food production requires an efficient transfer of energy and exchange of nutrients between soil, plant, animal and microorganism. The relationship can be exploited for short-term gains or managed for long-term sustenance. It can be ignored only at our peril.

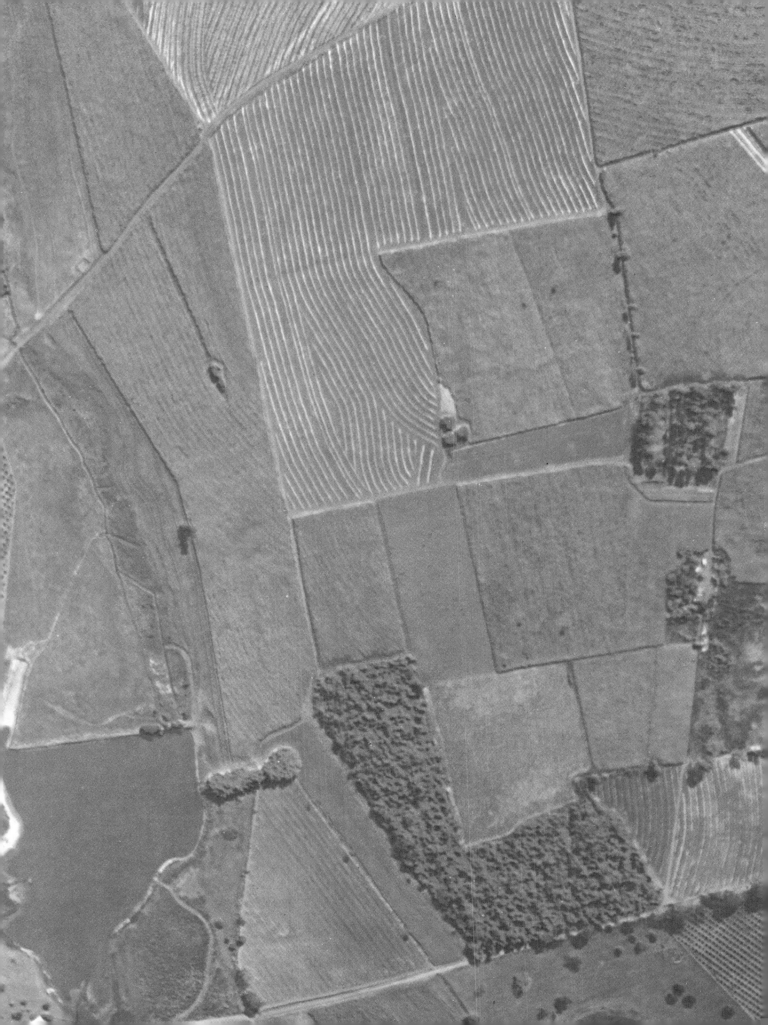

5

Human Food Production as a Process in the Biosphere

by Lester R. Brown
September 1970

*Human population growth is mainly the result of
increases in food production. This relation raises
the question: How many people can the biosphere
support without impairment of its overall operation?*

Throughout most of man's existence his numbers have been limited by the supply of food. For the first two million years or so he lived as a predator, a herbivore and a scavenger. Under such circumstances the biosphere could not support a human population of more than 10 million, a population smaller than that of London or Afghanistan today. Then, with his domestication of plants and animals some 10,000 years ago, man began to shape the biosphere to his own ends.

As primitive techniques of crop production and animal husbandry became more efficient the earth's food-producing capacity expanded, permitting increases in man's numbers. Population growth in turn exerted pressure on food supply, compelling man to further alter the biosphere in order to meet his food needs. Population growth and advances in food production have thus tended to be mutually reinforcing.

It took two million years for the human population to reach the one-billion mark, but the fourth billion now being added will require only 15 years: from 1960 to 1975. The enormous increase in the demand for food that is generated by this expansion in man's numbers, together with rising incomes, is beginning to have disturbing consequences. New signs of stress on the biosphere are reported almost daily. The continuing expansion of land under the plow and the evolution of a chemically oriented modern agriculture are producing ominous alterations in the biosphere not just on a local scale but, for the first time in history, on a global scale as well. The natural cycles of energy and the chemical elements are clearly being affected by man's efforts to expand his food supply.

Given the steadily advancing demand for food, further intervention in the biosphere for the expansion of the food supply is inevitable. Such intervention, however, can no longer be undertaken by an individual or a nation without consideration of the impact on the biosphere as a whole. The decision by a government to dam a river, by a farmer to use DDT on his crops or by a married couple to have another child, thereby increasing the demand for food, has repercussions for all mankind.

The revolutionary change in man's role from hunter and gatherer to tiller and herdsman took place in circumstances that are not well known, but some of the earliest evidence of agriculture is found in the hills and grassy plains of the Fertile Crescent in western Asia. The cultivation of food plants and the domestication of animals were aided there by the presence of wild wheat, barley, sheep, goats, pigs, cattle and horses. From the beginnings of agriculture man naturally favored above all other species those plants and animals that had been most useful to him in the wild. As a result of this favoritism he has altered the composition of the earth's plant and animal populations. Today his crops, replacing the original cover of grass or forest, occupy some three billion acres. This amounts to about 10 percent of the earth's total land surface and a considerably larger fraction of the land capable of supporting vegetation, that is, the area excluding deserts, polar regions and higher elevations. Two-thirds of the cultivated cropland is planted to cereals. The area planted to wheat alone is 600 million acres—nearly a million square miles, or an area equivalent to the U.S. east of the Mississippi. As for the influence of animal husbandry on the earth's animal populations, Hereford and Black Angus cattle roam the Great Plains, once the home of an estimated 30 to 40 million buffalo; in Australia the kangaroo has given way to European cattle; in Asia the domesticated water buffalo has multiplied in the major river valleys.

Clearly the food-producing enterprise has altered not only the relative abundance of plant and animal species but also their global distribution. The linkage of the Old and the New World in the 15th century set in motion an exchange of crops among various parts of the world that continues today. This exchange greatly increased the earth's capacity to sustain human populations, partly because some of the crops trans-

EXPERIMENTAL FARM in Brazil, one of thousands around the world where improvements in agricultural technology are pioneered, is seen as an image on an infrared-sensitive film in the aerial photograph on the opposite page. The reflectance of vegetation at near-infrared wavelengths of .7 to .9 micron registers on the film in false shades of red that are proportional to the intensity of the energy. The most reflective, and reddest, areas (*bottom*) are land still uncleared of forest cover. Most of the tilled fields, although irregular in shape, are contour-plowed. Regular patterns (*left and bottom right*) are citrus-orchard rows. The photograph was taken by a National Aeronautics and Space Administration mission in cooperation with the Brazilian government in a joint study of the assessment of agricultural resources by remote sensing. The farm is some 80 miles northwest of São Paulo.

ported elsewhere turned out to be better suited there than to their area of origin. Perhaps the classic example is the introduction of the potato from South America into northern Europe, where it greatly augmented the food supply, permitting marked increases in population. This was most clearly apparent in Ireland, where the population increased rapidly for several decades on the strength of the food supply represented by the potato. Only when the potato-blight organism (*Phytophthora infestans*) devastated the potato crop was population growth checked in Ireland.

The soybean, now the leading source of vegetable oil and principal farm export of the U.S., was introduced from China several decades ago. Grain sorghum, the second-ranking feed grain in the U.S. (after corn), came from Africa as a food store in the early slave ships. In the U.S.S.R. today the principal source of vegetable oil is the sunflower, a plant that originated on the southern Great Plains of the U.S. Corn, unknown in the Old World before Columbus, is now grown on every continent. On the other hand, North America is indebted to the Old World for all its livestock and poultry species with the exception of the turkey.

To man's accomplishments in exploiting the plants and animals that natural evolution has provided, and in improving them through selective breeding over the millenniums, he has added in this century the creation of remarkably productive new breeds, thanks to the discoveries of genetics. Genetics has made possible the development of cereals and other plant species that are more tolerant to cold, more resistant to drought, less susceptible to disease, more responsive to fertilizer, higher in yield and richer in protein. The story of hybrid corn is only one of many spectacular examples. The breeding of short-season corn varieties has extended the northern limit of this crop some 500 miles.

Plant breeders recently achieved a historic breakthrough in the development of new high-yielding varieties of wheat and rice for tropical and subtropical regions. These wheats and rices, bred by Rockefeller Foundation and Ford Foundation scientists in Mexico and the Philippines, are distinguished by several characteristics. Most important, they are short-statured and stiff-strawed, and are highly responsive to chemical fertilizer. They also mature earlier. The first of the high-yielding rices, IR-8, matures in 120

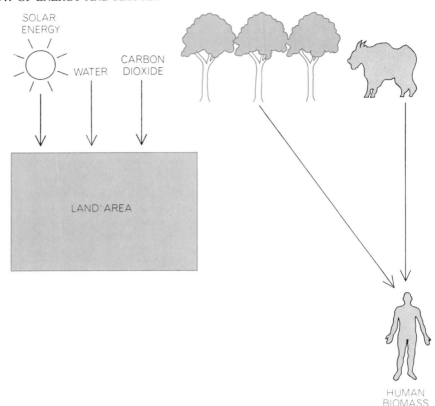

SOLAR ENERGY

WATER   CARBON DIOXIDE

LAND AREA

HUMAN BIOMASS

IMPACT OF THE AGRICULTURAL REVOLUTION on the human population is outlined in these two diagrams. The diagram at left shows the state of affairs before the invention of agriculture: the plants and animals supported by photosynthesis on the total land area could support a human population of only about 10 million. The diagram at right shows

days as against 150 to 180 days for other varieties.

Another significant advance incorporated into the new strains is the reduced sensitivity of their seed to photoperiod (length of day). This is partly the result of their cosmopolitan ancestry: they were developed from seed collections all over the world. The biological clocks of traditional varieties of cereals were keyed to specific seasonal cycles, and these cereals could be planted only at a certain time of the year, in the case of rice say at the onset of the monsoon season. The new wheats, which are quite flexible in terms of both seasonal and latitudinal variations in length of day, are now being grown in developing countries as far north as Turkey and as far south as Paraguay.

The combination of earlier maturity and reduced sensitivity to day length creates new opportunities for multiple cropping in tropical and subtropical regions where water supplies are adequate, enabling farmers to harvest two, three and occasionally even four crops per year. Workers at the International Rice Research Institute in the Philippines regularly harvest three crops of rice per

year. Each acre they plant yields six tons annually, roughly three times the average yield of corn, the highest-yielding cereal in the U.S. Thousands of farmers in northern India are now alternating a crop of early-maturing winter wheat with a summer crop of rice, greatly increasing the productivity of their land. These new opportunities for farming land more intensively lessen the pressure for bringing marginal land under cultivation, thus helping to conserve precious topsoil. At the same time they increase the use of agricultural chemicals, creating environmental stresses more akin to those in the advanced countries.

The new dwarf wheats and rices are far more efficient than the traditional varieties in their use of land, water, fertilizer and labor. The new opportunities for multiple cropping permit conversion of far more of the available solar energy into food. The new strains are not the solution to the food problem, but they are removing the threat of massive famine in the short run. They are buying time for the stabilization of population, which is ultimately the only solution to the food crisis. This "green revolution"

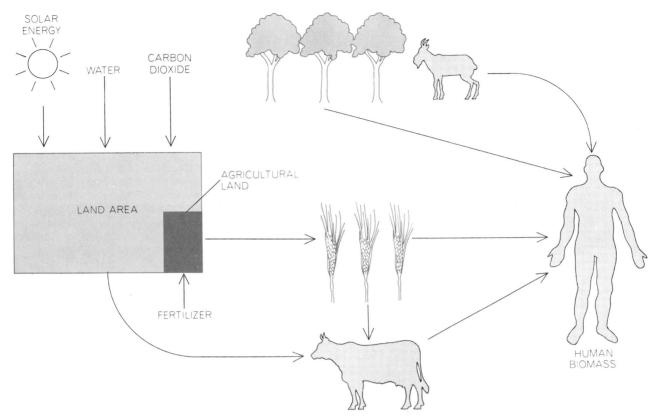

the state of affairs after the invention of agriculture. The 10 percent of the land now under the plow, watered and fertilized by man, is the primary support for a human population of 3.5 billion. Some of the agricultural produce is consumed directly by man; some is consumed indirectly by first being fed to domestic animals. Some of the food for domestic animals, however, comes from land not under the plow (curved arrow at bottom left). Man also obtains some food from sources other than agriculture, such as fishing.

may affect the well-being of more people in a shorter period of time than any technological advance in history.

The progress of man's expansion of food production is reflected in the way crop yields have traditionally been calculated. Today the output of cereals is expressed in yield per acre, but in early civilizations it was calculated as a ratio of the grain produced to that required for seed. On this basis the current ratio is perhaps highest in the U.S. corn belt, where farmers realize a four-hundred-fold return on the hybrid corn seed they plant. The ratio for rice is also quite high, but the ratio for wheat, the third of the principal cereals, is much lower, possibly 30 to one on a global basis.

The results of man's efforts to increase the productivity of domestic animals are equally impressive. When the ancestors of our present chickens were domesticated, they laid a clutch of about 15 eggs once a year. Hens in the U.S. today average 220 eggs per year, and the figure is rising steadily as a result of continuing advances in breeding and feeding. When cattle were originally domesticated, they probably did not produce more than 600 pounds of milk per year,

barely enough for a calf. (It is roughly the average amount produced by cows in India today.) The 13 million dairy cows in the U.S. today average 9,000 pounds of milk yearly, outproducing their ancestors 15 to one.

Most such advances in the productivity of plant and animal species are recent. Throughout most of history man's efforts to meet his food needs have been directed primarily toward bringing more land under cultivation, spreading agriculture from valley to valley and continent to continent. He has also, however, invented techniques to raise the productivity of land already under cultivation, particularly in this century, when the decreasing availability of new lands for expansion has compelled him to turn to a more intensive agriculture. These techniques involve altering the biosphere's cycles of energy, water, nitrogen and minerals.

Modern agriculture depends heavily on four technologies: mechanization, irrigation, fertilization and the chemical control of weeds and insects. Each of these technologies has made an important contribution to the earth's in-

creased capacity for sustaining human populations, and each has perturbed the cycles of the biosphere.

At least as early as 3000 B.C. the farmers of the Middle East learned to harness draft animals to help them till the soil. Harnessing animals much stronger than himself enabled man to greatly augment his own limited muscle power. It also enabled him to convert roughage (indigestible by humans) into a usable form of energy and thus to free some of his energy for pursuits other than the quest for food. The invention of the internal-combustion engine and the tractor 5,000 years later provided a much greater breakthrough. It now became possible to substitute petroleum (the product of the photosynthesis of aeons ago) for oats, corn and hay grown as feed for draft animals. The replacement of horses by the tractor not only provided the farmer with several times as much power but also released 70 million acres in the U.S. that had been devoted to raising feed for horses.

In the highly mechanized agriculture of today the expenditure of fossil fuel energy per acre is often substantially greater than the energy yield embodied in the food produced. This deficit in the output is of no immediate consequence, because the system is drawing on energy in the bank. When fossil fuels become scarcer, man will have to turn to some other source of motive energy for agriculture: perhaps nuclear energy or some means, other than photosynthesis, of harnessing solar energy. For the present and for the purposes of agriculture the energy budget of the biosphere is still favorable: the supply of solar energy—both the energy stored in fossil fuels and that taken up daily and converted into food energy by crops—enables an advanced nation to be fed with only 5 percent of the population directly employed in agriculture.

The combination of draft animals and mechanical power has given man an enormous capacity for altering the earth's surface by bringing additional land under the plow (not all of it suited for cultivation). In addition, in the poorer countries his expanding need for fuel has forced him to cut forests far in excess of their ability to renew themselves. The areas largely stripped of forest include mainland China and the subcontinent of India and Pakistan, where much of the population must now use cow dung for fuel. Although statistics are not available, the proportion of mankind using cow dung as fuel to prepare meals may

far exceed the proportion using natural gas. Livestock populations providing draft power, food and fuel tend to increase along with human populations, and in many poor countries the needs of livestock for forage far exceed its self-renewal, gradually denuding the countryside of grass cover.

As population pressure builds, not only is more land brought under the plow but also the land remaining is less suited to cultivation. Once valleys are filled, farmers begin to move up hillsides, creating serious soil-erosion problems. As the natural cover that retards runoff is reduced and soil structure deteriorates, floods and droughts become more severe.

Over most of the earth the thin layer of topsoil producing most of man's food is measured in inches. Denuding the land of its year-round natural cover of grass or forest exposes the thin mantle of life-sustaining soil to rapid erosion by wind and water. Much of the soil ultimately washes into the sea, and some of it is lifted into the atmosphere. Man's actions are causing the topsoil to be removed faster than it is formed. This unstable relationship between man and the land from which he derives his subsistence obviously cannot continue indefinitely.

Robert R. Brooks of Williams College, an economist who spent several years in India, gives a wry description of the process occurring in the state of Rajasthan, where tens of thousands of acres of rural land are being abandoned yearly because of the loss of topsoil: "Overgrazing by goats destroys the desert plants which might otherwise hold the soil in place. Goatherds equipped with sickles attached to 20-foot poles strip the leaves of trees to float downward into the waiting mouths of famished goats and sheep. The trees die and the soil blows away 200 miles to New Delhi, where it comes to rest in the lungs of its inhabitants and on the shiny cars of foreign diplomats."

Soil erosion not only results in a loss of soil but also impairs irrigation systems. This is illustrated in the Mangla irrigation reservoir, recently built in the foothills of the Himalayas in West Pakistan as part of the Indus River irrigation system. On the basis of feasibility studies indicating that the reservoir could be expected to have a lifetime of at least 100 years, $600 million was invested in the construction of the reservoir. Denuding and erosion of the soil in the watershed, however, accompanying a rapid growth of population in the area, has already washed so much soil into the reservoir that it is now expected to be completely filled with silt within 50 years.

A historic example of the effects of man's abuse of the soil is all too plainly visible in North Africa, which once was the fertile granary of the Roman Empire and now is largely a desert or near-desert whose people are fed with the aid of food imports from the U.S. In the U.S. itself the "dust bowl" experience of the 1930's remains a vivid lesson on the folly of overplowing. More recently the U.S.S.R. repeated this error, bringing 100 million acres of virgin soil under the plow only to discover that the region's rainfall was too scanty to sustain continuous cultivation. Once moisture reserves in the soil were depleted the soil began to blow.

Soil erosion is one of the most pressing and most difficult problems threatening the future of the biosphere. Each year it is forcing the abandonment of millions of acres of cropland in Asia, the Middle East, North Africa and Central America. Nature's geological cycle continuously produces topsoil, but its pace is far too slow to be useful to man. Someone once defined soil as rock on its way to the sea. Soil is produced by the weathering of rock and the process takes several centuries to form an inch of topsoil. Man is managing to destroy the topsoil

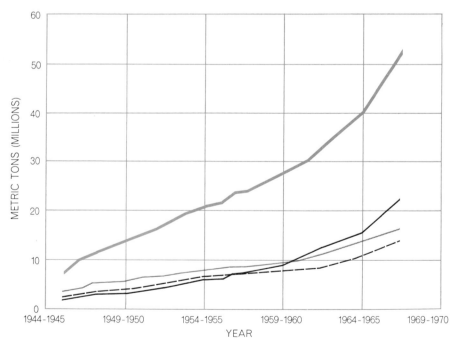

FERTILIZER CONSUMPTION has increased more than fivefold since the end of World War II. The top line in the graph (color) shows the tonnage of all kinds of fertilizers combined. The lines below show the tonnages of the three major types: nitrogen (black), now the leader, phosphate (gray) and potash (broken line). Figures, from the most recent report by the UN Food and Agriculture Organization, omit fertilizer consumption in China.

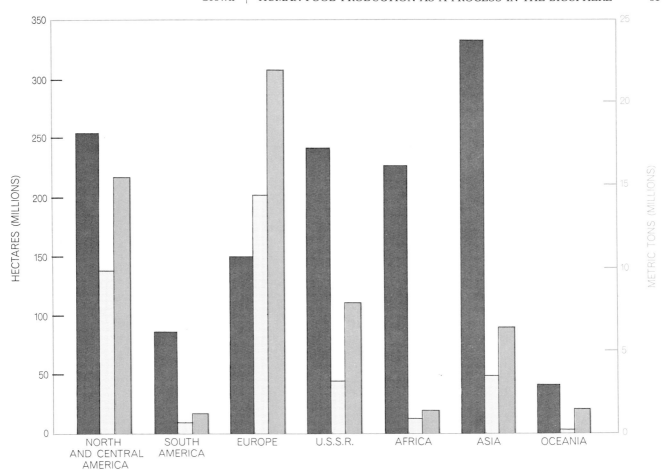

TONS OF FERTILIZER used in seven world areas are compared with the amount of agricultural land in each area. Two tonnages are shown in each instance: the amount used in 1962–1963 (*light color*) and the amount used in 1967–1968 (*solid color*). The great- est use of fertilizer occurs in Europe, the least fertilized area is Africa and the greatest percentage increase in the period was in Australia and New Zealand. Figures, from the Food and Agricul- ture Organization, omit China, North Korea and North Vietnam.

in some areas of the world in a fraction of this time. The only possible remedy is to find ways to conserve the topsoil more effectively.

The dust-bowl era in the U.S. ended with the widespread adoption of con- servation practices by farmers. Twenty million acres were fallowed to accumu- late moisture and thousands of miles of windbreaks were planted across the Great Plains. Fallow land was alternated with strips of wheat ("strip-cropping") to reduce the blowing of soil while the land was idle. The densely populated coun- tries of Asia, however, are in no position to adopt such tactics. Their food needs are so pressing that they cannot afford to take large areas out of cultivation; moreover, they do not yet have the finan- cial resources or the technical skills for the immense projects in reforestation, controlled grazing of cattle, terracing, contour farming and systematic manage- ment of watersheds that would be re- quired to preserve their soil.

The significance of wind erosion goes far beyond the mere loss of topsoil. As other authors in this issue have observed, a continuing increase in particulate mat- ter in the atmosphere could affect the earth's climate by reducing the amount of incoming solar energy. This particu- late matter comes not only from the technological activities of the richer countries but also from wind erosion in the poorer countries. The poorer coun- tries do not have the resources for un- dertaking the necessary effort to arrest and reverse this trend. Should it be es- tablished that an increasing amount of particulate matter in the atmosphere is changing the climate, the richer coun- tries would have still another reason to provide massive capital and technical as- sistance to the poor countries, joining with them to confront this common threat to mankind.

Irrigation, which agricultural man be- gan to practice at least as early as 6,000 years ago, even earlier than he harnessed animal power, has played its great role in increasing food production by bringing into profitable cultivation vast areas that would otherwise be un- usable or only marginally productive. Most of the world's irrigated land is in Asia, where it is devoted primarily to the production of rice. In Africa the Volta River of Ghana and the Nile are dammed for irrigation and power pur- poses. The Colorado River system of the U.S. is used extensively for irrigation in the Southwest, as are scores of rivers elsewhere. Still to be exploited for irri- gation are the Mekong of southeastern Asia and the Amazon.

During the past few years there has been an important new irrigation devel- opment in Asia: the widespread installa- tion of small-scale irrigation systems on individual farms. In Pakistan and India, where in many places the water table is close to the surface, hundreds of thou- sands of tube wells with pumps have been installed in recent years. Interest- ingly, this development came about partly as an answer to a problem that had been presented by irrigation itself.

Like many of man's other interventions in the biosphere, his reshaping of the hydrologic cycle has had unwanted side effects. One of them is the raising of the water table by the diversion of river water onto the land. Over a period of time the percolation of irrigation water downward and the accumulation of this water underground may gradually raise the water table until it is within a few feet or even a few inches of the surface. This not only inhibits the growth of plant roots by waterlogging but also results in the surface soil's becoming salty as water evaporates through it, leaving a concentrated deposit of salts in the upper few inches. Such a situation developed in West Pakistan after its fertile plain had been irrigated with water from the Indus for a century. During a visit by President Ayub to Washington in 1961 he appealed to President Kennedy for help: West Pakistan was losing 60,-000 acres of fertile cropland per year because of waterlogging and salinity as its population was expanding 2.5 percent yearly.

This same sequence, the diversion of river water into land for irrigation, followed eventually by waterlogging and salinity and the abandonment of land,

had been repeated many times throughout history. The result was invariably the decline, and sometimes the disappearance, of the civilizations thus intervening in the hydrologic cycle. The remains of civilizations buried in the deserts of the Middle East attest to early experiences similar to those of contemporary Pakistan. These civilizations, however, had no one to turn to for foreign aid. An interdisciplinary U.S. team led by Roger Revelle, then Science Adviser to the Secretary of the Interior, studied the problem and proposed among other things a system of tube wells that would lower the water table by tapping the ground water for intensive irrigation. Discharging this water on the surface, the wells would also wash the soil's salt downward. The stratagem worked, and the salty, waterlogged land of Pakistan is steadily being reclaimed.

Other side effects of river irrigation are not so easily remedied. Such irrigation has brought about a great increase in the incidence of schistosomiasis, a disease that is particularly prevalent in the river valleys of Africa and Asia. The disease is produced by the parasitic larva of a blood fluke, which is harbored by aquatic snails and burrows into the flesh

of people standing in water or in water-soaked fields. The Chinese call schistosomiasis "snail fever"; it might also be called the poor man's emphysema, because, like emphysema, this extremely debilitating disease is environmentally induced through conditions created by man. The snails and the fluke thrive in perennial irrigation systems, where they are in close proximity to large human populations. The incidence of the disease is rising rapidly as the world's large rivers are harnessed for irrigation, and today schistosomiasis is estimated to afflict 250 million people. It now surpasses malaria, the incidence of which is declining, as the world's most prevalent infectious disease.

As a necessity for food production water is of course becoming an increasingly crucial commodity. The projected increases in population and in food requirements will call for more and more water, forcing man to consider still more massive and complex interventions in the biosphere. The desalting of seawater for irrigation purposes is only one major departure from traditional practices. Another is a Russian plan to reverse the flow of four rivers currently flowing northward and emptying into the Arctic Ocean. These rivers would be diverted southward into the semiarid lands of southern Russia, greatly enlarging the irrigated area of the U.S.S.R. Some climatologists are concerned, however, that the shutting off of the flow of relatively warm water from these four rivers would have far-reaching implications for not only the climate of the Arctic but also the climatic system of the entire earth.

The growing competition for scarce water supplies among states and among various uses in the western U.S. is also forcing consideration of heroic plans. For example, a detailed engineering proposal exists for the diversion of the Yukon River in Alaska southward across Canada into the western U.S. to meet the growing need for water for both agricultural and industrial purposes. The effort would cost an estimated $100 billion.

Representing an even greater intervention in the biosphere is the prospect that man may one day consciously alter the earth's climatic patterns, shifting some of the rain now falling on the oceans to the land. Among the steps needed for the realization of such a scheme are the construction of a comprehensive model of the earth's climatic system and the development of a computational facility capable of simulating

FOOD GRAINS

LIVESTOCK PRODUCTS (EXCLUDING FATS)

TUBERS

OTHER VEGETABLES, FRUITS

FATS AND OILS

SUGAR

FISH

0   25   50   75   100
PERCENT

WORLDWIDE FOOD ENERGY comes in different amounts from different products. Cereals outstrip other foodstuffs; wheat and rice each supply a fifth of mankind's food energy.

and manipulating the model. The required information includes data on temperatures, humidity, precipitation, the movement of air masses, ocean currents and many other factors that enter into the weather. Earth-orbiting satellites will doubtless be able to collect much of this information, and the present generation of advanced computers appears to be capable of carrying out the necessary experiments on the model. For the implementation of the findings, that is, for the useful control of rainfall, there will of course be a further requirement: the project will have to be managed by a global and supranational agency if it is not to lead to weather wars among nations working at cross purposes. Some commercial firms are already in the business of rainmaking, and they are operating on an international basis.

The third great technology that man has introduced to increase food production is the use of chemical fertilizers. We owe the foundation for this development to Justus von Liebig of Germany, who early in the 19th century determined the specific requirements of nitrogen, phosphorus, potassium and other nutrients for plant growth. Chemical fertilizers did not come into widespread use, however, until this century, when the pressure of population and the disappearance of new frontiers compelled farmers to substitute fertilizer for the expansion of cropland to meet growing food needs. One of the first countries to intensify its agriculture, largely by the use of fertilizers, was Japan, whose output of food per acre has steadily risen (except for wartime interruptions) since the turn of the century. The output per acre of a few other countries, including the Netherlands, Denmark and Sweden, began to rise at about the same time. The U.S., richly endowed with vast farmlands, did not turn to the heavy use of fertilizer and other intensive measures until about 1940. Since then its yields per acre, assisted by new varieties of grain highly responsive to fertilizer, have also shown remarkable gains. Yields of corn, the production of which exceeds that of all other cereals combined in the U.S., have nearly tripled over the past three decades.

Experience has demonstrated that in areas of high rainfall the application of chemical fertilizers in conjunction with other inputs and practices can double, triple or even quadruple the productivity of intensively farmed soils. Such levels of productivity are achieved in Japan and the Netherlands, where farmers apply up to 300 pounds of plant nutrients per acre per year. The use of chemical fertilizers is estimated to account for at least a fourth of man's total food supply. The world's farmers are currently applying 60 million metric tons of plant nutrients per year, an average of nearly 45 pounds per acre for the three billion acres of cropland. Such application, however, is unevenly distributed. Some poor countries do not yet benefit from the use of fertilizer in any significant amounts. If global projections of population and income growth materialize, the production of fertilizer over the remaining three decades of this century must almost triple to satisfy food demands.

Can the projected demand for fertilizer be met? The key ingredient is nitrogen, and fortunately man has learned how to speed up the fixation phase of the nitrogen cycle [see "The Nitrogen Cycle," by C. C. Delwiche, SCIENTIFIC AMERICAN Offprint 1194]. In nature the nitrogen of the air is fixed in the soil by certain microorganisms, such as those present in the root nodules of leguminous plants. Chemists have now devised various ways of incorporating nitrogen from the air into inorganic compounds and making it available in the form of nitrogen fertilizers. These chemical processes produce the fertilizer much more rapidly and economically than the growing of leguminous-plant sources such as clover, alfalfa or soybeans. More than 25 million tons of nitrogen fertilizer is now being synthesized and added to the earth's soil annually.

The other principal ingredients of chemical fertilizer are the minerals potassium and phosphorus. Unlike nitrogen, these elements are not replenished by comparatively fast natural cycles. Potassium presents no immediate problem; the rich potash fields of Canada alone are estimated to contain enough potassium to supply mankind's needs for centuries to come. The reserves of phosphorus, however, are not nearly so plentiful as those of potassium. Every year 3.5 million tons of phosphorus washes into the sea, where it remains as sediment on the ocean floor. Eventually it will be thrust above the ocean surface again by geologic uplift, but man cannot wait that long. Phosphorus may be one of the first necessities that will prompt man to begin to mine the ocean bed.

The great expansion of the use of fertilizers in this century has benefited mankind enormously, but the benefits are not unalloyed. The runoff of chemical fertilizers into rivers, lakes and underground waters creates two important hazards. One is the chemical pollution

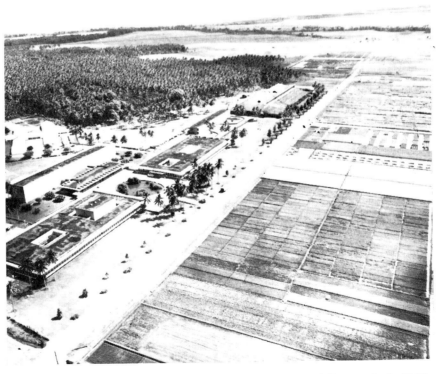

EXPERIMENTAL PLANTINGS at the International Rice Research Institute in the Philippine Republic are seen in an aerial photograph. IR-8, a high-yield rice, was bred here.

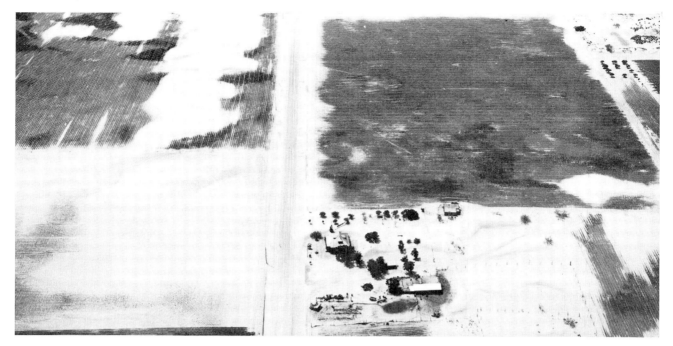

RUINED FARM in the "dust bowl" area of the U.S. in the 1930's is seen in an aerial photograph. The farm is near Union in Terry County, Tex. The wind has eroded the powdery, drought-parched topsoil and formed drifts among the buildings and across the fields.

of drinking water. In certain areas in Illinois and California the nitrate content of well water has risen to a toxic level. Excessive nitrate can cause the physiological disorder methemoglobinemia, which reduces the blood's oxygen-carrying capacity and can be particularly dangerous to children under five. This hazard is of only local dimensions and can be countered by finding alternative sources of drinking water. A much more extensive hazard, profound in its effects on the biosphere, is the now well-known phenomenon called eutrophication.

Inorganic nitrates and phosphates discharged into lakes and other bodies of fresh water provide a rich medium for the growth of algae; the massive growth of the algae in turn depletes the water of oxygen and thus kills off the fish life. In the end the eutrophication, or overfertilization, of the lake slowly brings about its death as a body of fresh water, converting it into a swamp. Lake Erie is a prime example of this process now under way.

How much of the now widespread eutrophication of fresh waters is attributable to agricultural fertilization and how much to other causes remains an open question. Undoubtedly the runoff of nitrates and phosphates from farmlands plays a large part. There are also other important contributors, however. Considerable amounts of phosphate, coming mainly from detergents, are discharged into rivers and lakes from sewers carrying municipal and industrial

wastes. And there is reason to believe that in some rivers and lakes most of the nitrate may come not from fertilizers but from the internal-combustion engine. It is estimated that in the state of New Jersey, which has heavy automobile traffic, nitrous oxide products of gasoline combustion, picked up and deposited by rainfall, contribute as much as 20 pounds of nitrogen per acre per year to the land. Some of this nitrogen washes into the many rivers and lakes of New Jersey and its adjoining states. A way must be found to deal with the eutrophication problem because even in the short run it can have damaging effects, affecting as it does the supply of potable water, the cycles of aquatic life and consequently man's food supply.

Recent findings have presented us with a related problem in connection with the fourth technology supporting man's present high level of food production: the chemical control of diseases, insects and weeds. It is now clear that the use of DDT and other chlorinated hydrocarbons as pesticides and herbicides is beginning to threaten many species of animal life, possibly including man. DDT today is found in the tissues of animals over a global range of life forms and geography from penguins in Antarctica to children in the villages of Thailand. There is strong evidence that it is actually on the way to extinguishing some animal species, notably predatory birds such as the bald eagle and the peregrine falcon, whose capacity for using calcium is so impaired by DDT

that the shells of their eggs are too thin to avoid breakage in the nest before the fledglings hatch. Carnivores are particularly likely to concentrate DDT in their tissues because they feed on herbivores that have already concentrated it from large quantities of vegetation. Concentrations of DDT in mothers' milk in the U.S. now exceed the tolerance levels established for foodstuffs by the Food and Drug Administration.

It is ironic that less than a generation after 1948, when Paul Hermann Müller of Switzerland received a Nobel prize for the discovery of DDT, the use of the insecticide is being banned by law in many countries. This illustrates how little man knows about the effects of his intervening in the biosphere. Up to now he has been using the biosphere as a laboratory, sometimes with unhappy results.

Several new approaches to the problem of controlling pests are now being explored. Chemists are searching for pesticides that will be degradable, instead of long-lasting, after being deposited on vegetation or in the soil, and that will be aimed at specific pests rather than acting as broad-spectrum poisons for many forms of life. Much hope is placed in techniques of biological control, such as are exemplified in the mass sterilization (by irradiation) of male screwworm flies, a pest of cattle that used to cost U.S. livestock producers $100 million per year. The release of 125 million irradiated male screwworm flies weekly in the U.S. and in adjoining areas of Mexico (in a cooperative effort with the Mexican government) is holding the fly population to a negligible level. Efforts are now under way to get rid of the Mexican fruit fly and the pink cotton bollworm in California by the same method.

Successes are also being achieved in breeding resistance to insect pests in various crops. A strain of wheat has been developed that is resistant to the Hessian fly; resistance to the corn borer and the corn earworm has been bred into strains of corn, and work is in progress on a strain of alfalfa that resists aphids and leafhoppers. Another promising approach, which already has a considerable history, is the development of insect parasites, ranging from bacteria and viruses to wasps that lay their eggs in other insects. The fact remains, however, that the biological control of pests is still in its infancy.

I have here briefly reviewed the major agricultural technologies evolved to meet man's increasing food needs, the problems arising from them and some possible solutions. What is the present balance sheet on the satisfaction of human food needs? Although man's food supply has expanded several hundredfold since the invention of agriculture, two-thirds of mankind is still hungry and malnourished much of the time. On the credit side a third of mankind, living largely in North America, Europe, Australia and Japan, has achieved an adequate food supply, and for the remaining two-thirds the threat of large-scale famine has recently been removed, at least for the immediate future. In spite of rapid population growth in the developing countries since World War II, their peoples have been spared from massive famine (except in Biafra in 1969–1970) by huge exports of food from the developed countries. As a result of two consecutive monsoon failures in India, a fifth of the total U.S. wheat crop was shipped to India in both 1966 and 1967, feeding 60 million Indians for two years.

Although the threat of outright famine has been more or less eliminated for the time being, human nutrition on the global scale is still in a sorry state. Malnutrition, particularly protein deficiency, exacts an enormous toll from the physical and mental development of the young in the poorer countries. This was dramatically illustrated when India held tryouts in 1968 to select a team to represent it in the Olympic games that year. Not a single Indian athlete, male or female, met the minimum standards for qualifying to compete in any of the 36

track and field events in Mexico City. No doubt this was partly due to the lack of support for athletics in India, but poor nutrition was certainly also a large factor. The young people of Japan today are visible examples of what a change can be brought about by improvement in nutrition. Well-nourished from infancy, Japanese teen-agers are on the average some two inches taller than their elders.

Protein is as crucial for children's mental development as for their physical development. This was strikingly shown in a recent study extending over several years in Mexico: children who had been severely undernourished before the age of five were found to average 13 points lower in I.Q. than a carefully selected control group. Unfortunately no amount of feeding or education in later life can repair the setbacks to development caused by undernourishment in the early years. Protein shortages in the poor countries today are depreciating human resources for at least a generation to come.

Protein constitutes the main key to human health and vigor, and the key to the protein diet at present is held by grain consumed either directly or indirectly (in the form of meat, milk and eggs). Cereals, occupying more than 70 percent of the world's cropland, provide 52 percent of man's direct energy intake. Eleven percent is supplied by livestock products such as meat, milk and eggs, 10 percent by potatoes and other tubers, 10 percent by fruits and vegetables, 9 percent by animal fats and vegetable oils, 7 percent by sugar and 1 percent by fish. As in the case of the total quantity of the individual diet, however, the composition of the diet varies greatly around the world. The difference is most marked in the per capita use of grain consumed directly and indirectly.

The two billion people living in the poor countries consume an average of about 360 pounds of grain per year, or about a pound per day. With only one pound per day, nearly all must be consumed directly to meet minimal energy requirements; little remains for feeding to livestock, which may convert only a tenth of their feed intake into meat or other edible human food. The average American, in contrast, consumes more than 1,600 pounds of grain per year. He eats only about 150 pounds of this directly in the form of bread, breakfast cereal and so on; the rest is consumed indirectly in the form of meat, milk and eggs. In short, he enjoys the luxury of the highly inefficient animal conversion

of grain into tastier and somewhat more nutritious proteins.

Thus the average North American currently makes about four times as great a demand on the earth's agricultural ecosystem as someone living in one of the poor countries. As the income levels in these countries rise, so will their demand for a richer diet of animal products. For the increasing world population at the end of the century, which is expected to be twice the 3.5 billion of today, the world production of grain would have to be doubled merely to maintain present consumption levels. This increase, combined with the projected improvement in diet associated with gains in income over the next three decades, could nearly triple the demand for grain, requiring that the food supply increase more over the next three decades than it has in the 10,000 years since agriculture began.

There are ways in which this pressure can be eased somewhat. One is the breeding of higher protein content in grains and other crops, making them nutritionally more acceptable as alternatives to livestock products. Another is the development of vegetable substitutes for animal products, such as are already available in the form of oleomargarine, soybean oil, imitation meats and other replacements (about 65 percent of the whipped toppings and 35 percent of the coffee whiteners now sold in U.S. supermarkets are nondairy products). Pressures on the agricultural ecosystem would thus drive high-income man one step down in the food chain to a level of more efficient consumption of what could be produced by agriculture.

What is clearly needed today is a cooperative effort—more specifically, a world environmental agency—to monitor, investigate and regulate man's interventions in the environment, including those made in his quest for more food. Since many of his efforts to enlarge his food supply have a global impact, they can only be dealt with in the context of a global institution. The health of the biosphere can no longer be separated from our modes of political organization. Whatever measures are taken, there is growing doubt that the agricultural ecosystem will be able to accommodate both the anticipated increase of the human population to seven billion by the end of the century and the universal desire of the world's hungry for a better diet. The central question is no longer "Can we produce enough food?" but "What are the environmental consequences of attempting to do so?"

II

MAN'S FOOD

II   MAN'S FOOD

INTRODUCTION

Early man ate what he could find. He hunted and gathered food, often wandering far from his home for this purpose. Hunting and gathering was a tedious and risky way to obtain an adequate diet. Humans practicing this life-style typically lived in small, scattered bands, shifting their campsites according to the cycle of the seasons and competing with other herbivores and predators for food. Diversity of diet could only be achieved by mastery of the local plant and animal lore and by systematic exploitation of all species known to be edible. And, in contrast to what may be believed, if he found enough food, early man had a balanced diet.

Today the hunting and gathering life-style is confined to a few peoples living in environments unsuitable for intensive agriculture—the pygmies of the equatorial rain forest of Africa, groups of Eskimos in the Arctic, and occasional bands of aborigines in the outback of Australia. For most of the peoples of the world, hunting and gathering has long since become obsolete, as a result of changes ushered in by the Agricultural Revolution.

With the Agricultural Revolution came plant and animal domestication, which led to profound and irreversible changes in human society as well as human nutrition. The new domesticates, when carefully sheltered from competing species, could support large, settled human populations. Improvement was undoubtedly brought about through rough genetic selection based on an intuitive understanding that "like breeds like." Thus, although the early plant and animal breeders were ignorant of genetic theory, they nonetheless managed to increase the productivity of their crops and herds from generation to generation. The result has been the growth of large human populations completely dependent upon one or a very few highly productive domesticated species for their continued survival. The anthropological, archeological, and biological origins of this situation are discussed by Jack Harlan in "The Plants and Animals that Nourish Man."

The mainstays of the human diet today are cereals, tubers, meat, fish, and poultry, together with a host of more localized plant and animal products that have been adopted as foods by particular peoples. Carbohydrate yields the bulk of the calories required for survival, and most societies rely upon a single kind of grain-bearing grass or tuber as their primary source of carbohydrate. The history and present status of the most widely cultivated grass is discussed in the article "Wheat" by Paul Mangelsdorf.

The first food of all young mammals, including the human infant, is milk. Milk derived from domesticated animals persists in the diet of certain peoples throughout adult life. The domestication of one milk- and meat-producing animal is discussed in "Cattle" by Ralph Phillips. The articles "Milk" by Stuart Patton (as well as "Lactose and Lactase" by Norman Kretchmer in Section III) describes the processes involved in the biologic synthesis and utilization of this food.

All foods were originally limited in distribution. Some foods are still used solely by certain people or in a single geographic locale. The edible snail enjoyed by the French, the dog or monkey consumed by the Chinese, the termite used as a source of protein in Zaire, and the seaweed used by the Japanese are all examples. Once a food has been discovered by one group of humans, it may be transported far from its site of origin and become established in the diet of distant peoples in radically different cultures. The manner of distribution of one little-known food is delightfully described by Richard Howard in "Captain Bligh and the Breadfruit."

The articles in this section acquaint the reader with the possibility that the availability of food sources change over time. Continuous progress in technology, beginning with the Agricultural Revolution and accelerating rapidly in the past century, has greatly enhanced our capacity for production, storage, and distribution of food. These advances in food technology have provided for a wider range of food products than ever before.

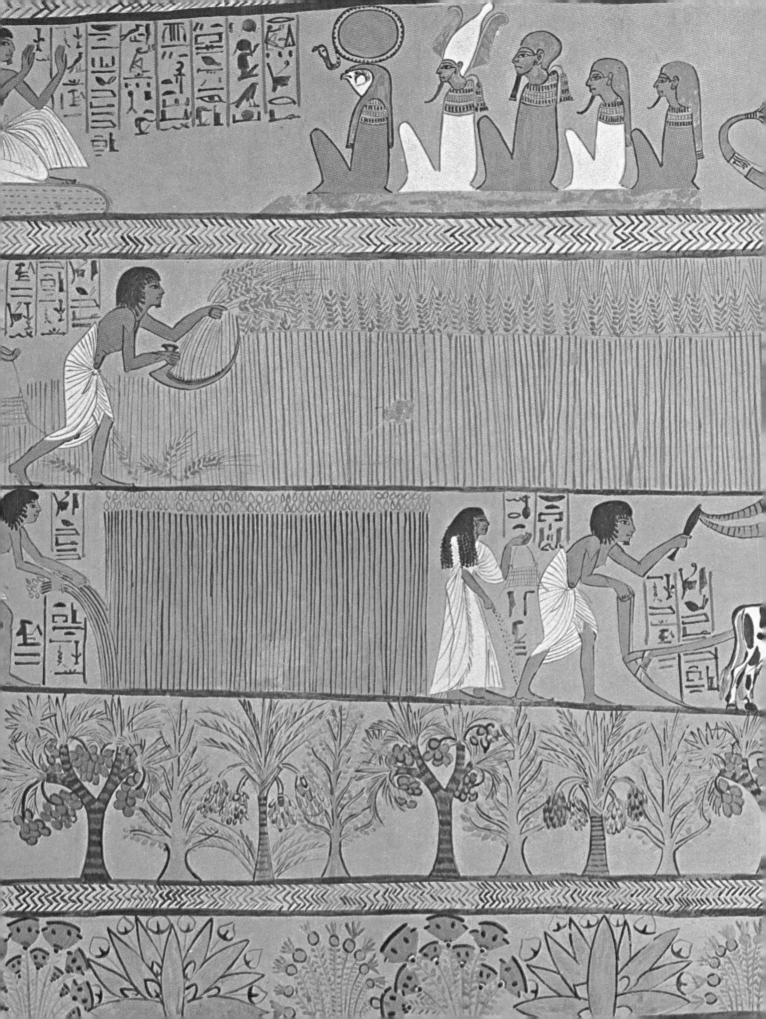

6

The Plants and Animals That Nourish Man

by Jack R. Harlan
September 1976

Over the past 10,000 years man has chosen a relatively small number of plants and animals for domestication. The process made the domesticated species and man mutually dependent

Man once enjoyed a highly varied diet. He has used for food several thousand species of plants and several hundred species of animals. Only a relatively small number of these species were ever domesticated. With the beginnings of agriculture there was a tendency to concentrate on the species that were the more productive and the most rewarding in terms of labor and capital invested. When towns and cities emerged, the list of food sources was narrowed somewhat as farmers sold the most profitable crops and animals to the urban population. In the past few centuries the trend has accelerated with industrialization and the rise of cash economies. The supermarket and quick-food services have drastically restricted the human diet in the U.S., and their influence is beginning to be felt abroad.

The trend for more and more people to be nourished by fewer and fewer plant and animal food sources has reached the point today where most of the world's population is absolutely dependent on a handful of species [*see illustration on next page*]. The four crops at the head of the list contribute more tonnage to the world total than the next 26 crops combined. This is a relatively recent phenomenon and was not characteristic of the traditional subsistence agricultures abandoned over the past few centuries. As the trend intensifies, man becomes ever more vulnerable. His food supply now depends on the success

of a small number of species, and the failure of one of them may mean automatic starvation for millions of people. We have wandered down a path toward heavy dependence on a few species, and there seems to be no return.

Where, when and how did man begin this long and fateful journey? Twenty years ago the "where" was an easy question to answer. If one wanted to locate the origin of a domesticated plant, all one needed to do was to look it up in the writings of N. I. Vavilov, the geneticist who directed the All-Union Institute of Plant Industry in Leningrad from 1920 to 1940. Vavilov organized plant-collecting expeditions on a global scale, assembled masses of material, analyzed the collections and identified geographic "centers of origin" on the basis of the patterns of variation observed in both domestic crops and their wild relatives. He concluded that eight such centers existed, six of them in the Old World and two in the New.

Vavilov's work was monumental, and its impact on students of agriculture around the world was enormous. Studies since his time have shown, however, that the history of plant domestication is much more complicated than had been supposed. The weight of today's evidence is that many crops either did not originate in the centers Vavilov indicated or originated in more than one center. Some crops seem to have evolved over vast regions; there is no evidence at all

for a center of origin. Others cannot be pinned down with any precision for lack of suitable evidence.

In Vavilov's day scholars looked on agriculture as a revolutionary system of food procurement that had evolved on one or two hearths and diffused over the face of the earth, replacing the older hunting-gathering systems. The deliberate rearing of plants and animals for food was regarded as a discovery or invention so radical and so complex that it could have developed only once (or possibly twice), after which the system spread by stimulus diffusion. Hunting peoples coming into contact with farmers would instantly see and appreciate the enormous advantages of agriculture and hasten to go and do likewise. The evidence that has accumulated in recent years, particularly in the past decade, tends to suggest an almost opposite view. Agriculture is not an invention or a discovery and is not as revolutionary as we had thought; furthermore, it was adopted slowly and with reluctance.

The current evidence indicates that agriculture evolved through an extension and intensification of what people had already been doing for a long time. As we examine the domestication of plants and animals in more detail what once seemed to be well-defined centers tend to fade or to become vague and indistinct. My own viewpoint has changed with the evidence, and what I thought and wrote 20 years ago bears little resemblance to my present assessment of the situation.

The innovative pattern that now emerges is complex, diffuse and not easy to describe. For example, evidence for the domestication of pigs is found all the way from Europe to the Far East. Cattle of various kinds were tamed over most of the same range. With respect to plants, much the same is true of rice in Asia, of sorghum in Africa and of beans

CROPS OF EGYPT in the latter half of the second millennium B.C. appear in the painting on the opposite page; the original painting is in a tomb near the royal capital of Thebes. Areas with a herringbone pattern represent water. The tan grain being reaped with a sickle is an early species of wheat, emmer, the common wheat of Egypt until the fourth century B.C. The tall green crop in the panel below is flax; it is being uprooted, the usual harvesting method. To the right a plowman is cutting a furrow. A pair of oxen draw the plow, and the plowman's wife follows, dropping seed into the furrow. In the next panel the trees with clusters of small fruits are date palms and those with larger fruits are doum palms; the pale green trees between them are a species of fig, *Ficus sycomorus,* the sycamore of the Bible. Bottom panel shows water plants.

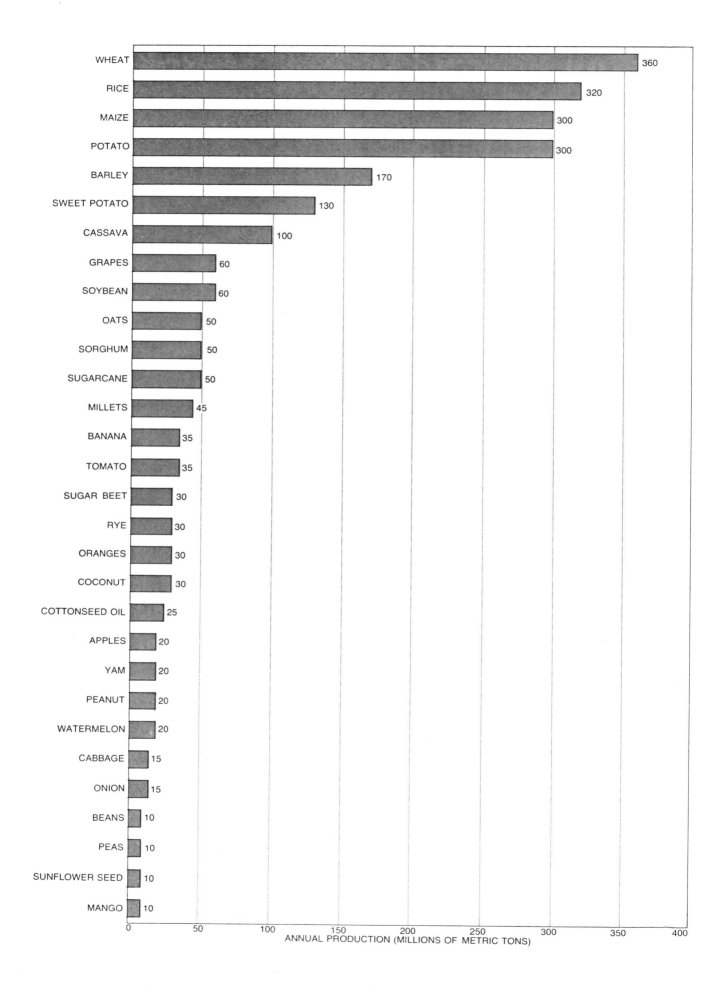

ANNUAL PRODUCTION (MILLIONS OF METRIC TONS)

in the Americas [*see top illustration on next two pages*]. The wild progenitors of these food plants are widely distributed and were manipulated by various peoples over their entire range. Each may have been repeatedly domesticated at different times in different places or may have been brought into the domestic fold in several regions simultaneously. At least we cannot point with any confidence or precision to a single center of origin for these particular plants and animals.

By the same token, if the plant or animal under investigation never spread very far or did so only in recent historical times, the picture is usually rather clear and we can assign it an origin with some assurance. For example, two species of oxen, the mithan (*Bos gaurus*) and the yak (*Bos grunniens*), have rather modest ranges, and it seems likely they were domesticated within their present distribution: the mithan among the hill tribes of northwestern Burma, Assam and Bhutan, and the yak in Tibet and the adjacent highland regions. The sunflower was a rather minor crop grown by the Indians of what is now the U.S. It became a major oil crop in eastern Europe only recently. The African oil palm is another plant that has become important on the world scene only in the past few decades; its history is easily traced.

The possibility of independent domestications clearly complicates matters greatly. In some cases the evidence is nonetheless fairly clear. For example, it seems likely that the large-seed lima bean was domesticated in South America and the small-seed sieva bean in Mexico. One species of rice was domesticated in Asia and another in Africa. One species of cotton was domesticated in either India or Africa, another in South America and a third in Mesoamerica. Five species of squash and five of *Capsicum* peppers were domesticated over a geographic range that extends from Mexico to Argentina. Different species of yams were domesticated in West Africa, in Southeast Asia and in tropical America. Different races of radishes were independently domesticated in Japan, Indonesia, India and Europe. Where the species and races are clearly distinguishable we can usually unravel their history. Where we cannot clearly separate the races of a wild progenitor, however, the evidence for origins may be vague indeed. Moreover, in many instances the evidence is inadequate be-

THIRTY MAJOR CROPS include seven with annual harvests of 100 million or more metric tons. The total tonnage of the top seven crops is more than twice the tonnage of the remaining 23. Cane sugar and beet sugar are listed separately here but millets are combined. Crops with an annual yield of less than 10 million metric tons have been omitted.

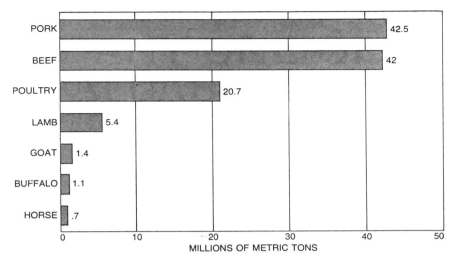

SEVEN MAJOR SOURCES provided a total of more than 110 million metric tons of meat worldwide in 1974, according to statistics from the Food and Agriculture Organization of the United Nations. The world pig population made the major contribution: 42.5 million tons. Beef and veal combined were in second place; chicken, duck and turkey combined were third.

cause we have failed to conduct serious investigations into the matter.

Such is probably the case for several crops with obscure origins. Old World cotton and the oilseed sesame could have either African or Indian origins or both. We do not know where, if anywhere, the bottle gourd genuinely grows wild. Indeed, it is often difficult to distinguish genuinely wild races from weedy escapes or naturalized races. In a few instances the original distribution patterns may have become so obscure that the evidence has disappeared.

Among the major food crops shown in the illustration on the opposite page several were of minor importance on the world scene until recently. The potato was restricted largely to the Andean highlands until the Europeans arrived there in the 16th century. It was brought to Europe soon afterward but was poorly adapted to local growing conditions and entered a period of acclimatization, particularly to the long-day regime characteristic of summers in Europe. Finally the potato found a congenial home and became so productive in northern Europe that it was credited by some historians with provoking something of a population explosion. From the world point of view such crops as sugarcane, the sugar beet, soybeans, citrus fruits, the tomato, the peanut, the sweet potato and the sunflower are all relatively recent major contributors to the food supply. Cottonseed as a major source of edible oil is a product of this century.

A point to be kept in mind when dealing with the "where" of domestication is that plants and animals under domestication change radically with time, and the forms familiar to us today may be strikingly different from the forms of the ancient progenitors. Wheat provides

a good example. Three kinds of wheat were originally domesticated from wild grasses; all three are so obsolete today that they are hardly grown at all. One was a diploid (that is, a plant with seven pairs of chromosomes) called einkorn. It was probably domesticated in southeastern Turkey, and it was always a minor crop. Einkorn did spread to western Europe, but it never reached Egypt, and it did not move eastward from its point of origin.

The second wheat was a tetraploid (that is, it had 14 pairs of chromosomes) called emmer. It was in its day by far the most successful of the three. Our best guess is that it originated in Palestine and/or southeastern Turkey. For some millenniums it was the dominant wheat. It spread across Europe and North Africa, Egypt and Arabia and reached Ethiopia, where it is still grown on a considerable scale. Emmer was the wheat of Egypt until it was replaced by bread wheat after Alexander the Great conquered Egypt in the fourth century B.C. Outside Ethiopia emmer lingers on as a relict crop in Yugoslavia and southern India.

The third domesticated wheat was also a tetraploid. It was so trivial that there is no common name for it; scientifically it is called *Triticum timopheevii*. It originated in Transcaucasian Georgia and has spread only as a collector's item for genetic studies.

The wheat we grow today is none of these three early domesticates. All three are known as glume wheats because the spike, or seed-bearing head, breaks up when it is threshed, leaving each seed enclosed in a hard, shell-like glume, or husk. The seeds must then be processed further, usually by pounding in a mortar, to free them of the husks. Some time after emmer was domesticated a mutation occurred that caused the base of the

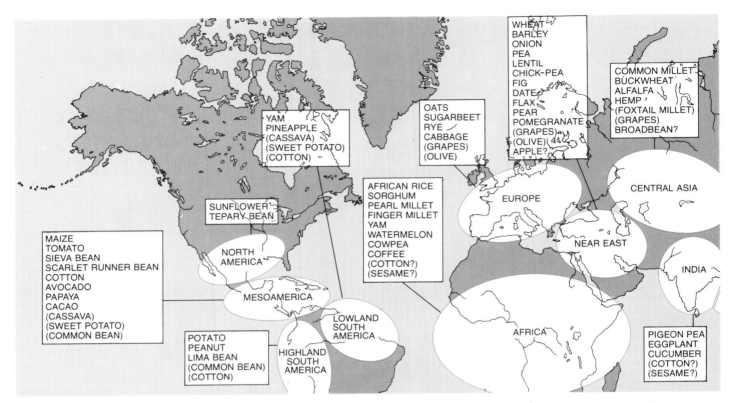

AREAS WHERE PLANTS WERE DOMESTICATED are indicated on this map; area boundaries have been generalized. Except for wheat, where different genera or species were independently domesticated in different areas, the name appears in each area; cotton, yams and the millets are examples. Where the same species was certainly or probably domesticated independently the name appears enclosed in parentheses in each area; among the examples are the common bean, the sweet potato, olive and grapes. Where the area of domesti-

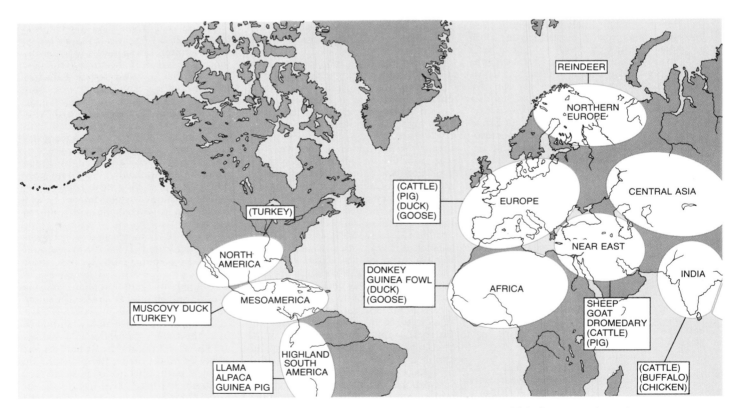

AREAS WHERE ANIMALS WERE DOMESTICATED are indicated on this map; as with the map showing plant domestication the area boundaries are generalized. In addition to the six species of mammals and the three species of birds that are man's most numerous domesticates, a number of animals valued for food, for work or for transport are also shown. The names of animals that were cer-

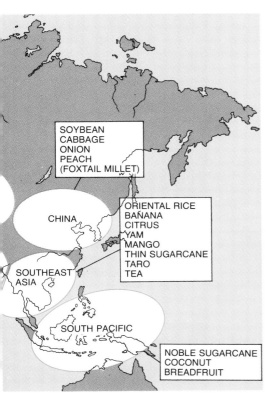

cation is in doubt a question mark follows the plant name. Several crops with an annual yield below 10 million metric tons are included; examples are lentils, coffee and tea.

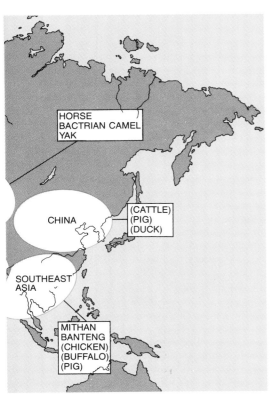

tainly or probably domesticated independently in more than one area are in parentheses: examples include pigs, cattle and chickens.

glume to collapse at maturity, freeing the seed. At the same time the spike became tough, so that it did not fall apart as the ancestral spikes had done. The mutated, free-threshing emmer is the ancestor of our durum or macaroni wheats.

The major wheat species of the world, and the one that contributes most to the annual harvest of 360 million metric tons, is still another kind, known generally as bread wheat. It is a hexaploid, that is, it has 21 pairs of chromosomes, and it arose long after the initial domestication of the three primitive glume wheats. Its extra set of chromosomes was contributed by a wild goat grass called *Triticum tauschii,* and the distribution of the wild progenitor suggests that the hybridization may have taken place somewhere near the southern end of the Caspian Sea. *T. tauschii* is the only species of goat grass with a continental distribution, and it may have contributed the adaptation that makes it possible for bread wheat to be grown on the dry steppes of the world. As a wild grass *T. tauschii* is essentially worthless, but as a contributor of genetic characteristics it literally made a billion-dollar crop out of a million-dollar one.

The word wheat, then, has several meanings. Modern wheats are quite different from the primitive glume wheats that were first domesticated. We can assign the origin of wheat to the Near East as long as we do not restrict the area too narrowly. The early evolution of wheat took place in a zone extending from Palestine to the Caucasus and the southern Caspian. Like all other domestic plants, however, wheat is still evolving and changing wherever it grows today.

It is now possible to list in similar fashion other major domesticated plants and animals, along with our best guess as to their geographic origins. In a number of cases, however, it is necessary to include the same species in more than one region because of diffuse patterns of domestication, and in some instances we must resort to question marks because of ignorance.

We are not much better off with our answers to the "when" of domestication, although each year brings some new knowledge. For example, it has often been said that the dog was the first animal to be domesticated. Until recently we had no firm evidence for this belief, but the jaws and teeth of domestic dogs have now been identified and dated to about 12,000 B.C. in the Old World (Iraq) and to about 11,000 B.C. in the New World (Idaho). Dogs have been eaten by man on every continent, but they were probably never considered a major meat animal except in parts of the New World before the arrival of the Europeans.

Apart from the two dog dates we see little evidence for animal domestication until about 9000 B.C. Even here the data are rather tenuous and not conclusive. Zawi Chemi Shanidar is an archaeological site in Iraq that was excavated by Ralph S. Solecki in the 1960's; the animal bones unearthed there were analyzed by Dexter Perkins, Jr. Now, if one finds the right bones, it is possible to distinguish between sheep and goats that are less than a year old and those that are more than a year old. Near the bottom of Solecki's excavations the remains of both sheep and goats less than a year old made up about 25 percent of the sample. Toward the top, where the remains were more recent, there was a shift to a higher ratio of sheep bones to goat bones, and about 50 percent of the sheep were less than a year old. The implication is that the people at Shanidar had acquired considerable control over the sheep population but not over the goat population.

It is also possible, given the right bones, to determine the sex of an animal. At some archaeological sites it has been found that the bones of a high percentage of young male animals are present. This does not in itself prove domestication; similarly displaced sex and age ratios are found among the remains of red deer in European Mesolithic sites and the remains of gazelles at Near Eastern sites. Both are considered game animals, but both can be tamed. Evidence for domestication is difficult to obtain from bones unless changes in morphology are involved. Such findings do, however, suggest manipulation of some kind, and they certainly indicate that as far back as the Mesolithic man had both the capacity and the technique for selective slaughtering. This in turn was probably a first step in an increasingly intimate interaction of man with his food animals.

A second Near Eastern archaeological site, Ali Kosh in Iran, may have been occupied as early as 7500 B.C. The dating of its lower levels is uncertain, but the skull of a hornless female sheep was unearthed in one of the lowest. In wild sheep both sexes have horns, so that the hornless skull is taken to mean that domestic sheep were present at Ali Kosh. Goat bones are much more abundant at the site than sheep bones, and a high percentage represent young males.

Çayönü, an early farming village in Turkey, was first excavated by Robert J. Braidwood and Halet Çambel in 1964. It was first inhabited perhaps a little before 7000 B.C.; the bones of domestic sheep, pigs, dogs and probably goats were present. Remains of domestic goats with twisted horns are present at the site of Jarmo in Iraq, a site dating to about 6750 B.C. Twisted horns are characteristic of domesticated breeds and not of wild goats.

The earliest remains of domesticated

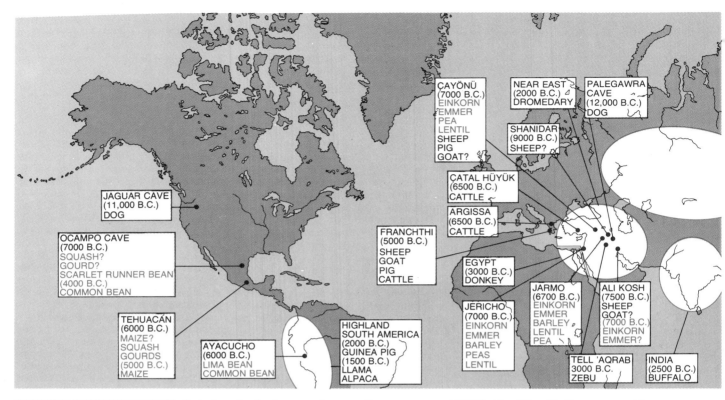

EARLIEST DOMESTICATIONS of plants and animals appear to have taken place at roughly the same time around the world. Shown on the map are general Old World and New World areas or specific archaeological sites where the remains of plants (*color*) and animals

cattle now known come from Greece and date to about 6500 B.C. By then this species of animal apparently had long been worshiped. At Çatal Hüyük, a Turkish site excavated by James Mellaart and dated about 6500 B.C., more than 50 shrines were uncovered; most of them were decorated with bull's heads and horns. The humped cattle we associate with India today are represented by Mesopotamian figurines dating back to about 3000 B.C.; they are not recorded in India until about 2500 B.C. We have no information on the antiquity of other bovids, such as the banteng (*Bos javanicus*) of Malaysia, the mithan and the yak. The water buffalo was known as a domesticate in India by 2500 B.C., but it could have been a source of draft power, meat and milk long before then.

The donkey was known as a domesticate in Egypt by 3000 B.C. and may have been exploited well before that; it has not been used much as a food animal. The horse, in contrast, has been an important source of meat and milk for many peoples. Fermented mare's milk is still popular in Asia, and half a million metric tons of horsemeat are eaten worldwide each year [*see illustration on page 63*]. The horse is thought to have first been tamed in central Asia or southern Russia about 3000 B.C. The reindeer, a domesticate now commonest in Scandinavia and the U.S.S.R., was probably herded at a very early date, but we have

no firm evidence for it. Among the camelids our best guesses suggest 2000 B.C. for the one-humped dromedary and 1500 B.C. for the two-humped Bactrian camel; about the same time range probably applies to the New World camelids, the llama and the alpaca. The guinea pig of the Andes was probably a tamed food animal by 2000 B.C.

Many Near Eastern sites have also yielded early plant remains. None appear at Shanidar, but Ali Kosh yielded grains of einkorn and emmer wheats that date back to about 7000 B.C. and barley that is somewhat younger. Seeds of einkorn, emmer, pea, lentil, vetch and flax were found at Çayönü. Jarmo had einkorn, emmer, barley, pea, lentil and vetch, and a similar array of plant foods was found in the prepottery Neolithic levels at Jericho, which are also dated at about 7000 B.C. Other sites document rather clearly a progression of farming into Greece and the Balkans and thereafter a fanning out over Europe.

The bias in our data has led many to conclude that the Near East was the center of Old World plant and animal domestication. We have a fairly respectable body of information for that part of the world and an even better record for Europe. Some caution is advisable, however; no other parts of the world have been as well explored (except North America, where agriculture ar-

rived comparatively late). For example, we have almost no archaeological information from Africa of the kind that is available from the Near East and Europe. Plant remains have been unearthed in Africa, including those of sorghum, pearl millet and finger millet, but all the sites are too recent to tell us much. Indirect evidence, such as the discovery of mortars and grinding stones and of flint blades with a particular kind of sheen or gloss, which might have been used to reap grasses, appears in the Nile Valley by about 12,000 B.C., but we do not know what plants were being processed.

The situation is much the same in India, where a number of sites have yielded plant materials but where most of the finds are too recent to yield information on the beginnings of agriculture. Wheat and barley from the west, rice from the east and sorghum and millets from Africa have all been found in India, but no firm evidence of early indigenous Indian domestications has yet appeared.

The Chinese Neolithic has been studied on a modest scale. The Yang Shao culture is now fairly well known, and some sites, such as Pan P'o, have yielded plant materials. This Neolithic village was first inhabited, however, only around 4000 B.C. Moreover, it contains some rather elegant pottery and appears much too large, complex and sophisticated to represent the beginnings of ag-

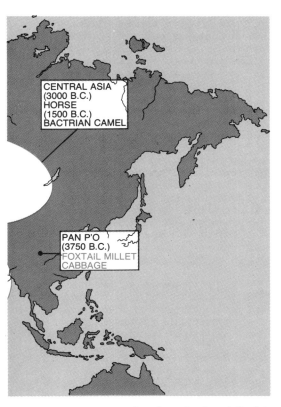

CENTRAL ASIA
(3000 B.C.)
HORSE
(1500 B.C.)
BACTRIAN CAMEL

PAN P'O
(3750 B.C.)
FOXTAIL MILLET
CABBAGE

suggest or confirm domestication at the date indicated. Data imply independent invention.

riculture in the Far East. Foxtail millet was the chief food crop of that time and place.

Work in Southeast Asia has for all practical purposes just begun. Early plant materials have been found at sites in Thailand, and there is even evidence for early landform manipulation in remote New Guinea. At present the body of information is too meager and fragmentary to allow the drawing of definite conclusions. Nevertheless, there are hints that the inhabitants of the region were manipulating plants quite as early as the people of the Near East.

The situation in the Americas is not much better and not much different. Enormous quantities of beautifully preserved plant materials are available from coastal Peru, but this is not a likely region for agricultural innovation. Excavations in Tamaulipas and in the Tehuacán valley in Mexico by Richard S. MacNeish have given us sequences of deposits suggesting plant manipulation about 7000 B.C., and some later material on domesticates, possibly dating back to 6000 B.C. and surely to 5000 B.C. Maize was apparently a crop in Tehuacán by then, along with squash and gourds, and beans appeared before 3000 B.C. Tehuacán is too dry, however, to have been a center of agricultural developments. It seems more likely that events taking place elsewhere were sometimes recorded there and that the valley itself was

outside the mainstream of agricultural innovation. MacNeish's investigations at Ayacucho in Peru are perhaps more revealing. Although he failed to find evidence of early agriculture in the Andean highlands, he did find plant materials in the intermontane valleys. By 6000 B.C. fully domesticated beans and lima beans were being cultivated there. Thus agriculture could well be as ancient a tradition in South America as it is in the Near East and in Southeast Asia, although conclusive evidence of it is not available at present.

On balance, then, the evidence for "when," such as it is, seems to be as diffuse and imprecise as the evidence for "where." This is only partly owing to inadequate investigation. Some of the uncertainties are surely the result of the way domestication took place. For reasons we can only speculate about, people in various parts of the world all seem to have begun the processes of domestication at roughly the same time. That time was not long after the final Pleistocene glaciation, when the great ice sheets had melted and the seas had risen to approximately their present levels. It would not be appropriate to pursue the various speculations here; it is enough to say that the picture now emerging in terms of both time and place turns out to be far more complex and diffuse than we used to think.

With both the where and the when of domestication left somewhat up in the air, what is there to say about how? One can begin by pointing out that plant cultivation and plant domestication are often confused. Cultivation refers to man's efforts to care for plants; in this sense it is perfectly possible to cultivate wild plants. Domestication, from *domus,* the Latin for house, means to bring into the household, and hence it implies far more than cultivation. Domestication involves genetic changes that make the plants better suited to the conditions of man-made environments and less well adapted to the conditions of natural environments. In a similar way one can tame a wild animal without domesticating it. The genetic alteration that is involved in the process of domestication, however, is often carried to the point where a fully domesticated plant or animal is fitted exclusively to an artificial environment and cannot survive in the wild.

Horses, cattle and camels have escaped from domestication in western North America in historic times and have thrived. Sheep that escape from domestication, on the other hand, have little chance of survival unless they are protected from predators. Goats that escape thrive in the absence of predators, as when they escape to an island; when predators are present, they fare poor-

ly. Similarly, the domesticated races of maize, wheat, rice, potato, sweet potato and most other crops would all die out without human intervention.

Because domestication is an evolutionary process it is variable in degree, and one finds an entire range of intermediate states from wild races to fully domesticated races that depend entirely on man for survival. Indeed, all these intermediate states may be found in the same species. There are wild, weedy and domesticated races of most of our crops. The wild ones can survive without man, the weedy races survive because of man (and in spite of his efforts to get rid of them) and the domesticated races demand care and cultivation for survival. Weeds are species or races that thrive in man-made habitats; most of our crops have weed races somewhere. There are weed races of wheat, rice, maize, potato, barley and so on, all the way down the list. They readily propagate themselves, but they require habitats that are disturbed by man.

This kind of adaptation is not confined to plants. Cats, dogs and pigs readily become feral. The statuary pigeon, the house sparrow and the starling thrive even in the face of intense human disturbance, as they do in cities. The house mouse, the sewer rat, the housefly and the fruit fly all do well in the artificial habitats created by man. Indeed, what species thrives in man-made habitats better than *Homo sapiens?* We are the weediest of all.

Recent studies of weed races show that their origins may be diverse. Even genuinely wild plants can show weedy tendencies; after all, many natural environments such as shorelines, riverbanks, the margins of glaciers and steep talus slopes are unstable, whereas others are subject to disturbances such as forest fires, blowdowns, avalanches and the like. Many wild species occupy these niches, and some of our crop plants are derived from wild plants with just such colonizer tendencies. Other weeds are derived from natural crosses between wild and domesticated races and still others come from the escape of half-domesticated plants. Hybridization between cultivated plants and related weed races has played a role in crop evolution by increasing diversity and developing efficient population structures. Similar genetic interactions of domestic animals and their wild relatives were probably an important element in the early days of animal husbandry. The process is now relatively uncommon because the related wild races have become rare or extinct, but in Southeast Asia chickens still mate with jungle fowl and in New Guinea tame sows are frequently serviced by wild boars.

The process of plant domestication presumably began with man's intensive use of and at least partial dependence on the plant in question. The relationship inevitably increased in intimacy. For example, man's harvesting of seeds from wild plants would have had relatively little effect on the genetic structure of the wild plant populations until man himself sowed what he had reaped. Once seed is deliberately planted the composition of the next plant generation depends on what man harvests, and so some genetic changes become virtually automatic. The most common genetic response in crops valued for their edible seed is a shift toward nonshattering, that is, a shift away from natural seed dispersal. Cereal panicles and spikes become tough and do not break apart at maturity. Pods and capsules no longer burst open to disperse their seeds when they are ripe. Once the natural mechanism for seed dispersal is lost the plants become dependent on man for survival. They are domesticated, or at least partly so. The genetic change may be very simple and is frequently controlled by a single gene.

Other changes also take place more or less automatically. The seeds of wild plants are often dormant at maturity,

and even if conditions are favorable for germination, they will not germinate until the proper season. This is an elegant adaptation for wild species, but it may not be at all suitable for agriculture. When this is the case, selection for nondormancy, or at least for a dormancy that breaks down by the next planting time, is automatic. By the same token automatic selection for larger seeds will occur in the seedbeds if there is competition between seedlings. Large seeds have larger food reserves and are likely to produce more vigorous seedlings; the first plants to come up and those with the greatest seedling vigor are likely to contribute the most seed to the next generation. Still other automatic selection pressures adapt plants to field conditions. A disruptive selection is set up: natural selection causes the wild populations to maintain tneir adaptations, but repeated sowing and reaping modify the cultivated populations in the direction of adaptation to field and garden. Genetic divergence is easily maintained even when there is considerable crossing between the wild and the cultivated populations.

In addition to the automatic selection

pressures, man intervenes by deliberate and intentional processes of selection. These processes may aim in different directions and may be capricious, to say the least. Man selects corn for boiling, for popping, for roasting in the ear, for flour quality, for making hominy, for beer, for unfermented beverages, for dyes and even for ceremonial and religious purposes. He selects nonglutinous and glutinous rice, long-grained and short-grained rice, red rice, white rice and aromatic rice. He selects barley for food, for beer, for livestock feed, for processing in his grinding equipment and for ease of harvesting. Man delights in bright colors and in curious and unusual variants, and so he preserves plant forms that would have no chance of survival under natural conditions.

The part of the plant of greatest interest to man is the part that is modified the most. If the crop is a tuber, the greatest variation and the greatest deviation from the wild type will be in the tuber. If it is a cereal, the parts most modified will be the inflorescence and the grains borne on it. A striking example is the kale species, *Brassica oleracea,* which as a result of man's influence has been modified in half a dozen ways. The species has a remarkable capacity for developing starch-storage organs on demand. In the familiar cabbage the storage organ is the terminal bud, in the cauliflower it is the inflorescence, in kohlrabi the stem, in Brussels sprouts the lateral buds, in broccoli the stems and flowers and in kale the leaves. All evolved by selection from the wild *B. oleracea.* Different as these plants are in appearance, they are all the same species and are fully fertile when they are hybridized. Kale is closer to the wild type than the others.

Beets provide another example: the garden beet, the mangel or fodder beet, the sugar beet and the leafy green Swiss chard are all derivative forms of *Beta vulgaris.* Some peoples selected for the leaves, some for the roots and some for the sugar. Still other examples are legion. The variation in lettuces in a neighborhood market in Italy is surprising to those of us who see only the lettuces offered in an American supermarket. Selection strategies in beans have taken two major forms: dry beans and green beans. The strategies in peas include not only dry and green forms but also pod (or snow) peas. The end result of such intense and divergent selection pressures is the production of morphological monsters that are completely dependent on man for survival; these plants are fully domesticated.

The domestication of animals is no different in principle. The process begins with an intimate relation between man and an animal and a partial dependence of man on the animal. This may involve a selective kind of hunting or the

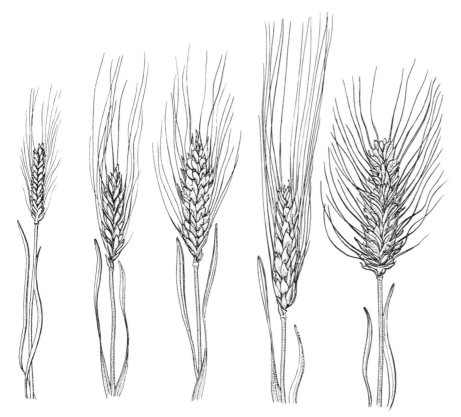

SPECIES OF WHEAT include, from left to right, the three earliest domesticates: einkorn (*Triticum monococcum*), once grown in Turkey and Europe, emmer (*T. dicoccum*), once grown in the Near East, Africa and Europe, and a third with no common name, *T. timopheevii*. Next are the principal modern wheats: macaroni wheat (*T. durum*), a descendant of a mutated emmer, and bread wheat (*T. aestivum*), a cross between emmer or macaroni wheat and goat grass.

management of a herd. Sooner or later the animals are tamed. It is usually not difficult. Young animals that are raised in or near the household often become tame for life. Some animal species are recalcitrant and difficult to tame, but many that have never been domesticated prove to be quite tractable. In the course of domestication there has doubtless been some selection for genes conferring docility. In cattle and pigs selection led to smaller animals that were easier to handle, and dwarf breeds of several other domestic animals have also been developed.

Recent experience may serve as a model of what probably happened in the deep past. For example, the musk-ox has been tamed to allow access to its extraordinarily fine wool. The project was designed to provide income for Eskimos and other northern populations whose traditional hunting cultures had been disrupted. In spite of a reputation for belligerency the musk-ox has proved to be tractable and docile under artificial husbandry. As another example, about a century ago the African eland was introduced into Russia on a trial basis. It adapted to confinement very well, and selection for milk production resulted in a more than 400 percent increase over the production of animals in the wild state. The milking eland could be called a modern domesticate.

Selective breeding of tamed or confined animals leads eventually to domesticated races and lineages that cannot survive in nature even if the species itself could manage without the aid of man. Extreme types such as the Pekingese dog, the bubble-eyed goldfish, chickens with five-meter feathers, pouter pigeons, waltzing mice and for that matter most strains of laboratory mice, rats, rabbits and mutant stocks of fruit flies have been genetically modified to the point where they depend on man for survival and are fully domesticated.

If total dependence is a consequence of domestication, what is one to say of the human condition? Man likes to think that he is in charge of the plants and animals he first began to bring into his household several thousand years ago, but the fact is that he has been domesticated by them. Many of them cannot now survive without man, but certainly they are essential to man's survival. More precisely, man and his domesticates have been bound together for some millenniums in an adaptive coevolution. Human evolution, in its peculiar way, is largely social and cultural, whereas the evolution of man's plant and animal domesticates has involved notable genetic changes and the development of striking new morphologies. Although man must care for his domesticates, the human population of the world eats or starves according to the performance of those few plants and animals that nourish man.

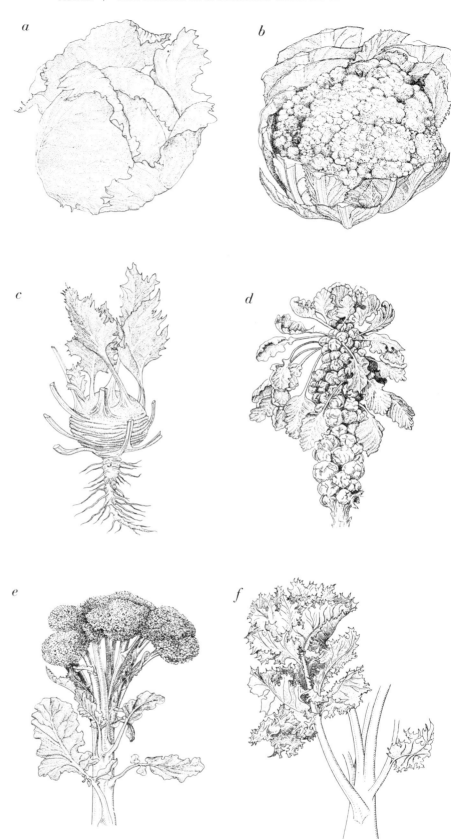

PRESSURE OF SELECTION has produced six separate vegetables from a single species, *Brassica oleracea*, **a mustard with a remarkable capacity for developing starch-storage organs on demand. Selection for enlarged terminal buds produced the cabbage (*a*); for inflorescences, the cauliflower (*b*); for the stem, kohlrabi (*c*); for lateral buds, Brussels sprouts (*d*); for the stem and flowers, broccoli (*e*), and for leaves, kale (*f*). Kale most closely resembles the wild plant.**

7 Wheat

Paul C. Mangelsdorf
July 1953

The grass that bears our daily bread is synonymous with European civilization. What is the basis of its usefulness, and what is the origin of modern wheat?

WHEAT is the world's most widely cultivated plant. The wheat plants growing on the earth may even outnumber those of any other seed-bearing land species, wild or domesticated. Every month of the year a crop of wheat is maturing somewhere in the world. It is the major crop of the U. S. and Canada and is grown on substantial acreages in almost every country of Latin America, Europe and Asia.

Apparently this grain was one of the earliest plants cultivated by man. Carbonized kernels of wheat were found recently by the University of Chicago archaeologist Robert Braidwood at the 6,700-year-old site of Jarmo in eastern Iraq, the oldest village yet discovered—a village which may have been one of the birthplaces of man's agriculture. Through the courtesy of Dr. Braidwood I have had an opportunity to study some of these ancient kernels and compare them with modern kernels, carbonized to simulate the archaeological specimens. The resemblance between the ancient and modern grains is remarkable. There were two types of kernels in the Jarmo site; one turned out to be almost identical with a wild wheat still growing in the Near East, and the other almost exactly like present-day cultivated wheat of the type called einkorn. Evidently there has been no appreciable change in these wheats in the 7,000 years since Jarmo.

When he domesticated wheat, man laid the foundations of western civilization. No civilization worthy of the name has ever been founded on any agricultural basis other than the cereals. The ancient cultures of Babylonia and Egypt, of Rome and Greece, and later those of northern and western Europe, were all based upon the growing of wheat, barley, rye and oats. Those of India, China and Japan had rice for their basic crop. The pre-Columbian peoples of America —Inca, Maya and Aztec—looked to corn for their daily bread.

What are the reasons for this intimate relation between the cereals and civiliza-

tion? It may be primarily a question of nutrition. The grain of cereal grasses, a nutlike structure with a thin shell covering the seed, contains not only the embryo of a new plant but also a food supply to nourish it. Cereal grains, like eggs and milk, are foodstuffs designed by nature for the nutrition of the young of the species. They represent a five-in-one food supply which contains carbohydrate, proteins, fats, minerals and vitamins. A whole-grain cereal, if its food values are not destroyed by the over-refinement of modern processing methods, comes closer than any other plant product to providing an adequate diet. Man long ago discovered this fact and learned to exploit it. Guatemalan Indians manage to subsist fairly well on a diet which is 85 per cent corn. In India people sometimes live on almost nothing but rice. Such diets do not meet the approval of modern nutritionists, but they are better than those made up too largely of starchy root crops such as potatoes, sweet potatoes or cassava, or of proteinaceous legumes such as beans, peas and lentils.

Perhaps the relationship between cereals and civilization is also a product of the discipline which cereals impose upon their growers. The cereals are grown only from seed and must be planted and harvested in their proper season. In this respect they differ from the root crops, which in mild climates can be planted and harvested at almost any time of the year. Root-crop agriculture can be practiced by semi-nomadic peoples who visit their plantations only periodically. The growing of cereals has always been accompanied by a stable mode of life. Moreover, it forced men to become more conscious of the seasons and the movements of the sun, moon and stars. In both the Old World and the New the science of astronomy was invented by cereal growers, and with it a calendar and a system of arithmetic. Cereal agriculture in providing a stable food supply created leisure, and leisure in turn fostered the arts, crafts and

sciences. It has been said that "cereal agriculture, alone among the forms of food production, taxes, recompenses and stimulates labor and ingenuity in an equal degree."

From Grain-chewing to Bread

Today wheat is the cereal *par excellence* for breadmaking, and it is used almost exclusively for that purpose. But it is quite unlikely that breadmaking, a complex and sophisticated art, came suddenly into full flower with the domestication of wheat. Man may have begun by merely parching or popping the grain to make it edible. Primitive wheats, like other cereals, were firmly enclosed in husks, called glumes. Heating makes the glumes easy to rub off and allows the kernel itself to be more easily chewed or ground into meal. The scorching and parching of grains is still practiced on unripened cereals in parts of the Near East. In Scotland until recently barley glumes were sometimes removed by setting fire to the unthreshed heads. The Chippewa Indians still prepare wild rice by heating the unhusked kernels and tramping on them in a hollow log.

Hard-textured cereal grains with a certain moisture content explode and escape from their glumes when heated. In America the first use of corn was undoubtedly by popping. The earliest known corn had small vitreous kernels, and archaeological remains of popped corn have been found in early sites in both North and South America. In India certain varieties of rice are popped by stirring the kernels in hot sand. Many villages in India have a village popper who performs this service for his neighbors and provides himself with food by taking his toll of the product.

The botanical as well as archaeological evidence, though meager, indicates that wheat was first used as a parched cereal. The dwellings at Jarmo contain ovens which prove that this primitive economy knew the controlled use of heat. All the very ancient prehistoric kernels so far found are carbonized as if they had been over-parched. In itself this evidence is not telling, since only carbonized grains would be preserved indefinitely, but it is in harmony with other evidence. Finally, the most ancient wheats are species whose kernels would not be removed from the husks merely by threshing. The simplest method of husking them to make them edible would have been parching.

Probably the second stage in progress was to grind the parched grains and soak the coarse meal in water to make a gruel. For the toothless, both old and young, this must have been a life-saving invention. Gruel or porridge is well known as a primitive form of food. A gruel prepared from parched barley was the principal food of the common people of ancient Greece. American Indians prepared a kind of porridge from corn, which has its modern counterpart in "mush" and "polenta."

A gruel allowed to stand for a few days in a warm dwelling would become infected with wild yeasts. Fermenting the small amounts of sugar in cereal, the yeasts would have produced a mild alcoholic beverage. This would have pointed the way to leavened bread. It is questionable which art developed first— brewing or breadmaking. Some students believe that brewing is older even than agriculture, but there is no supporting archaeological or historical evidence. On the contrary, the earliest Egyptian recipes for beer described a process in which the grain was first made into half-baked loaves, which then became the raw material for beer-making. There is no doubt that brewing and the making of leavened bread are closely related arts, both depending upon fermentation by yeasts.

Modern breadmaking, however, had to await the appearance of new types of wheat. It is as much a product of the evolution of wheat as it is one of human ingenuity.

From Wild Grass to Wheat

Wheat differs from most cultivated plants in the complexity of its variations. True, the other major cereals, rice and corn, are each differentiated into thousands of varieties, but these form a continuous spectrum of variation and hence are classed as a single botanical species. Wheat is separated into distinct groups which differ from one another in many ways and are therefore classified as separate species under the single Old World genus *Triticum*. The domesticated wheats and their wild relatives have been studied more intensively than any other group of plants, cultivated or wild, and from these studies, truly international in scope, a picture is beginning to emerge of the evolution of wheat under domestication.

Authorities differ on the number of distinct species of wheat. This article follows the classification of Nikolai Vavilov, the Russian geneticist and botanist who, with his colleagues, brought together for study more than 31,000 samples of wheat from all parts of the world. Vavilov recognized 14 species; other botanists have recognized fewer or more. All authorities agree, however, that the wheat species, whatever their number, fall into three distinct groups, determined by the number of chromosomes in their cells. The chromosome numbers (in the reproductive cells) of the three types are, respectively, 7, 14 and 21. They were discovered by T. Sakamura in Japan in 1918 and slightly later, but independently, by Karl Sax in the U. S. The numbers are closely associated with differences in anatomy, morphology, resistance to disease, productiveness and milling and baking qualities. It is interesting to note that August Schulz, a German botanist, had arranged the wheats into these three groups in 1913, well before their chromosome numbers were known.

The 14- and 21-chromosome wheats have all arisen from 7-chromosome wheat and related grasses, through hybridization followed by chromosome doubling. The cultivated wheats are the most conspicuous example of this "cataclysmic evolution," described by G. Ledyard Stebbins, Jr., in his article in SCIENTIFIC AMERICAN of April, 1951. It is the only known mechanism by which new true-breeding species can be created almost overnight.

Since different wild grasses have been involved in wheat's evolution, the species differ not only in the number but also in the nature of their chromosomes. Relationships of different sets of chromosomes are determined by studying the degree of chromosome pairing in the reproductive cells of hybrids. If the pairing is complete, or almost so, the chromosome sets (genoms) of the parents are regarded as identical or closely related. If there is no pairing, the parental genoms are considered to be distinct. Four different genoms, each comprising seven chromosomes, designated A, B, D

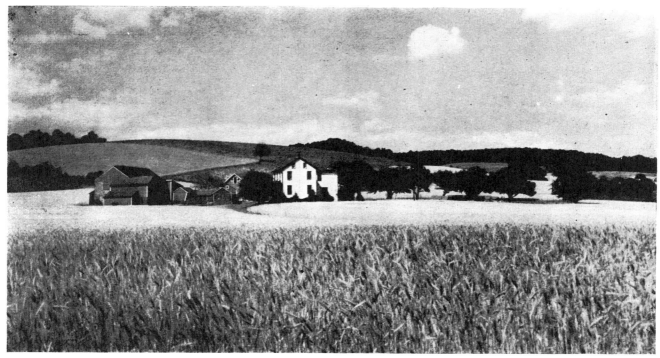

Wheat field and farm buildings

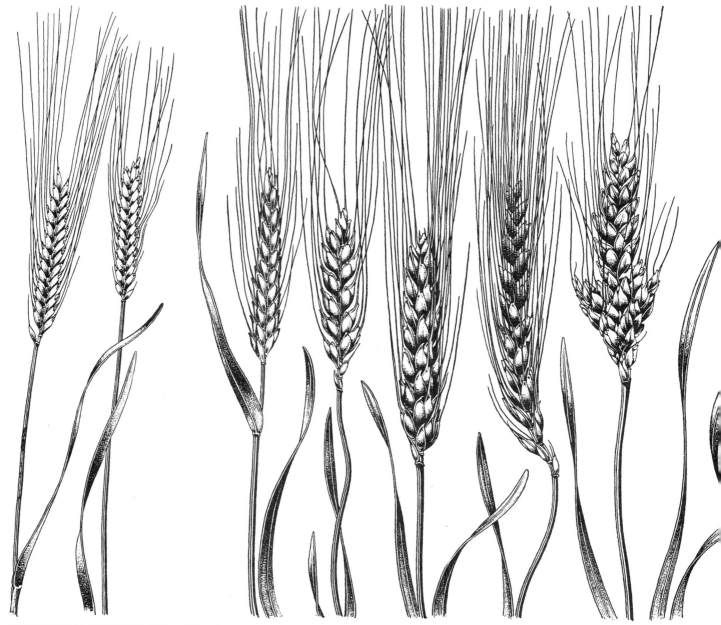

FOURTEEN SPECIES OF WHEAT are shown actual size. From left to right they are *Triticum aegilopoides* (wild einkorn), *T. monococcum* (einkorn), *T. dicoc-* *coides* (wild emmer), *T. dicoccum* (emmer), *T. durum* (macaroni wheat), *T. persicum* (Persian wheat), *T. turgidum* (rivet wheat), *T. polonicum* (Polish wheat), *T.*

and G, are recognized in wild and cultivated wheats.

Another important difference in wheats is in their heads. Primitive cereals and many wild grasses have heads whose central stem is brittle and fragile, breaking apart when mature and providing a natural mechanism for seed dispersal. When such cereals are threshed, the heads break up into individual spikelets (clusters of one or more individual grass flowers) in which the kernels remain firmly enclosed in their husks. Under domestication this characteristic, so essential to perpetuation of the species in the wild, has been lost. New forms have evolved, not only in wheat but in other

cereals, in which the stems are tough and the heads remain intact when mature. In such cereals threshing alone removes the kernels from their glumes. The cereals with free-threshing, naked grains are much more useful to man, especially for milling and baking, than those that cling stubbornly to their husks. In wheats, therefore, the naked varieties have almost completely superseded the primitive forms.

Ancestors

The 7-chromosome wheats, probably the most ancient, consist of two species: *T. aegilopoides* and *T. monococcum*,

known as wild einkorn and einkorn. Carbonized kernels of both were found at Jarmo, but whether they are the only wheats occurring in this ancient village site remains to be seen. Both species of einkorn have fragile stems and firm-hulled seeds. Their spikelets contain but a single seed, hence their name. Each has the same set of chromosomes, genom A, and they hybridize easily together to produce highly fertile offspring. Cultivated einkorn has slightly larger kernels than the wild form and a slightly tougher stem. Its heads do not fall apart quite so easily when ripe. Except for these slight differences the two species are essentially identical, and einkorn is

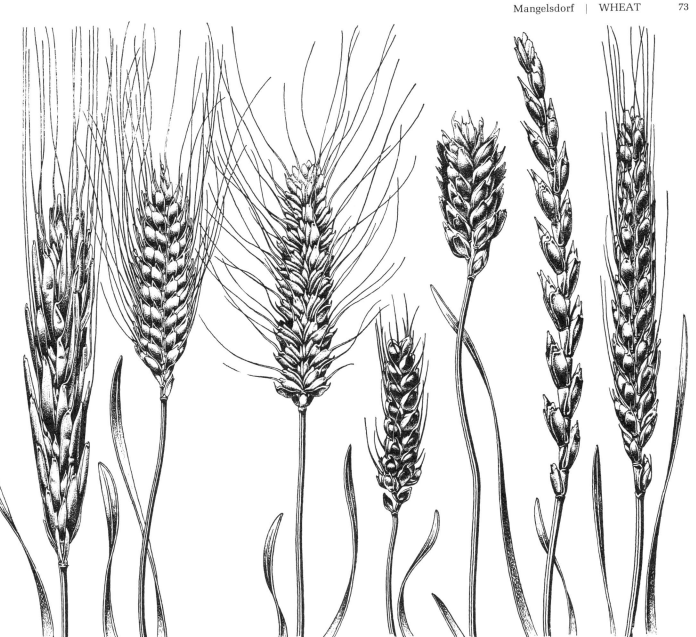

timopheevi (which has no common name), *T. aestivum* (common wheat), *T. sphaerococcum* (shot wheat), *T. compactum* (club wheat), *T. spelta* (spelt) and *T. macha* (macha wheat). The first two species have 7 chromosomes; the following seven, 14 chromosomes; the last five, 21 chromosomes (*see table on next two pages*).

undoubtedly the domesticated counterpart of the wild species. Apparently little significant change has been wrought in them over the centuries.

Wild einkorn has its center of distribution in Armenia and Georgia of the Soviet Union, and in Turkey. It also occurs in the eastern Caucasus and in western Iran. Westward from Asia Minor it is a common grass on the sides of low hills in Greece and Bulgaria and a weed in the well-drained vineyards of southern Yugoslavia. Cultivated einkorn originated, according to Vavilov, in the mountains of northeastern Turkey and the southwestern Caucasus. However, if my identification of the kernels at Jarmo is correct, and if Jarmo represents the beginnings of agriculture, einkorn may have been domesticated first slightly farther south in eastern Iraq. Certainly it is an ancient cereal. Carbonized grains of it have been found in neolithic deposits of the lake-dwellers and in many other sites in central and northeastern Europe. Impressions of einkorn have been identified in neolithic pottery in Britain and Ireland. There are no records of its prehistoric occurrence in India, China or Africa.

Einkorn is still grown in some parts of Europe and the Middle East, usually in hilly regions with thin soils. Its yields are low, usually not more than 8 to 15 bushels per acre. A bread, dark brown in color but of good flavor, can be made from it if it is husked, but it is more commonly used as a whole grain, like barley, for feeding cattle and horses. Einkorn's importance lies not in its present use but in its progeny. It is the ancestor of all other cultivated wheats, with the possible exception of the type called emmer. Einkorn's descendants all have in common the set of seven chromosomes called genom A.

Second Stage

In the next stage of evolution are the 14-chromosome species, of which Vavilov recognized seven. All these have come from the hybridization and chromosome doubling of a 7-chromosome wheat with a 7-chromosome related wild grass. The wheat parent in each case was undoubtedly einkorn, or possibly in one instance its wild relative, since all the species possess the genom A. But the wild-grass parent remains to this day unidentified and is the chief botanical mystery in the origin of cultivated wheats. This parent contributed a genom B to all in the group except one species. Edgar McFadden and Ernest Sears of the U. S. Department of Agriculture have suggested that genom B may have been derived from a species of *Agropyron*, a genus of weedy grasses which includes the pernicious couch grass of the northeastern U. S. Only one of the 14-chromosome wheats is found wild. This species, which is called wild emmer, is indigenous to southern Armenia, northeastern Turkey, western Iran, Syria and northern Palestine.

Closely resembling wild emmer, and possibly derived directly from it by domestication, is emmer, the oldest of 14-chromosome cultivated wheats and once the most widely grown wheat of all. An alternative possibility, however, is that emmer is the product of hybridization between einkorn and a 7-chromosome wild relative. The fact that crosses of wild and cultivated emmer are sometimes partly sterile indicates that the two forms may not be closely related and that one may be the product of an ancient hybridization and the other of a more recent one. There is at least no doubt about the antiquity of emmer. Well-preserved spikelets scarcely different from those of modern emmer have been found in Egyptian tombs of the Fifth Dynasty. Emmer may well have been the chief cereal of the Near East from very early times to the Greco-Roman period, for until the Jarmo find it was the only wheat found archaeologically in early sites of that region. Remains or impressions of it have also been common in neolithic sites in continental Europe, Britain and Ireland.

Emmer, like einkorn, has a fragile stem and clinging hull. Good bread and fine cake and pastry can be made from it, but most emmer today is fed to livestock. Some varieties are quite resistant to stem and leaf rust, the principal diseases of wheat, and have been useful in plant breeding.

The 14-chromosome wheats were the first to produce species with tough stems and with kernels that thresh free from their glumes. Four such species are known: *durum* (macaroni), *persicum* (Persian), *turgidum* (rivet) and *polonicum* (Polish). All have a more recent history than einkorn or emmer. The oldest, durum, first appeared in the Greco-Roman period about the first century B.C. One of the most recent, Polish

wheat, unique for its massive heads and long, hard kernels, did not appear until the 17th century. None of these wheats except durum is of great commercial importance today. Durum wheat, the best variety for the manufacture of macaroni, spaghetti and other edible paste products, is grown fairly extensively in Italy, Spain and parts of the U. S. Rivet wheat is of some interest because it is the tallest-growing (four to six feet high) and under ideal conditions one of the most productive. However, its grains are soft, yielding a weak flour unsuitable for breadmaking unless mixed with stronger wheats. One variety of rivet called "miracle" or "mummy" wheat, with massive branched heads, has been persistently exploited as a rare and valuable wheat claimed to have been propagated from prehistoric grains discovered in ancient Egyptian tombs, usually in the wrappings of a mummy. The story in all of its versions is a complete fabrication. Wheat kernels, like seeds of other plants, are living metabolic systems with a maximum life expectancy of about 10 years. Furthermore, there is no evidence that rivet wheat was ever known in ancient Egypt.

One additional 14-chromosome wheat, *T. timopheevi*, which has no common name, deserves mention. This species was discovered in this century by Russian botanists and is known only in western Georgia, where it is grown on a few thousand acres. The species is of botanical interest because its second set of seven chromosomes, designated genom G, is different from that of any of the

other 14-chromosome wheats. It is also of great practical interest because it is resistant to virtually all diseases attacking other cultivated wheats, including rusts, smuts and mildews. In the hands of skilled wheat breeders it may become the ancestor of improved wheats for the next century.

Third Stage

The 21-chromosome wheats, of which there are five, are as a group the most recently evolved and the most useful today. All are cultivated; none has ever been known in the wild. All are products of the hybridization of 14-chromosome wheats containing the genoms A and B with a wild 7-chromosome relative of wheat (almost certainly a grass species of the genus *Aegilops*) containing the genom D. All are believed to have arisen from such hybridization after man, spreading the revolutionary art of agriculture, exposed his earlier cultivated wheats to hybridization with native grasses.

Two of the 21-chromosome wheats, *T. spelta* (spelt) and *T. macha*, are, like einkorn and emmer, hard-threshing species. *T. macha*, like *T. timopheevi*, is confined to western Georgia, where it is grown on not more than a few thousand acres. Spelt was once the principal wheat of central Europe. No archaeological remains of it have been found in the Near East or any part of Asia. There is no doubt about the hybrid origin of spelt, for it has now been synthesized by McFadden and Sears and independ-

| LATIN NAME | COMMON NAME | CHROMOSOMES | | GROWTH | GRAINS |
		NUMBER	GENOMS		
T. AEGILOPOIDES	WILD EINKORN	7	A	WILD	HULLED
T. MONOCOCCUM	EINKORN	7	A	CULTIVATED	HULLED
T. DICOCCOIDES	WILD EMMER	14	AB	WILD	HULLED
T. DICOCCUM	EMMER	14	AB	CULTIVATED	HULLED
T. DURUM	MACARONI WHEAT	14	AB	CULTIVATED	NAKED
T. PERSICUM	PERSIAN WHEAT	14	AB	CULTIVATED	NAKED
T. TURGIDUM	RIVET WHEAT	14	AB	CULTIVATED	NAKED
T. POLONICUM	POLISH WHEAT	14	AB	CULTIVATED	NAKED
T. TIMOPHEEVI		14	AG	CULTIVATED	HULLED
T. AESTIVUM	COMMON WHEAT	21	ABD	CULTIVATED	NAKED
T. SPHAEROCOCCUM	SHOT WHEAT	21	ABD	CULTIVATED	NAKED
T. COMPACTUM	CLUB WHEAT	21	ABD	CULTIVATED	NAKED
T. SPELTA	SPELT	21	ABD	CULTIVATED	HULLED
T. MACHA	MACHA WHEAT	21	ABD	CULTIVATED	HULLED

SOME CHARACTERISTICS of the 14 species, as well as their distribution and antiquity, are given in this table. The genoms are sets of inherited charac-

ently by H. Kihara in Japan. In both cases the researchers concluded that the botanical characteristics to be sought in the unknown 7-chromosome parent of spelt were possessed by *Aegilops squarrosa*, a completely useless wild grass which grows as a weed in wheat fields from the Balkans to Afghanistan. Both researchers hybridized this wild grass with wild emmer. McFadden and Sears doubled the chromosome number by treatment with colchicine; Kihara was fortunate in discovering a case of natural doubling. The hybrid was highly fertile and similar in characteristics to cultivated spelt. As a final step in a brilliant piece of inductive reasoning and genetic experimentation, McFadden and Sears crossed their synthesized spelt with natural spelt and obtained fully fertile hybrids. The results leave no doubt that the wild grass used in this experiment is one of the parents of cultivated spelt, and they suggest strongly that the other four 21-chromosome wheats are likewise hybrids in which the genom D has been derived from the same grass or a species close to it.

These experiments suggest that cultivated spelt originated in the region where the species of wild grass and wild emmer overlap. But the primitive hulled form of spelt has not been found there. An alternate possibility is that the wild grass hybridized not with wild emmer but with the cultivated species, which has had a much wider distribution. Vavilov concluded that hulled spelt originated in southern Germany. Earlier Elisabeth Schiemann, Germany's leading student of cereals, had placed it in Switzerland and southwest Germany. Both centers are not far from the northeastern limits of the area in which cultivated emmer and the wild grass are known to have occurred together. Thus the botanical and historical evidence are not far apart in indicating a central European origin.

The remaining three species of 21-chromosome wheats are *T. aestivum* (common), *sphaerococcum* (shot) and *compactum* (club). They are the true bread wheats, accounting for about 90 per cent of all the wheat grown in the world today. The three are closely related and easily intercrossed. Whether they are the product of three different hybridizations between 14-chromosome wheats and wild grasses, or of three diverging lines of descent from a single hybridization, is not known. Club and shot wheat differ from common wheat in a number of details whose inheritance is governed by a relatively small number of genes. It is possible, therefore, that the three species are descended from a single hybrid ancestor. Common wheat or something very like it has recently been produced by Kihara by crossing 14-chromosome Persian wheat with the wild grass used to synthesize spelt. Its chromosome number has not yet been doubled, but its botanical characteristics are those of common wheat.

Where and when the modern bread wheat first occurred are still matters for conjecture. Since Persian wheat is known only in a limited area in northeastern Turkey and the adjoining states of the Soviet Union, common wheat very probably originated there. Kernels of shot wheat have been found at the most ancient site in India, Mohenjo-Daro, dated about 2500 B.C. A wheat found in neolithic store-chambers in Hungary has been identified as club wheat. Impressions of grains of bread wheat, either common or club, have been found in the neolithic Dolmen period, dated between 300 and 2300 B.C. The earliest archaeological wheat in Japan, dated in the third century, is regarded by Kihara as a bread wheat. And since the 14-chromosome wheats evidently are recent introductions in China, it is possible that the wheat described in the Chinese classics for the Chou period (about 1000 B.C.) is a 21-chromosome bread wheat. All these items, none in itself conclusive, indicate that the bread wheats originated before the time of Christ but later than einkorn or emmer. A conservative guess would put their origin at approximately 2500 B.C.

A Historic Explosion

Whether the bread wheats originated earlier than this or later, and whether they had one hybrid origin or three, they represent today the most rapid increase in geographical range and numbers of any species of seed-plant in history. They are now grown in all parts of the world from the Equator to the Arctic Circle. Originating probably not more than 5,000 years ago in the general region of Asia Minor, the new species have increased at an average rate of

GEOGRAPHICAL DISTRIBUTION	EARLIEST EVIDENCE
WESTERN IRAN, ASIA MINOR, GREECE, SOUTHERN YUGOSLAVIA	PRE-AGRICULTURAL
EASTERN CAUCASUS, ASIA MINOR, GREECE, CENTRAL EUROPE	4750 B. C.
WESTERN IRAN, SYRIA, NORTHERN PALESTINE, NORTHEASTERN TURKEY, ARMENIA	PRE-AGRICULTURAL
INDIA, CENTRAL ASIA, NORTHERN IRAN, GEORGIA, ARMENIA, EUROPE, MEDITERRANEAN AREA, ABYSSINIA	4000 B. C.
CENTRAL ASIA, IRAN, MESOPOTAMIA, TURKEY, ABYSSINIA, SOUTHEASTERN EUROPE, U.S.	100 B. C.
DAGESTAN, GEORGIA, ARMENIA, NORTHEASTERN TURKEY	NO PREHISTORIC REMAINS
ABYSSINIA, SOUTHERN EUROPE	NO PREHISTORIC REMAINS
ABYSSINIA, MEDITERRANEAN AREA	17TH CENTURY
WESTERN GEORGIA	20TH CENTURY
WORLD WIDE	NEOLITHIC PERIOD
CENTRAL AND NORTHWESTERN INDIA	2500 B. C.
SOUTHWESTERN ASIA, SOUTHEASTERN EUROPE, U.S.	NEOLITHIC PERIOD
CENTRAL EUROPE	BRONZE AGE
WESTERN GEORGIA	20TH CENTURY

teristics, or combinations of sets. The chromosome number is a clue to the evolution of wheat. The species with larger chromosome numbers descended from those with smaller by hybridization and chromosome doubling.

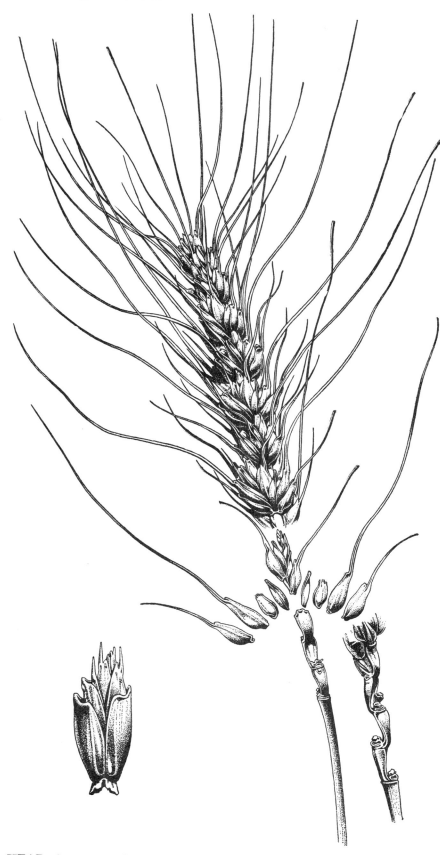

HEAD of common wheat is dissected to show the rachis (*lower right*) which bears the spikelets. Enclosing each kernel is a bearded glume. In some varieties the beard is absent. At lower left is a single spikelet of spelt, which during threshing remains intact and attached to a joint of the rachis.

about 75,000 acres per year until they now occupy almost 400 million acres. Their evolution and dispersal have been explosive phenomena in which man's principal part has been to recognize their usefulness and to open up new agricultural areas for their culture.

The particular value of the bread wheats lies not only in their productiveness and in their free-threshing, naked kernels, but in the peculiar quality of their gluten, the protein component. Of all the cereals only the bread wheats are capable of producing the light, fluffy, leavened breads we know today.

All known species of cultivated wheat, except einkorn and possibly emmer, came into existence spontaneously. Man played no part in their origin except as he spread their culture and their opportunities for natural hybridization over the earth. There is no evidence that ancient man gave much attention to selection of superior forms, or if he did, no evidence that he succeeded. The cultivated einkorn of today is scarcely different from the einkorn of millennia ago, and it, in turn, is no great improvement over wild einkorn. Essentially the same can be said about emmer. Consequently, to speak of primitive man as a plant breeder is to attribute more purposefulness to his activities than the evidence warrants.

Within the past century, especially since the rediscovery of Mendel's laws of inheritance in 1900, vast programs of wheat improvement have been undertaken in almost all the wheat-growing regions of the world. These have been especially successful in the U. S. and Canada, where a constant succession of new varieties has been introduced. Scarcely any state of the Union today grows extensively the principal varieties of wheat grown 50 years ago.

Early in the century the most common method of wheat breeding was "pure-line" selection as invented by Wilhelm Johannsen, a Danish botanist and geneticist. Johannsen had concluded from experiments on garden beans that self-fertilized plants such as beans, peas and cereals are racial mixtures of many pure lines, differing from one another in many characteristics but each genetically uniform. Continuous selection can have no effect in changing the characters of a genetically pure line, but a mixture of lines can be separated into its component parts and improvements effected by propagating the superior lines.

In practice the wheat breeder selects hundreds of individual heads from a variety, threshes each one separately and grows the progeny of each in a short row called a head row. In succeeding generations more and longer rows are grown, and the pure lines, each originating from a single head, are compared in productiveness and other characteristics. Among wheat breeders in the

U. S. It is standard procedure at this stage to use rows 16 feet long and one foot apart. Rows of this length and spacing simplify computation, since the yield of grain in grams can be converted to a bushel yield per acre by simply pointing off one decimal place. The more promising lines are increased still further in field plots and eventually one is chosen as the best, is named and is distributed to farmers.

The two outstanding U. S. varieties produced by pure-line selection are both Kansas products. The first, Kanred (Kansas Red), was selected by Herbert Roberts of the Kansas Agricultural Experiment Station from Crimean, a hard, red, winter-type wheat introduced from Russia by Mark Carleton. The first head selections were made in 1906, and the improved pure line first distributed for commercial growing in 1917. By 1925 Kanred wheat, the product of a single head only 19 years earlier, was grown on nearly five million acres in Kansas, Nebraska, Colorado, Oklahoma and Texas. The second Kansas wheat, Blackhull, is the product of a single head selection made in 1912 from a field of Turkey wheat by Earl Clark, a farmer and plant breeder. Blackhull, like Kanred, was first distributed in 1917. By 1929 it occupied almost six million acres, principally in Kansas and Oklahoma.

The Hybrid Wheats

Pure-line selection merely sorts out from a variety the superior lines already there; it creates no new genetic combinations. To form a new variety the breeder employs hybridization. He selects as parents two varieties with the characteristics he seeks to combine. For example, one parent may be chosen for its superior milling and baking qualities, the other for its resistance to disease. To cross these two the breeder first emasculates one of them by removing the anthers, the male pollen-containing organs, with delicate forceps when these organs are full-grown but not yet ripe. Then he covers the emasculated head with a small glassine bag to prevent uncontrolled pollination. A few days later, when its female organs, the stigmas, have become receptive, the operator pollinates them with ripe anthers taken from the second parent.

Such pollinations produce seeds that grow into first-generation hybrid plants. These are quite uniform and nothing is accomplished by practicing selection among them. But in the second and subsequent generations genetic segregation creates new combinations as numerous and diverse as the hands in a shuffled deck of cards. The opportunities for creative selection are enormous. It is in the early generations following a cross that the plant breeder shows his skill, for at this stage he must select for propagation

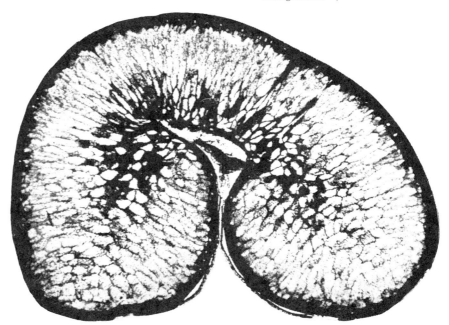

KERNEL of common wheat is photographed in cross section at the Northern Regional Research Laboratory of the U. S. Department of Agriculture. The interior of the kernel is the endosperm, from which flour is made.

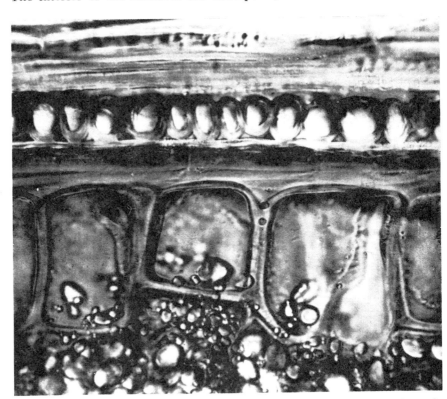

BRAN, or outer layer of the kernel, is shown in this photomicrograph made at the Northern Regional Research Laboratory. At the bottom of the photomicrograph, which enlarges these structures 600 times, is the endosperm.

those combinations which approach most closely the ideal wheat he has in mind and discard those which do not meet his specifications. Eventually genetic segregation produces pure lines.

One of the earliest and greatest achievements in hybrid wheat was the development of the Marquis strain. This variety, a hybrid of early-growing Hard Red Calcutta from India and Red Fife from Poland, was produced in Canada by Charles Saunders, cerealist for the Dominion from 1903 to 1922. The cross from which Marquis wheat was derived

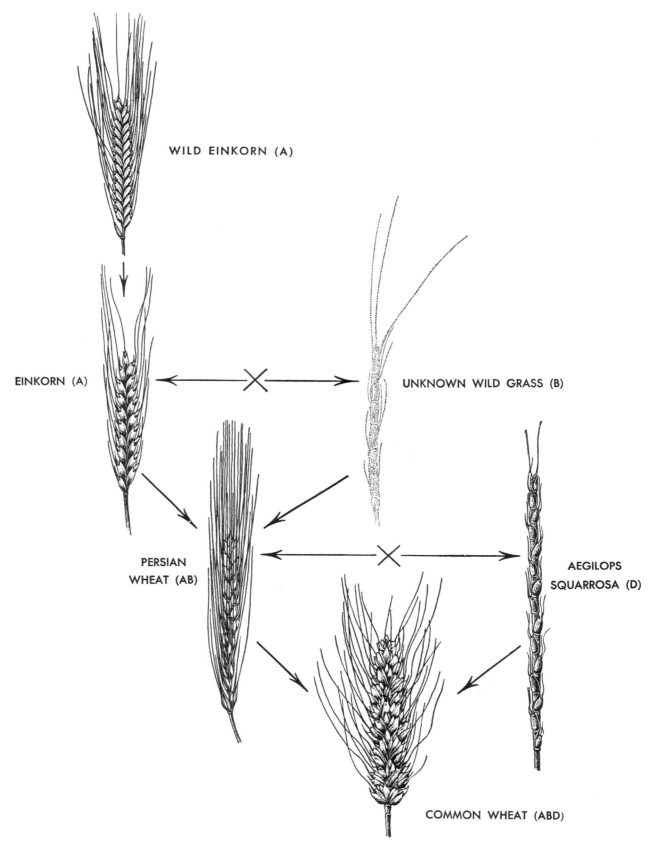

WILD EINKORN (A)

EINKORN (A) × UNKNOWN WILD GRASS (B)

PERSIAN
WHEAT (AB) × AEGILOPS
SQUARROSA (D)

COMMON WHEAT (ABD)

EVOLUTION of common wheat is outlined. Wild einkorn (7 chromosomes, genom A) evolved into einkorn,
which, crossed with a wild grass (genom B), gave rise
to Persian wheat (14 chromosomes, genom AB). When
this wheat was crossed with another grass (genom D),
common wheat (21 chromosomes, genom ABD) resulted.

had been made in 1892 by his brother Arthur under the direction of his father, William Saunders, who had been hybridizing wheats since 1888. The new hybrid was promising from the beginning. It was a few days earlier than the spring-planted varieties then commonly grown in Canada, thus often avoiding the first frosts. The grain yielded a cream-colored, strongly elastic dough with strong gluten and excellent baking qualities. Marquis wheat later set new standards for baking quality. By 1907, four years after the initial head selection, there were 23 pounds of seed. Distribution to farmers began in the spring of 1909. News of the new wheat spread swiftly from the prairie provinces down into our own spring-wheat belt. By 1913 Marquis seed was being imported into Minnesota and the Dakotas at the rate of 200,000 bushels per year. In 1918 more than 300 million bushels were produced, and the superiority of this variety over those previously grown was a factor in meeting the food shortage of World War I, just as 25 years later hybrid corn was a similar factor in World War II.

For 20 years Marquis was the "king of wheats" in Canada and the U. S., and during this period it served as a standard both in the field and in the milling and baking laboratory. Marquis was also used extensively as a parent in new hybrids and is the ancestor of many improved wheats, including Tenmarq, developed in Kansas by John Parker; Ceres, produced in North Dakota by L. R. Waldron, and Thatcher and Newthatch, bred by Herbert K. Hayes and his associates in Minnesota.

Today most new wheat varieties are produced by controlled hybridization rather than by pure-line selection, which is little used. The modern wheat breeder has many objectives. Usually his principal one is productiveness, but involved in this are many factors, including resistance to diseases and tolerance of unfavorable environmental conditions. To test new wheats for these characteristics, breeders have invented devices and methods for subjecting wheat to artificial drought, cold and epidemics of disease.

Breeders v. Fungi

Breeding for disease resistance is especially important because wheat is a self-fertilized plant which, except for natural hybridization and occasional mutations, tends to remain genetically uniform. A field of wheat of a single variety, especially one originating from a single head, contains millions of plants which are genetically identical. If the variety happens to be susceptible to a disease, it serves as a gigantic culture medium for the propagation of the disease organism, usually a fungus. Thus the growing of new varieties over large acreages increases the hazards from those diseases to which they are susceptible. The result is a never-ending battle between the wheat breeders and the fungi.

The breeding of wheat for resistance to stem rust, a devastating disease, is a prime example. There are many kinds of stem rust. Pathologists, led by Elvin Stakman of the University of Minnesota, have devised ingenious methods of identifying them by inoculation of different hosts. The wheat breeder then develops a new variety which is resistant to the predominating races of stem rust. This is distributed to farmers and its acreage increases rapidly. But while the wheat breeder is hybridizing wheats, nature is hybridizing rusts. The reproductive stage of stem rusts occurs not on wheat but on an alternate host, the common barberry. On this plant new races of rust are constantly created. Although most of them probably die out, one that finds susceptible wheat varieties may multiply prodigiously and in a few years become the predominating race. The wheat breeder then searches the world for wheats resistant to the new hazard and again goes through all the stages of producing a new hybrid variety. The competition between man and the fungi for the wheat crop of the world is a biological "cold war" which never ends.

A wheat breeder must seek not only disease resistance and productiveness but also milling and baking quality. In modern mass-production bakeries with high-speed mixing machinery, dough undergoes stresses and strains which it was never called on to endure when kneaded by hand in the home. As a result wheat breeders have been compelled to subject their new productions to elaborate milling and baking tests which simulate the processes of commercial bakeries. A new wheat that proves superior in the field may be rejected in the laboratory.

In spite of the difficulties involved, the development of more productive varieties of wheat is one of the surest ways of increasing the food supply and raising living standards. When Mussolini drained the Pontine swamp in Italy, the Italian wheat breeder Alzareno Strampelli produced new varieties of wheat which flourished in the fertile soils newly opened to cultivation. An important part of the well-publicized Etawah Village Improvement Program in India is the growing of improved varieties of wheat developed by British and Indian geneticists. Mexico's agricultural program, sponsored by the Rockefeller Foundation in cooperation with the Mexican Government, owes much of its success to new rust-resistant varieties of wheat. Crossing the old varieties of Mexican wheat with rust-resistant wheats from the U. S., South America, Australia and New Zealand, the U. S. breeder Norman Borlaug and his associates, working closely with Mexican technologists, have bred new varieties so resistant to rust that they can be grown in Mexico's summer rainy season as well as in the winter dry season, heretofore its only season for growing wheat. The bulk of Mexico's wheat acreage is now devoted to new hybrids developed since 1943, while acreage and production have expanded substantially.

Hybridization among wheats is usually confined to varieties of one species, but interspecific hybrids also are employed and sometimes are successful. A notable example is the development of Hope wheat by McFadden from a cross of Marquis with Yaroslav emmer, a 14-chromosome wheat extremely resistant to stem rust, leaf rust and several other diseases. From this hybrid, which was partly sterile, McFadden succeeded in developing a 21-chromosome wheat which has a high degree of resistance to many races of stem and leaf rust. Unfortunately Hope wheat has a grain somewhat lacking in milling and baking qualities and the variety has never become important commercially. It has, however, been the parent of many modern varieties of wheat which are commercially grown, including Newthatch in Minnesota, Austin in Texas and several of the new varieties developed in Mexico.

New Cereals

A future possibility in wheat breeding is the creation of wholly new types of cereals by species hybridization followed by artificial chromosome doubling, a man-made counterpart of wheat's earlier evolution in nature. In the U.S.S.R. and the U. S. wheat has been crossed with rye to produce a fertile, true-breeding hybrid cereal which combines the chromosomes of both. The hybrid, neither a wheat nor a rye, is more resistant to cold than wheat is, but less useful as a bread-making cereal. It has not become popular. Wheat has been crossed with a perennial wild grass to produce a new perennial cereal for which Russian agronomists have made fantastic claims. A field of this wheat, once planted, will, according to the Russians, yield a crop of grain year after year with little or no further attention except to gather the annual harvest. It turns out that this perennial "wheat" may have some promise as a forage grass for livestock, but so far little bread has been made from it and few people have been fed by it.

The idea of producing new cereal species by hybridization and chromosome doubling is, however, quite sound, and the possibilities inherent in it are far from exhausted. Some day new wheat species consciously created by man may replace those which arose spontaneously in nature.

Cattle

Cattle

8

Ralph W. Phillips
June 1958

They can convert otherwise useless vegetation into milk and meat. Physiology and genetics are now showing how they can be made to do so more efficiently in widely varying environments

Cattle stand first among the animals serving man. They are outnumbered, it is true, by sheep, and they are outranked in man's esteem by the horse and the dog, but no other domestic animal renders such a variety of important services to human well-being. To the American or European consumer, cattle represent beef, veal, milk, butter, cheese and leather; behind the scenes in the packing house they yield in addition hormones and vitamin extracts, bone meal for feed and fertilizer and high-protein concentrates for livestock feeding. This does not exhaust the catalogue of their utility. More than a third of the world's 800 million cattle are engaged primarily in the generation of brute energy for the tasks of plowing, hauling and milling.

Considered as machines for converting vegetable matter into human food, cattle are not particularly efficient. The best such machine is the pig, which converts about a fifth of what it eats into food for human consumption. A dairy cow converts less than a sixth, a beef steer no more than a twentieth. Even these figures refer to animals bred for food production and raised by up-to-date techniques; the cattle of Asia and Africa, bred mainly for work, are less efficient. Cattle, however, convert foodstuffs which are otherwise useless to man. The efficient pig must subsist almost entirely on concentrated carbohy-

drates and proteins; its food could, at least in theory, be consumed directly by human beings. But cattle, though they need more food than pigs to yield the same number of calories, feed in part on cellulose, which they digest with the help of certain microorganisms in their enormous stomachs. By using cattle as intermediaries we can process the vegetation of semi-arid grasslands which cannot be farmed in any other way. Recent studies suggest that some day we may even use cattle to produce food from sawdust [see "The Metabolism of Ruminants," by Terence A. Rogers; Scientific American, February].

But if the world's food problem is to be solved, we must find ways to improve

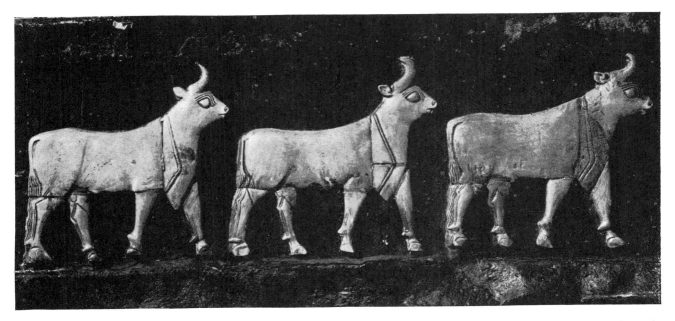

IMPORTANCE OF CATTLE early in human history is shown by their recurrence in wall paintings and sculptures such as this Sumerian frieze. In early civilizations cattle were used not for food but mainly for work, as in most of Africa and Asia today.

the efficiency with which cattle convert fodder, of whatever sort, into meat and milk. Selective breeding of cattle to this end has been going on for several centuries in western Europe. There, and more recently in America, cattle breeders have achieved remarkably good results considering the empirical methods they have relied upon. Only during the past 20 or 30 years have scientific physiology and genetics come into play. Though many important questions remain unanswered, scientists have already done much to help cattlemen improve existing breeds and develop new breeds which can produce efficiently in unfavorable environments.

Breeds

We do not know when or where cattle were first domesticated. Cave paintings and bits of charred bone tell us that primitive man in Europe and Asia hunted wild cattle of various species, and our domestic cattle must be descended from one or more of these. In Europe the wild species are all extinct, though one of them, the aurochs, survived in remote parts of eastern Europe as late as the 17th century. Similar wild species still roam the forests and savannas of southeast Asia. The Americas have no native cattle, nor does Australia. Our best guess is that cattle were domesticated at least 10,000 years ago somewhere in central or southern Asia by nomadic tribesmen who raised them for meat and milk. As agricultural and urban societies developed, cattle came to be used primarily as draft animals. So great was their economic importance in this role that the Egyptians, Assyrians and other ancient peoples worshipped them as gods. Indeed, until the coming of steam they were man's main source of power other than his own muscles; the heavy draft horse is a relatively recent development.

Even in ancient times herdsmen seem to have practiced some sort of selective breeding. The Mosaic law specifically provides that "thou shalt not let thy cattle gender with a diverse kind." Jacob, under his shrewdly drawn contract with Laban, succeeded in making his fortune by judicious cattle breeding. As the 30th chapter of Genesis records, he relied in part on superstition, but he also employed the perfectly sound genetic principle that like tends to produce like. His "speckled and spotted" cattle produced calves of like coloring.

Thousands of years of domestication have produced dozens of more or less distinct breeds of cattle [see drawings on page 84 to 87]. Almost all of them, however, seem to stem from two species: European cattle (*Bos taurus*) and Indian or zebu cattle (*Bos indicus*).

From the original European species breeders in western Europe and especially in the British Isles developed all but one or two of the popular milk and beef breeds in the world today. Their distribution on the world map [see below] follows that of the European settlers who took them along to the Temperate Zones of the Americas, New Zealand and Australia. In addition some minor breeds are found in northern and eastern Asia.

The beef breeds, including the white-faced Herefords and the black Aberdeen Angus of our midwestern and plains states, are typically low-set and blocky in appearance, with a relatively small percentage of bone and a good deal of fat. Dairy cattle, by contrast, are lean and angular, bred to turn every possible bit of feed into milk. Their udders are, of course, much larger than those of the beef breeds, and their swollen mid-sections bespeak a digestive tract capable of handling large quantities of grass.

The most important dairy breeds are the Holstein, the Jersey and the Guernsey. The Holstein, largest of the three, is also the most copious producer, but the other two give richer milk and are favored by dairymen who specialize in butter production and farmers who keep a few "family cows" to produce butter and cream as well as milk. The Ayrshire, perhaps the original "friendly cow, all

1. AYRSHIRE
2. WEST HIGHLAND
3. ANGUS
4. SHORTHORN
5. HEREFORD
6. JERSEY
7. HOLSTEIN
8. CHAROLAIS
9. BROWN SWISS
10. CHIANINI
11. BLANCO OREJINEGRO
12. WEST AFRICAN SHORTHORN
13. KANKREJ
13a. BRAHMAN
14. ONGOLE
15. SAHIWAL
16. KANGAYAM
17. BORAN
18. MADAGASCAR
19. AFRICANDER
20. SANTA GERTRUDIS
21. EGYPTIAN
22. ANKOLE
23. CHINESE "YELLOW COW"

CATTLE OF EUROPEAN TYPE

NATIVE ZEBU CATTLE

CATTLE OF INTERMEDIATE TYPE

INTRODUCED ZEBU CATTLE

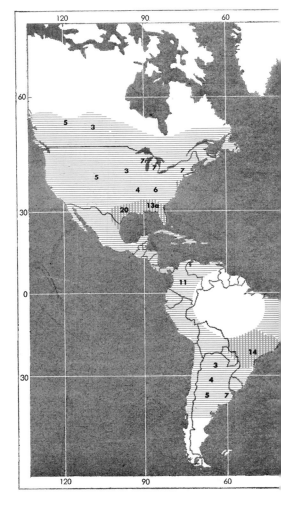

WORLD DISTRIBUTION of the two main species of cattle indicates their adaptation to different climates. European cattle (*Bos taurus*) are found in most temperate regions; they

red and white," is less well known, though it is a good milk producer.

A number of European breeds are dual- or triple-purpose animals, used for milk and meat or for milk, meat and work. The Shorthorn is generally considered a dual-purpose breed, though different strains have been selected primarily for meat or for milk production. The Brown Swiss and the Simmenthal, also a Swiss breed, are triple-purpose animals in their native country. Many other European countries have developed their own dual- and triple-purpose breeds, but few of these have spread to other lands.

The Zebu

The zebu, the other great species of domestic cattle, probably originated in India but long ago spread, or was brought by man, into Africa and parts of southeast Asia. Thousands of years of natural selection have inured it to tropical conditions. In recent decades it has been successfully introduced into Brazil, the U. S. Gulf Coast and other tropical and semitropical regions.

The zebu differs from European cattle most obviously in having a large hump on its shoulders and a heavy dewlap. The biological function of these organs is uncertain. Until recently it was believed that by increasing the animal's surface area they helped to dissipate heat. But recent experiments indicate that even when these parts of its anatomy are surgically removed the zebu remains heat-tolerant. The hump apparently does not provide any important food reserve for the animal, as the camel's does; the zebu's hump does not shrink much when the animal has to get along on sparse food rations. Zebus are generally more alert and more active than European cattle. They do not moo or bellow but emit a kind of coughing grunt.

The zebus of the Indian peninsula have evolved into many breeds, most of which inhabit fairly limited areas. The great majority are work animals, but several rather similar breeds found in Pakistan and India are known for their milking qualities. The best of these milking breeds, the Sahiwal, has been introduced into Jamaica; another, the Gir, is used extensively in Brazil. Experiments with the Sindhi breed are being carried on in the U. S. The "Brahman" cattle of our Gulf States are a mixture of several Indian working breeds, chiefly the Kankrej; their beef qualities have

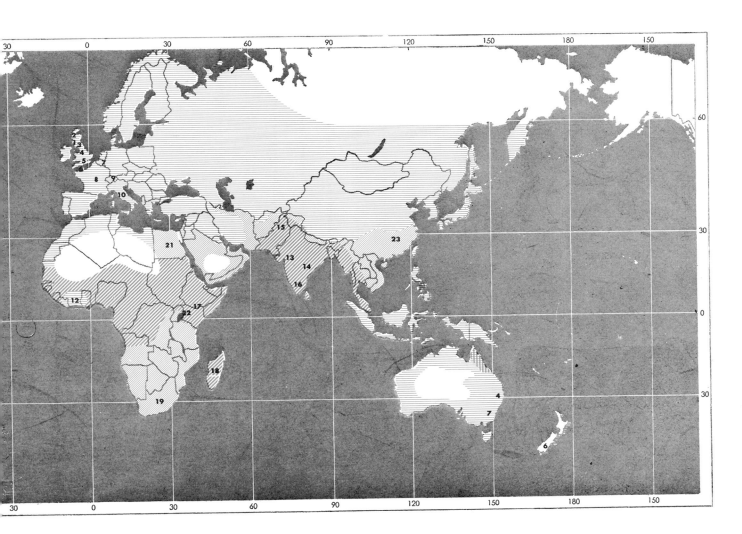

seldom do well in the tropics. Zebu cattle (*Bos indicus*) originated in India and have spread or been introduced into other hot regions. Numbers suggest the distribution of some important breeds, which are depicted in drawings on the next four pages.

been considerably improved by selection.

In addition to the more or less improved breeds, the zebu cattle of India and Pakistan include large numbers of small and relatively unproductive "village cattle" and "hill cattle"; the latter sometimes are only about the size of a large dog.

As one might expect, zebus have been crossbred with European cattle where the two species have come in contact. Cattle breeds in southern China, the Near East and some along the northeast shore of the Mediterranean as far west as Italy show evidences of zebu ancestry. In Africa centuries of tribal migrations have so mixed the two species as to make classification difficult. Some African breeds, such as the Ankole, differ from European and zebu cattle in possessing enormous, bulbous horns. Broadly speaking, the cattle of northwest Africa stem from the European species or some similar humpless type; zebus in-

habit a wide belt across Madagascar and central Africa; elsewhere the two species have mingled to produce bewildering variety. European cattle, zebus, and their intermixtures account for almost all the cattle in the world. The only significant additions are two close relatives, the bantin of Java and the gayal of Assam and upper Burma, which have been domesticated on a small scale.

We should not, however, overlook a distant cousin which has great economic importance in some parts of the world— the water buffalo. India, with some 140 million cattle, also has more than 40 million buffaloes; Thailand actually has more buffaloes than cattle. In some countries, such as China, buffaloes are used primarily for work; elsewhere, as in India and Egypt, they are kept mainly for milk. Surplus animals are slaughtered for meat almost everywhere, though the meat is of poor quality by our standards. Buffaloes are particularly useful in the tropics because they seem to be better

able than cattle to digest the crude fiber that forms a large part of much tropical vegetation. Curiously, however, they resist heat less well than even European cattle. Buffaloes apparently have no sweat glands, except in their muzzles. For this reason and possibly others, their heat-regulating mechanism is inadequate, and in hot weather they must be drenched with water periodically or allowed to wallow in water or mud if their working or milk-producing capacity is to be maintained.

It stands to reason that cattle bred for work will be inefficient producers of food. In the underdeveloped countries of the world, where the food problem is most acute, the usefulness of cattle is still further reduced by primitive slaughtering methods. The hides, too, are often damaged by knife-cuts or are poorly tanned. In India, of course, Hindu religious taboos generally forbid the slaughtering of cattle. A similar situation prevails among the tribal cultures of

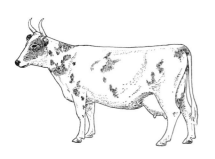

1. AYRSHIRE

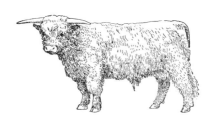

2. WEST HIGHLAND

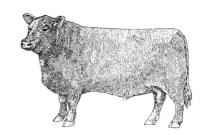

3. ANGUS

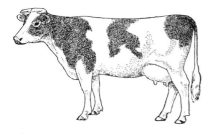

7. HOLSTEIN

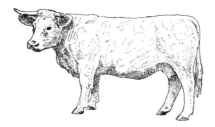

8. CHAROLAIS

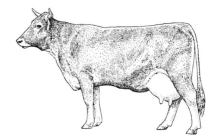

9. BROWN SWISS

EUROPEAN CATTLE include almost all the specialized dairy (1, 6, 7) and beef (3, 5, 8) breeds. Shorthorns are used for both purposes; the Brown Swiss, a dairy breed in the U. S., is used for milk, meat and work in Switzerland. The Chianini, though unspe-

Africa and the Near East, where cattle, along with other livestock, are a kind of currency. (Our own word "pecuniary" comes from the Latin word *pecus*, meaning cattle.) Where a man's wealth is measured by the size of his herds, and the price of a wife is stated in cows, the tribesman will be concerned with the numbers rather than with the quality of his cattle. Some tribes have developed bizarre ways of getting food from cattle without killing them. The Masai of East Africa, for example, bleed their cattle periodically and drink the fresh blood or combine it with other foods.

Cattle Breeding

Systematic efforts to improve the productivity of cattle began in Great Britain during the 18th century with the work of Robert Bakewell, the great pioneer in animal husbandry. Bakewell and his successors in Britain and western Europe produced almost all of the dairy and beef breeds we know today. These early breeders, of course, knew nothing of scientific genetics. Their success in developing so many productive breeds testifies that they had a good grasp of the empirical principles and a certain amount of good luck.

Breeders have been most successful with dairy cattle, because the productivity of a milker is easily measured in pounds of milk and percentage of butterfat content. The best milkers could be chosen as breeding animals, and even bulls could be selected by the productivity of their daughters.

The productivity of beef cattle is more difficult to measure. How quickly they put on weight, which determines how quickly the cattleman can turn over his capital, can be measured fairly easily. But it takes an elaborate analysis of each carcass to judge qualities such as the ratio of meat to bone and the extent to which meat is "marbled" with fat. Lacking any simple measure of quality, breeders have tended to estimate animals by their appearance, selecting breeds with deep, wide bodies, well-developed loins and hindquarters (which contain the more expensive cuts) and a blocky, smooth exterior. Such visual criteria put emphasis on a thick layer of fat under the skin. Breeders have a saying: "Fat is a pretty color." Much of this pretty fat, however, is trimmed away on the butcher's block to please the American taste. Moreover, the amount of fat on the outside of the carcass seems to have little bearing on the fat inside, which makes for tender and juicy meat, or on the proportion of lean meat to bone.

A number of scientists have been working on better methods of evaluating beef cattle on the hoof. In one promising method certain harmless chemicals which are absorbed much more rapidly by fat than by muscle are injected into the animal's bloodstream. By taking blood samples at intervals one can

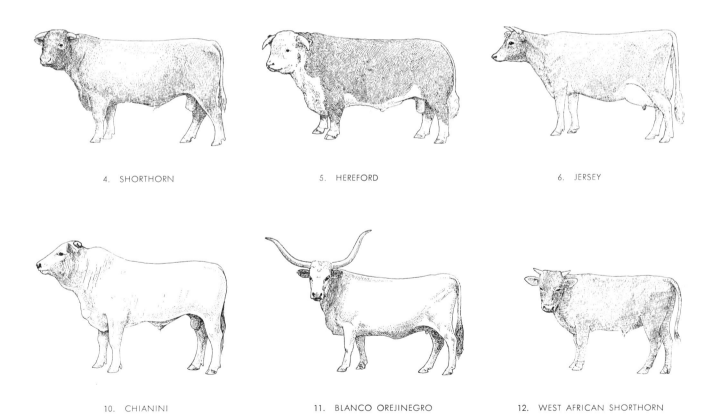

4. SHORTHORN   5. HEREFORD   6. JERSEY

10. CHIANINI   11. BLANCO OREJINEGRO   12. WEST AFRICAN SHORTHORN

cialized, is the best beef producer among Italian breeds. The West Highland is adapted to a cold, damp climate; the Blanco Orejinegro and West African Shorthorn (no relation to the Shorthorn) are among the few breeds of European type which thrive in the tropics.

measure the rate at which the chemicals are absorbed and thus estimate the amount of fat inside the carcass.

The most promising work in cattle improvement, however, is drawing upon the science of genetics. Although this is a new undertaking, it has moved ahead rapidly and is already showing results.

Genetic Traits

A few traits in cattle are known to be inherited by simple Mendelian principles. The black coat and hornlessness of the Aberdeen Angus and the white face of the Hereford are Mendelian dominants, controlled by single pairs of genes. These traits, however, are not of major economic importance. The more significant qualities of milk production, percentage of butterfat, rate of growth and efficiency of feed utilization involve many pairs of genes and are also powerfully influenced by environment. Nonetheless geneticists have made progress in estimating the relative weight of the genetic and environmental factors that determine these traits. By studying the extent to which related animals, such as half-brothers or half-sisters, are more alike than randomly selected animals reared under the same conditions, it is possible to estimate the degree to which a particular trait can be inherited and thus to predict how effective selection for that trait is likely to be.

In dairy cows, for example, butterfat production is about 30 per cent inheritable. That is, if we select a group of heifers whose butterfat production averages 100 pounds a year more than the herd-average and breed them to bulls of similar superior stock, the offspring will produce about 30 pounds a year above the average. According to studies by the U. S. Range Experiment Station at Miles City, Mont., the indications are that the birth weight of beef cattle is 53 per cent inheritable and the weight at 15 months (just before slaughtering) is 86 per cent inheritable. The grade of the carcass is estimated to be 33 per cent inheritable.

In the early 1940s the Miles City workers began to select cattle for rapid growth, and they have developed some superior strains. These results have been accomplished by selecting on the basis of performance tests rather than appearance. That looks can be deceiving was illustrated some time ago when a distinguished foreign visitor to the station, after being shown some very good performers, spied a herd of fat, blocky steers just as he was leaving. "Why didn't you show me these before?" he exclaimed. He was startled to learn that these seemingly superior cattle were in fact the poorest producers on the station!

With more experimental work of this sort breeders may soon be able to provide bulls which transmit to their offspring high feeding efficiency, optimum proportions of bone, muscle and fat, a rapid growth rate and perhaps even tenderer meat. For the general public

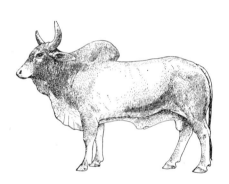

13. KANKREJ

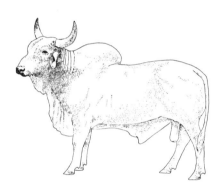

13a. BRAHMAN

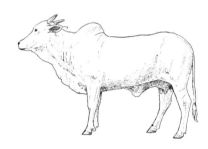

14. ONGOLE

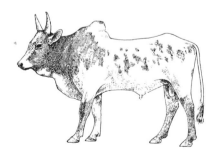

18. MADAGASCAR

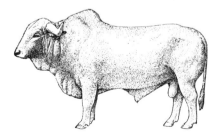

19. AFRICANDER

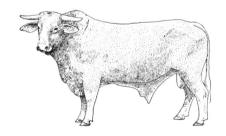

20. SANTA GERTRUDIS

ZEBU CATTLE (13-18) are mostly used for work; the few dairy breeds, such as the Sahiwal, produce far less than European milk cattle. The Brahman is a mixture of several Indian zebu breeds, mainly the Kankrej. Interbreeding between zebus and European

this will mean cheaper and better steaks and roasts.

Backward Areas

Work of this kind has been carried on so far in the Temperate Zone countries where levels of production are already high. Little or nothing has been done to improve the cattle in more needful regions of the world, even by empirical methods. Effective selection implies a sizable herd to select from, but the average farmer in these regions has only one or two cattle, and often these are work oxen which cannot breed. The farmers owning larger herds can seldom afford to purchase superior breeding stock, nor can the near-subsistence economies of these countries spare much money for large-scale breeding experiments.

Moreover, the attempts that have been made to improve the productivity of zebus have not been very fruitful so far, partly because too little is yet known about the genetic potential of the various strains and partly because in many areas the feeding and management of the cattle are not efficient enough to bring out their full possibilities. The best zebu performances have been far below those of European breeds. In India a few well-handled Sahiwal cows have produced somewhat more than 10,000 pounds of milk in a year. In the U. S., Holsteins have produced as much as 40,000 pounds. The high productivity of European cattle is the result of several centuries of selective breeding. Even assuming that the economic difficulties can be overcome, it would take a long time to raise the best zebu breeds, such as the Sahiwal, to similar levels.

Nor has much attention been given to improving the zebu as a work animal. Some agricultural leaders in the underdeveloped countries hold that such research is a waste of money, believing that draft cattle will soon be replaced by tractors. I myself am not so sure.

Small fields, a low economic level, the need for manure and, in rice-growing areas, the water-covered ground are all likely to delay the substitution of tractors for cattle.

It may be that the most rapid improvement of cattle in the underdeveloped areas of the world will be gained by crossing the European and zebu animals. The pure European breeds do not do well in these regions. Their digestive systems are not adapted to the coarse and often scanty grasses; parasites and disease are additional hazards. Worst of all is the heat. In hot climates European cattle suffer from the bovine equivalent of heat exhaustion. They eat poorly and do not seek food actively (as cattle must where pastures are sparse). Their fertility is lowered by poor nutrition and still further reduced by high body temperatures.

The zebu, of course, thrives in the tropics. Its skin, thicker than that of European cattle, can better resist ticks

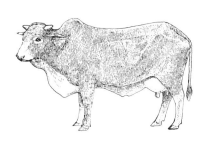

15. SAHIWAL

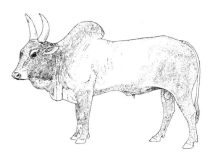

16. KANGAYAM

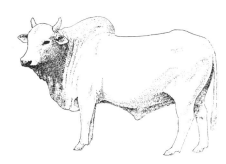

17. BORAN

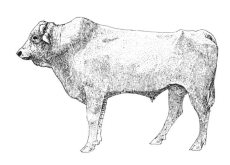

21. EGYPTIAN

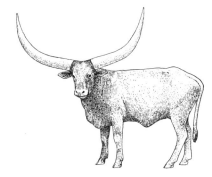

22. ANKOLE

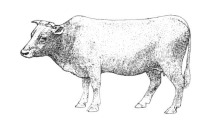

23. CHINESE "YELLOW COW"

cattle in many parts of the world has produced mixtures of quite varied appearances (19-23). The Santa Gertrudis, a recently developed breed based on a Brahman-Shorthorn cross, has in recent years become an important beef producer in the Gulf states.

and stinging flies. It can digest crude fodder, though not so well as the buffalo. And it keeps cool. For one thing, its coat is thinner than those of the European breeds; for another, most zebus are light-colored and absorb less sunlight. There are indications that the zebu may have more, or more effective, sweat glands than European cattle. Apparently the principal reason the zebu keeps cool is that it produces less body heat, even though it is typically more active than European cattle. How it manages this metabolic trick is a mystery which investigators are currently trying to unravel.

Efforts to combine the zebu's resistance to heat and the European breeds' high productivity have already achieved considerable success. An outstanding example is the Santa Gertrudis, a breed developed from a Brahman-Shorthorn cross, which during the past 20 years has become an important producer in our Gulf States. Crosses between Jerseys and various milking breeds of zebus also are yielding good results. The Jamaica Hope, a Jersey-Sahiwal cross, already approaches the U. S. average in milk production.

A less urgent but equally challenging objective is the development of breeds adapted to the cold climates of northern Canada and Siberia. The Mongolians and Tibetans have long crossed cattle with the yak to produce an animal combining some of the yak's hardiness with the cow's milking capacity. Unfortunately only the females of these crosses are fertile. The Canadian government has crossed cattle with bison to produce the "catalo," and has even bred a cattle-bison-yak, but neither of these combinations has yet shown any particular economic advantages.

Not very much is known about the cattle breeds in the underdeveloped areas of the world. It may well be that combinations of these types with the better-known breeds would produce more productive breeds of cattle for specific conditions. One obstacle to such experimentation is that infections such as the hoof-and-mouth disease and rinderpest are prevalent among cattle in many underdeveloped regions, and it is dangerous to import breeding animals or even semen from such areas. But we can hope that the obstacles will be overcome, so that better cattle and better raising methods will become available to meet the growing world population's need for protein food and to add more meat to the diet of the many peoples in underdeveloped countries who now get very little.

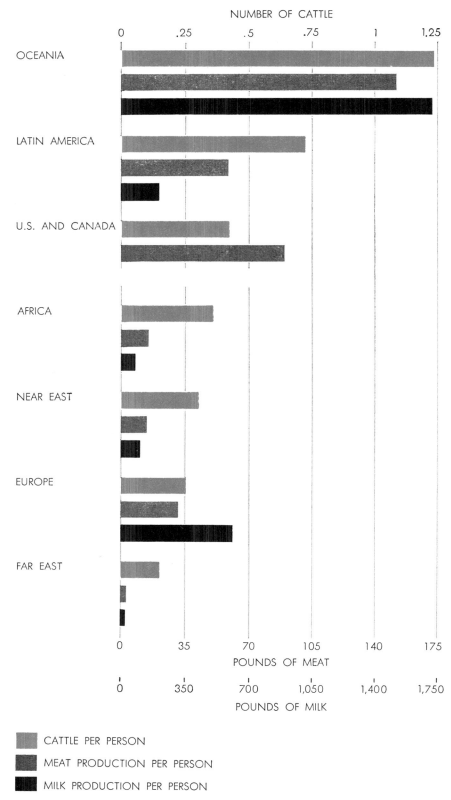

NUMBERS AND PRODUCTIVITY of cattle in proportion to population vary in different regions. High figures for Oceania reflect large cattle industries and low population of Australia and New Zealand. In Latin America dairying is much less important; cattle in most areas are of poor quality. U. S., Canada and Europe have fewer but more productive cattle. In Africa, Near East and Far East cattle are used mainly for work and produce little food.

Milk

9

Stuart Patton
July 1969

The fluid made by the mammary gland is a remarkable blend of complex biological molecules. How the gland does its work is the subject of active investigation

According to the census of manufactures taken in 1967 the production, distribution and sale of dairy products constituted the seventh largest industry in the U.S., exceeded in value of shipments only by the motor vehicle, steel, aircraft, meat, petroleum and industrial-chemical industries. The basic product of the dairy industry is of course milk, which in the year of the census was produced in the amount of 118,769,000,-000 pounds by 15,198,000 cows. As one might expect, the basic product has been studied intensively: nearly every state university has a program of dairy research, and the industry itself maintains a substantial research program. Notwithstanding these activities, much remains to be learned about milk. One reason is that milk is a remarkably complex substance; another is that the cellular processes whereby it is produced in the mammary tissue are highly intricate.

Milk's role, as a nearly complete food, in sustaining life processes is well known. Of equal importance is its role as a product of life processes. Milk is a record of the exquisite functioning of a cell, a fascinating cell that might be described as a factory, but a factory with the unusual property of becoming, to a certain extent, a product. Indeed, the lactating mammary cell ranks second in importance only to the photosynthesizing cell as a factor in sustaining life. For these reasons I shall focus here on the biology of milk, dealing to a lesser extent with its physical and chemical properties.

One's senses readily ascertain that cow's milk is a white, opaque liquid with characteristics of odor and flavor that are normally quite faint; a taste shows that it is slightly sweet and just perceptibly salty. One might go a step further and reason that rather large particles or molecules must be suspended in milk, because if all the constituents were fairly small dissolved molecules, milk would be as clear a solution as water is. Milk does have large components in suspension; they are mainly globules of fat and particles of protein.

Constituents of Milk

These observations indicate the gross composition of cow's milk: it is about 3.8 percent fat, 3.2 percent protein, 4.8 percent carbohydrate, .7 percent minerals and 87.5 percent water. Such an analysis, however, greatly oversimplifies cow's milk. For example, milk contains a large number of trace organic substances, some that pass through the mammary gland directly from the blood and others that result from the synthesis of milk in the mammary tissue. Moreover, the fat globules contain thousands of different molecules and are enclosed by a complex membrane acquired at the time of secretion. Milk protein was originally thought to have three components: casein, albumin and globulin. It is now known that there are four caseins, each with a number of genetic variants, and that albumin and globulin are actually a complex group of proteins known as the whey proteins. The number of proteins eventually discovered in this group probably will be limited only by the patience of the investigators and the sensitivity of the methods they apply. Only lactose, the sugar of milk, seems to be a pure and relatively simple compound.

The statements that can be made about cow's milk do not apply uniformly to the milk of other mammals, because there are large variations in the composition of milk. For example, the pinnipeds (the group of aquatic mammals including seals, sea lions and walruses) have milk that is often like heavy cream, containing 40 to 50 percent fat. In addition, depending on the species, pinniped milk contains little or no lactose. These variations can be explained in terms of their value in assisting the survival of the young of the species. A young pinniped is in special need of fat (in the form of blubber) as insulation against its cold environment, as an aid to buoyancy, as a source of energy and as a source of metabolic water in a salty environment.

A Closer Look

With the request that the reader keep in mind the important fact that milk differs substantially among mammalian species, I shall now be discussing milk in terms of cow's milk. Because of its commercial importance as a food and a raw material for foods, more is known about it than about the milk of other mammals. Moreover, the mechanisms of the synthesis of milk by the cow have been investigated closely because of the cow's importance as a unit of agriculture.

In addition to the major constituents already described, milk contains a large number of substances that occur in small amounts, ranging from .1 percent or so down to parts per billion. Among them are fatty acids, amino acids, sugars and sugar phosphates, proteoses, peptones, nitrogenous bases, gases and other volatiles. Many of these substances, such as the vitamins and minerals, play a key role in nutrition. Nonetheless, the most important components of milk are the lipids (fats), the proteins and the carbohydrate (lactose). A more precise description of them will lay a foundation for considering the remarkable processes of their synthesis and secretion by the cells of the mammary gland.

The term lipid specifies a broad group of fatty (greasy, waxy or oily) substances found in biological systems, including those used for food. The term fat is often used interchangeably with lipid, but in

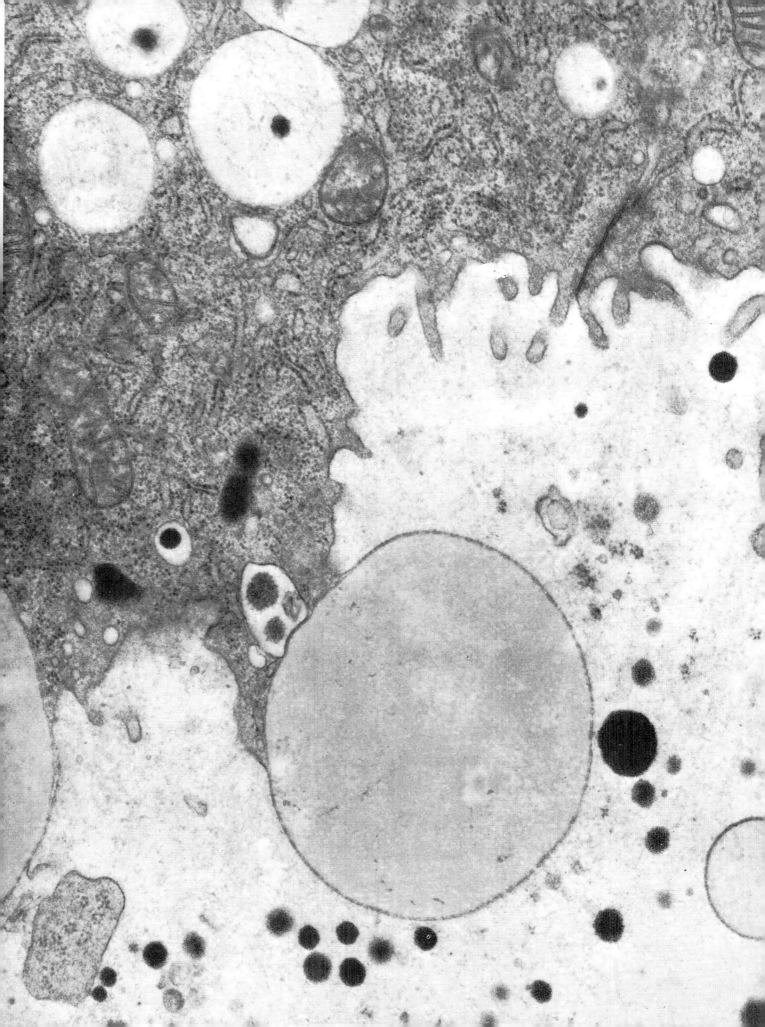

fact fat refers more narrowly to edible oils or the characteristically fatty tissue of the animal body. The lipids in milk are sometimes called its butterfat content; they exist as minute droplets or globules that under proper conditions will rise to form a layer of cream. The process known as homogenization reduces the globules in size and stabilizes their suspension, so that they no longer form a layer of cream. Agitation, in the form of churning, causes the globules to aggregate into granules that can be gathered and worked into butter. Butter is about 80 percent fat, and the part that is not fat is mainly water. If butter is melted, clarified and dried, it yields a product that is almost 100 percent fat and is known as butter oil; it is used commercially in the making of candy and baked goods.

The fat droplets in milk have an average diameter of three to four microns (about .00014 inch). A droplet consists of a membranous coat about .02 micron thick and a core that is virtually pure glyceride material. A glyceride is the ester, or product, resulting from the combination of glycerol with fatty acid. Because a molecule of glycerol has three reactive sites, it is possible to have monoglycerides, diglycerides or triglycerides, depending on how many molecules of fatty acid react with each molecule of glycerol. The lipids of milk are mostly triglycerides.

The fatty acids that are esterified with glycerol to form glycerides can vary in many ways. At least 150 different fatty acids can be found in the glycerides of milk, but only 10 of them occur consistently in amounts larger than 1 percent of the total. The principal ones are oleic acid, palmitic acid and stearic acid, which are also common in the glycerides of many other natural fats. The fat of cow's milk is unusual in that it contains the short-chain fatty acids, including butyric acid and caproic acid. Short-chain fatty acids are also found in the milk fat of other ruminants, such as the sheep and the goat. As I shall describe more fully below, the rumen, or first stomach, in these animals has a profound effect on their metabolism and on the composition of their milk fat. Another point to note in

passing is that the short-chain fatty acids are highly odorous, and when they are released from the glycerides by the enzymes known as lipases, they contribute significantly to the flavor of many kinds of cheese.

The membrane that forms the surface of the milk-fat droplet is derived from the outer membrane of the lactating mammary cell at the time of secretion. It also appears to include materials that were at the surface of the droplet while it was still in the cell. The structure and composition of the membrane are the subject of intensive study. It is known that the portion of lipids not accounted for in the triglyceride fraction is involved in the membrane. The membrane lipids include part of the milk's cholesterol, phospholipids and glycolipids and most if not all of the vitamin A and carotene (a yellow pigment). The membrane also comprises unique proteins and enzymes, and its structure seems to be an aggregate of lipoprotein subunits. All in all, the milk-fat globule—a droplet of fat wrapped in a membrane—is a remarkable biological package.

Proteins of Milk

As with proteins in general, the proteins of milk are fundamentally chains of amino acid units. Since there are 18 common amino acids, the number of protein chains that could be formed is very large indeed. About 80 percent of the protein in milk, however, is casein. No other natural protein is quite like it. One aspect of its uniqueness is that it contains phosphorus; it is known as a phosphoprotein. In milk the molecules of casein are marshaled in aggregates called micelles, which are roughly spherical in shape and average about 100 millimicrons in diameter.

Casein occurs in four distinct types called alpha, beta, gamma and kappa, respectively representing about 50, 30, 5 and 15 percent of this protein. The four types differ in molecular weight and in a number of other characteristics. Kappa casein is unique in that it contains a carbohydrate, sialic acid. Little is known about the internal organization of the casein micelle and its subunits. It is as-

sumed, however, that each subunit contains each of the four caseins.

The alpha, beta and gamma caseins can be made to aggregate by calcium ions, but kappa casein is highly resistant to such aggregation. Hence kappa casein serves as a protective colloid that keeps the casein micelles themselves from aggregating, which would give milk a curd-like consistency. In the making of cheese the enzyme rennin is added to milk to promote the formation of curds; the enzyme splits from kappa casein a peptide containing sialic acid, thereby destabilizing the casein micelles and giving rise to the formation of curds. After the resulting whey, or watery portion, has been drawn off, the curd can be used to make cheese.

Another protein unique to milk is beta-lactoglobulin, which accounts for about .4 percent of milk and is found in two common forms, A and B, and two uncommon ones, C and D. Beta-lactoglobulin contains a comparatively high proportion of the amino acid cysteine, which bears a reduced sulfur group (—SH). When milk is heated, these groups (starting at a temperature of about 70 degrees Celsius) are released from the protein as hydrogen sulfide; this is the source of the cooked flavor in heated milk.

Beta-lactoglobulin has much practical importance for the processing properties of milk proteins. If it is denatured beforehand, evaporated milk is stabilized against coagulating during sterilization by heat. On the other hand, if milk for cottage cheese is overheated so that the beta-lactoglobulin is denatured, an unsatisfactory soft curd is formed. Presumably the denatured protein is adsorbed on the surface of the casein micelles, thus hindering the action of rennin and the coalescence of the casein into a curd.

Enzymes are of course proteins too, and freshly secreted milk contains a great abundance of them. Robert D. McCarthy, working with radioactively labeled substances in our laboratory at Pennsylvania State University, has shown that enzymes in milk can incorporate fatty acids into glycerides and phospholipids and can convert stearic acid into oleic acid. It is also known that milk can synthesize lactose from added glucose. Such activities make it appropriate to describe milk as an unstructured tissue, in many ways resembling the enzymatically active solid tissues of the body.

The Carbohydrate of Milk

The substance responsible for the slightly sweet taste of milk is lactose, a

LACTATING CELL secretes a droplet of milk fat in the electron micrograph on the opposite page. The fat droplet is the large circular object at top center. The dark region from which it is emerging is the cell; the light region the droplet is entering is the lumen, or hollow portion, of an alveolus, one of the many pear-shaped structures that are basic units in lactation. The small dark circles visible in several places are granules of protein. The electron micrograph, which is of mammary tissue of a mouse, was made by S. R. Wellings of the University of Oregon Medical School; the enlargement is about 48,000 diameters.

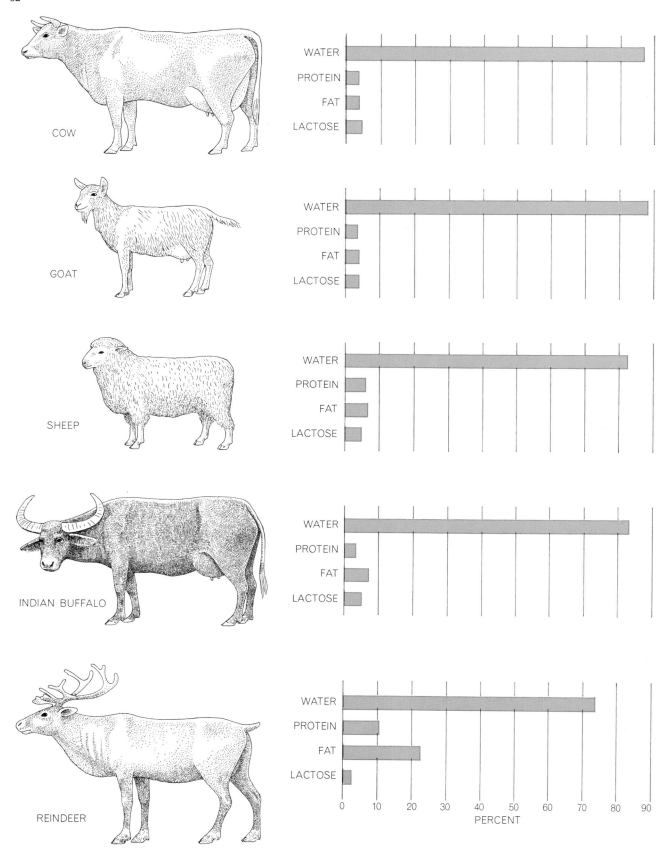

COMPOSITION OF MILK yielded by five kinds of animal is compared. In a few species the variation is even more marked; for example, the pinniped group, which includes seals and walruses, has milk that is about 50 percent fat and contains little or no lactose.

FAT

$$R-C-O-C-H$$

O H₂-C-O-C-R
‖
R-C-O-C-H   O
‖   ‖
O H₂-C-O-C-R

R = FATTY ACIDS INCLUDING
BUTYRIC C_3H_7COOH
CAPROIC $C_5H_{11}COOH$
PALMITIC $C_{15}H_{31}COOH$
OLEIC $C_{17}H_{33}COOH$
STEARIC $C_{17}H_{35}COOH$

PROTEIN

AMINO ACID

PROTEIN

CASEIN   ALBUMIN   GLOBULIN
ALPHA CASEIN
BETA CASEIN
GAMMA CASEIN
KAPPA CASEIN

LACTOSE

GALACTOSE   GLUCOSE

CONSTITUENTS OF COW'S MILK, exclusive of water and minerals, are portrayed with diagrams of basic chemical structure of its fat, protein and lactose. Casein is the major protein, and lactose the carbohydrate, of milk. Milk has many other fats and proteins.

carbohydrate with about a fifth the sweetness of ordinary sugar. Like casein, lactose is found only in milk. Lactose is composed of a molecule of galactose combined with a molecule of glucose, the simple sugar of the blood.

Since lactose is found only in milk, and only in the milk of certain species, one wonders why it is there. Indeed, it is reasonable to ask why milk contains carbohydrate of any kind, inasmuch as the most obvious role of lactose—providing a source of energy for the newborn—is filled by fat in milk from species such as the pinnipeds. The synthesis of lactose in the mammary gland does lock up molecules of glucose drawn from the blood, and since glucose is a highly active metabolite that might otherwise go elsewhere in the body or be metabolized in a different way, it may be that the synthesis of lactose provides a means of ensuring that glucose remains in the lactating cell and so becomes a part of the milk. Another possible role for lactose arises from its solubility; soluble molecules are important to the osmotic relations of cells, and lactose, which accounts for approximately 5 percent of milk, probably affects the osmotic relations of the lactating cell. Lactose may also be the carbohydrate of milk because it encourages certain desirable bacteria, which form lactic acid, to thrive in the intestine. Lactic acid is thought to promote the absorption of the calcium and phosphorus the young animal needs for the formation of bone. In any event, it would appear that the net effect of lactose from an evolutionary point of view was to promote the survival of the young, and so its synthesis was favored by natural selection.

A factor in the synthesis of lactose is the enzyme lactose synthetase, which is composed of two proteins. One of them, the B protein, was identified by Urs Brodbeck and Kurt E. Ebner of Oklahoma State University as alpha-lactalbumin. Thus for the first time a metabolic function for one of the principal milk proteins was identified. Then it was shown by a group at Duke University that the A protein is an enzyme that normally incorporates galactose into glycoproteins. In the presence of alpha-lactalbumin the enzyme has its specificity changed to the promotion of the reaction of galactose with glucose to form lactose. This seems to be the only case known where such a protein modifies the specificity of an enzyme. In subsequent work led by Roger W. Turkington the Duke group showed that organ cultures of mouse mammary gland, when pretreated with the hormones insulin and hydrocortisone, would produce both A and B proteins after treatment with the hormone prolactin. These three hormones are known to be necessary for the synthesis of milk in the mouse to begin.

In sum, the synthesis of lactose depends on enzymes, and the synthesis of the enzymes depends in turn on several hormones, which ultimately are also regulating the synthesis of the other components of milk. It is particularly interesting that lactose synthetase not only figures in the synthesis of lactose but also is present in the milk. This is evidence for my earlier observation that in milk production the factory becomes to a certain extent the product.

The Lactating State

In considering the synthesis of milk it is necessary to recognize that the process is related to all the other processes going on within the animal. It is an integral part of the animal's total metabolism. A case in point is the relation of milk fat to the other fats in the animal. Milk fat is immediately derived from two main sources: lipids circulating in the blood and synthesis from simple metabolites in the mammary gland. The origin of the simple metabolites traces back to the blood, to various sites in the body and ultimately to the food. The lipids circulating in the blood arise from all the many locations of lipid synthesis, transformation and storage in the body [see top illustration on page 194].

It is also necessary to consider metabolic activity at the cellular level. Clearly the lactating mammary cell, which is continuously turning out fat, protein, carbohydrate and many other substances, is not a resting cell—a cell that is simply maintaining itself. It is a busy place, with substances constantly moving in through the basal parts of the cell and out through the secreting parts. Some of the substances are used to maintain the cell and others are merely transported through the cell, but most of them are used by the lactating cell in the synthesis of the major constituents of milk.

Another consideration in the cow is the rumen, which is in effect a large fermentation tank ranging in capacity from 30 to 60 gallons depending on the size of the animal. Plant materials eaten by the cow are broken down in the rumen by a large and highly diverse population of bacteria and protozoa. The changes in the food are of major importance. Cellulose, which man cannot digest, is readily broken down in the rumen, and the products—acetate, propionate and butyrate—are prime metabolites in the bovine metabolic economy. Another sig-

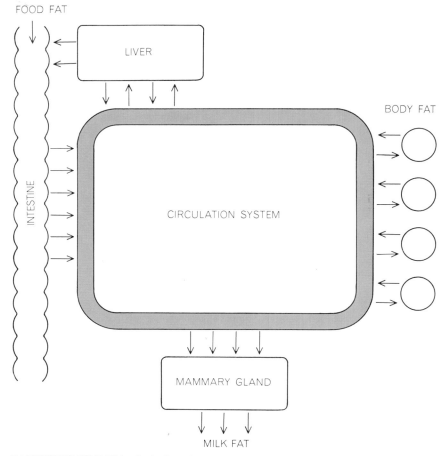

PATHWAYS OF FAT in the body indicate the sources of the fat in milk and thereby the mechanisms by which milk is synthesized. Fat from food enters the bloodstream through the intestines and also from the body's reserves of fat and from the liver. The mammary gland draws on these sources of raw material for the synthesis of the droplets of fat in milk.

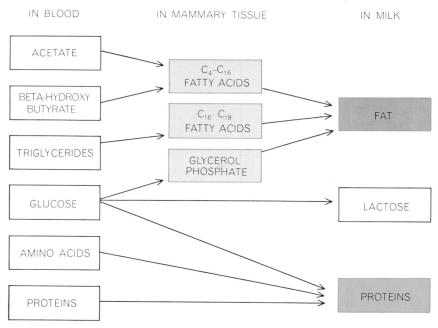

RAW MATERIALS of milk are depicted in a scheme showing the materials from the blood that are used by the mammary tissue in the synthesis of milk. Information on the materials going into the synthesis is obtained with radioactive tracers and by measuring changes in concentration of a substance between arterial and venous blood in mammary gland.

nificant change taking place in the rumen involves lipids. The lipids of plants are highly unsaturated, meaning that they have many free bonding sites where they can add more hydrogen molecules or form new chemical compounds. In the rumen the fatty acids are released enzymatically from such feed lipids and are then hydrogenated, so that they are converted into saturated fatty acids (mainly palmitic acid and stearic acid). These acids are subsequently absorbed and become part of the lipids of both meat and milk, which is why meat, milk and milk products of the ruminant animal contain saturated fats. In contrast, the milk fat of animals with a single stomach (such as human beings) will readily reflect dietary unsaturated fatty acids.

Another interesting fact about the rumen is that the microorganisms involved in fermentation become part of the milk as a result of subsequent digestion. Mark Keeney of the University of Maryland has estimated that at least 10 percent of the fatty acids of bovine milk are derived from the bacteria and protozoa in the rumen. Similarly, the amino acids used in the synthesis of milk proteins originate partly with microbes in the rumen.

Lactogenesis, the process that sets in motion the synthesis and secretion of milk, depends on the action of hormones. Hormonal changes in the female following conception lead to proliferation and differentiation of certain mammary cells. The organelles of the cell increase in size and quantity. Enzymes required to synthesize the various milk constituents appear in the cells, some gradually and some rather suddenly at about the time the animal gives birth. It is probably conservative to say that 100 enzymes are newly formed or greatly intensified in activity during the lactogenic transformation of tissue.

The mode of action of a hormone at the molecular level has not been established with certainty. As a result of work by Yale J. Topper and his colleagues at the National Institutes of Health, however, considerable progress has been made in determining what hormones are involved in lactogenesis and what effects they have at the cellular level. Working in vitro with mammary tissue from virgin mice, Topper's group has shown that the hormones insulin, hydrocortisone and prolactin, acting synergistically, are required to stimulate the synthesis of milk by the mammary tissue.

The hormone progesterone has an inhibitory effect on the differentiation of

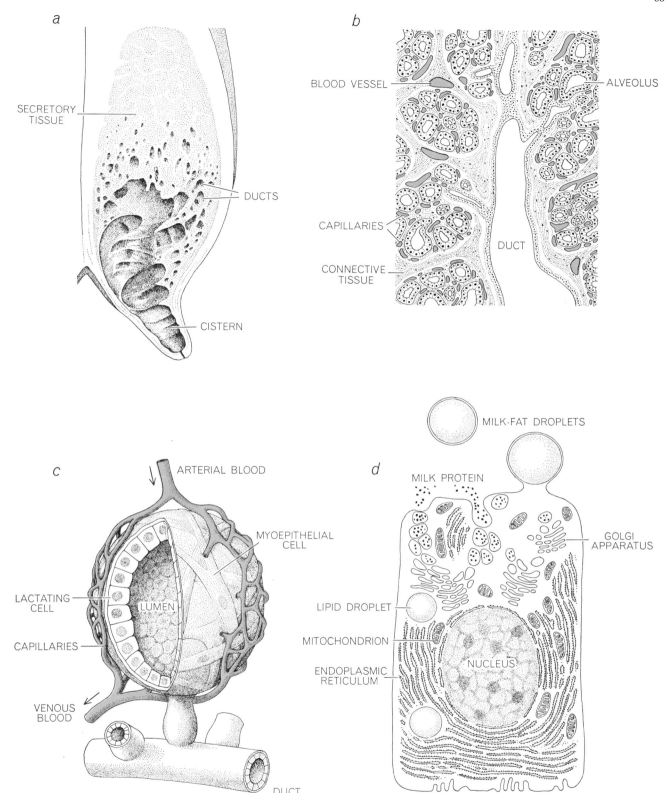

a

SECRETORY TISSUE

DUCTS

CISTERN

b

BLOOD VESSEL

ALVEOLUS

CAPILLARIES

CONNECTIVE TISSUE

DUCT

c

ARTERIAL BLOOD

MYOEPITHELIAL CELL

LACTATING CELL

LUMEN

CAPILLARIES

VENOUS BLOOD

DUCT

d

MILK-FAT DROPLETS

MILK PROTEIN

GOLGI APPARATUS

LIPID DROPLET

MITOCHONDRION

ENDOPLASMIC RETICULUM

NUCLEUS

MILK-PRODUCING TISSUE of a cow is shown at progressively larger scale. At (*a*) is a longitudinal section of one of the four quarters of the mammary gland. The boxed area is reproduced at (*b*), where the arrangement of the alveoli and the duct system that drains them is apparent. A single alveolus (*c*) consists of an elliptical arrangement of lactating cells surrounding the lumen, which is linked to the duct system of the mammary gland. A lactating cell (*d*), similar to the one in the electron micrograph on page 114, is shown as it discharges a droplet of fat into the lumen. Part of the cell membrane apparently becomes the membranous covering of the fat droplet. Dark circular bodies in the vacuoles of Golgi apparatus are granules of protein, which are discharged into the lumen.

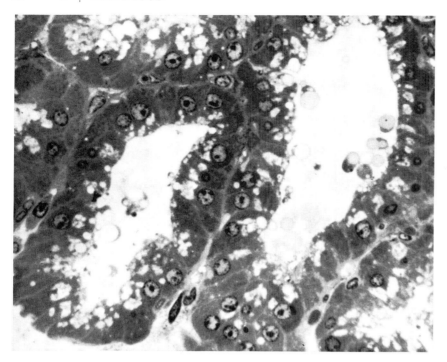

TWO ALVEOLI in the mammary gland of a lactating rat appear in a photomicrograph made by C. W. Heald in the laboratory of R. G. Saacke at the College of Agriculture of the Virginia Polytechnic Institute. The light areas are the lumens, which are surrounded by lactating cells. Between the two alveoli is a capillary. The enlargement is 2,500 diameters.

mammary tissue and the secretion of milk. Thus lactogenesis results in part from suppression of the activity of progesterone. Another important regulator of milk synthesis and secretion is the removal of milk from the mammary gland. Unless the milk is removed regularly, synthesis stops.

The Synthesis of Milk

Milk is produced by the vast number of cells that make up the mammary gland. The cells are formed into billions of pear-shaped, hollow structures called alveoli [see illustration on previous page]. Each cell in an alveolus discharges its milk into the lumen, which is the hollow part of the structure. When an alveolus is full, its outer cells contract under the influence of the hormone oxytocin, causing the alveolus to discharge its milk into a duct system that carries it to the cistern, or sac, that is the main collecting point.

In the present state of knowledge little more can be said about the precise mechanisms taking place within the lactating cell. It is possible, however, to describe to a certain extent the raw materials the cell draws from the blood and how they get from the blood into the cell. Much of the knowledge about the

raw materials or metabolites comes from painstaking experiments by John M. Barry of the University of Oxford and J. L. Linzell and E. F. Annison of the British Agricultural Research Council's Institute of Animal Physiology. The principle of their work has been that any compounds being used by the mammary gland will show a drop in concentration between the entering arterial blood and the departing venous blood. The British workers have measured such arteriovenous differences and also have amplified their findings through use of radioactive tracers. The metabolites include acetate, triglycerides, glucose, amino acids and proteins.

In order to reach the cell the metabolites must move through the walls of the blood-carrying capillaries, across the endothelium lining the capillaries, through intercellular spaces and into the alveolar epithelium where the milk is synthesized. For the transport of small ions from the blood there is a selective system, as is shown by the fact that compared with the blood serum milk is much reduced in sodium and chloride ions and much elevated in potassium ions. Molecules such as the amino acids, glucose and acetate could in principle simply diffuse through the system. In the light of the rapid, selective and continuing up-

take of these substances, however, it seems likely that here too there are special transport systems. The same is true for certain large molecules of protein that appear to pass unchanged from the blood into the milk. They include serum albumin and the immune globulins. Unless there are extremely large discontinuities in the cellular structure all the way from the blood to the milk, one is almost obliged to invoke special transport mechanisms for these large molecules. (Most of the milk proteins are made within the cell by the usual method of transcription by ribonucleic acid on the ribosomes of the cell.)

This question of how large particles can migrate through cell membranes without destroying the integrity of the cells arises for the exports of the lactating cells as well as for its imports. Indeed, the fat droplets steadily secreted by the cell are at times nearly as large as the cell itself. The first evidence of the remarkable biophysical mechanisms required for this task was supplied in 1959 by electron microscopy done in Germany by Wolfgang L. Bargmann and his coworkers at the University of Kiel. From their micrographs of mouse and hamster mammary tissue it was deduced that the fat droplets are secreted as a result of being progressively engaged in and enveloped by the limiting membrane at the apex of the cell [see illustration on page 190]. When a fat droplet is completely surrounded by the membrane in this way, it is effectively displaced from inside the cell out into the lumen of the alveolus. All that remains for completion of its secretion is for the slender membrane bridge to be pinched off. From our calculation of the sizable forces (as much as 100 atmospheres) involved in the attraction of the membrane to the surface of the droplet it is possible that once the droplet makes a close approach to the membrane it is quickly and forcefully snapped through.

Bargmann and his colleagues reported that their electron micrographs suggested the existence of milk-protein granules inside cell vacuoles that arise from the Golgi apparatus [see illustration on previous page]. According to the German workers the contents of the vacuoles were secreted by being emptied through the cell membrane. Our group believes the membrane processes in the two mechanisms of secretion (for fat droplets and protein granules) are related. The membrane around the Golgi vacuole carrying protein granules becomes continuous with the cell membrane at the time the vacuole empties its contents into the

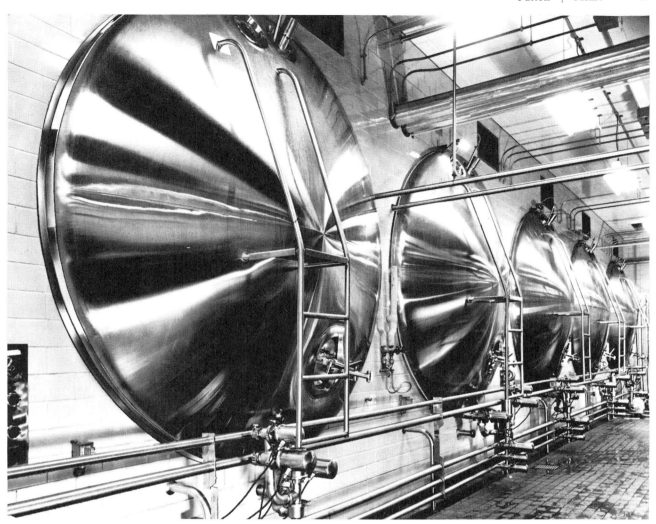

STORAGE TANKS in a milk and ice cream plant of the Borden Company in West Allis, Wis., hold 48,000 quarts each. Raw milk delivered to the plant from dairy farms is stored in the tanks at a temperature of about 37 degrees Fahrenheit until it is processed. The five slender pipes at bottom are used in loading and unloading the tanks. An inspection port and a gauge are at top of each tank.

lumen. The cell membrane then is engaged by the milk-fat droplet and becomes the membrane around the secreted milk-fat globule. Evidence from both electron microscopy and biochemical studies is tending to substantiate these mechanisms of secretion for the lipids and proteins of milk, but many questions of both a gross and a refined nature remain to be answered.

Further Questions

The basal portion of the lactating cell, as distinguished from its apical, or secreting, end, contains extensive membranous processes known as the endoplasmic reticulum. The evidence is convincing that these membranes are the sites of synthesis for the major constituents of milk: triglycerides, proteins and lactose. The means whereby the compo-

nents are gathered for secretion is not known. For example, it is not understood how all the triglyceride molecules are gathered into a droplet.

The precise operation of the Golgi apparatus is not established. The apparatus is defined as an organelle that accomplishes the differentiation of membranes and the "packaging" of materials for secretion, but just how it does these things in the lactating cell is unclear. It is now a reasonable assumption that alpha-lactalbumin, the B protein of lactose synthetase, joins the A protein in the Golgi apparatus, thus allowing the synthesis of lactose at that site. The lactose, milk protein and other constituents of milk serum are then packaged into Golgi vacuoles for secretion. One wonders, however, if the Golgi vacuoles are the vehicle of secretion for all the milk proteins. Electron micrographs show clearly that the gran-

ules the vacuoles contain have the appearance of casein micelles. Perhaps the other proteins are also present in the vacuoles but are not evident because they are transparent to electrons. We have suggested that these vacuoles, since they must carry some of the fluid of milk, may provide the vehicle for the secretion of milk-serum constituents such as lactose. Investigations of these questions and inferences are needed.

In sum, the lactating mammary cell, like all cells, is an almost incredible unit of organization and action. We are beginning to gain an understanding of this cell, which is so important to mammalian life, but the detailed revelation of its elegant mechanisms is still to come. The findings may lead to more and better food products. At the very least they will mean a deeper understanding of cellular processes and of life itself.

10 Captain Bligh and the Breadfruit

by Richard A. Howard
March 1953

The voyage of the Bounty, which ended in the celebrated mutiny, was undertaken for an almost forgotten purpose: to bring a plant from the South Seas to the West Indies

THE VOYAGE of the *Bounty*, Captain William Bligh commanding, has been celebrated in history and literature for its melodramatic end; not so widely known is the fact that its mission was as unusual as its conclusion was violent. Bligh was engaged in a project of considerable scientific and economic importance. He was attempting to transport live breadfruit trees from Tahiti, chief island of the Society group in the mid-South Pacific, to the British West Indies on the other side of the world.

The breadfruit project arose from the needs of the British planters in the West Indies. In the 18th century the islands of Jamaica, Barbados, St. Vincent, Grenada and Trinidad were planted extensively to sugar cane. The planters, regretting the amount of land and time occupied in raising food (cassava, taro and plantain) to feed their plantation slaves, thought they saw an answer in the breadfruit. News of this fabulous food had been brought to Europe by various South Seas explorers, including the adventurous Captain Cook. A British navigator, hydrographer and occasional buccaneer named William Dampier had written glowingly:

"The breadfruit (as we call it) grows on a large tree, as big and high as our largest apple-trees: It hath a spreading head, full of branches and dark leaves. The fruit grows on the boughs like apples; it is as big as a penny-loaf when wheat is at five shillings the bushel, it is of a round shape, and hath a thick tough rind. When the fruit is ripe it is yellow and soft, and the taste is sweet and pleasant. The natives at Guam use it for bread. They gather it, when full-grown, while it is green and hard; then they bake it in an oven, which scorcheth the rind and makes it black; but they scrape off the outside black crust, and there remains a tender thin crust; and the inside is soft, tender, and white like the crumb of penny-loaf. . . . The fruit lasts in season eight months in the year, during which the natives eat no other food of bread kind."

The West Indian planters were fascinated: the breadfruit crop would use relatively little land, and the plant spread rapidly, was not damaged by hurricanes, bore fruit almost the year around, required no cultivation and was well adapted to the Caribbean climate. The one serious difficulty was that the tree could not be grown from seed; it would have to be carried thousands of miles to be transplanted from the South Seas to the West Indies. This meant a voyage of several months around Cape Horn or the Cape of Good Hope, during which the delicate young tropical trees would have to be nurtured carefully and protected from the sea, the salt air and the cold of the low latitudes. The colo-

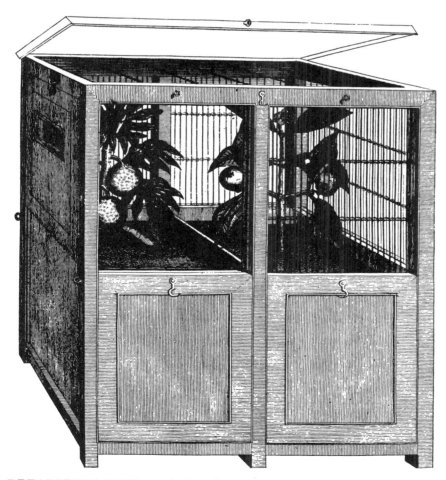

BREADFRUIT CAGE was designed to transport the plant from the South Seas. On the *Bounty*, however, most of the plants were carried in pots.

nists called upon the mother country for help in transporting the plant.

SIR JOSEPH BANKS, president of the Royal Society, who had been naturalist on Cook's first voyage to the South Seas and knew the breadfruit at first hand, took up their cause. He persuaded King George III to charter a ship and chose as its master Captain Bligh, who also had sailed with Cook and had a keen interest in natural history. To accompany Bligh as guardians of the trees, Sir Joseph selected two horticulturists of the Kew Gardens named David Nelson and William Brown. He drew up elaborate instructions to assist them. The master and crew of the ship, he said, would have to give up its best accommodations and put up with some inconvenience to care for the plants.

"It is necessary that the cabin be appropriated to the sole purpose of making a kind of greenhouse, and the key of it given to the custody of the gardener.... No dogs, cats, monkeys, parrots, goats or indeed any animal whatever must be allowed on board except the hogs and fowls for the Company's use; and they must be carefully confined to their coops. Every precaution must be taken to prevent or destroy rats as often as convenient. As poison will constantly be used to destroy them and cockroaches, the crew must not complain if some of them who may die in the ceiling make an unpleasant smell."

The *Bounty* sailed from England on October 15, 1787. She set off on the route around South America, but she failed to round Cape Horn; after 30 days of battle with the wind and currents, Bligh turned her about and sailed across the South Atlantic to go the other route around the tip of Africa. He reached the Cape of Good Hope on May 22. There he spent 40 days repairing and restocking the ship, took aboard some fruit trees and other plants and then sailed for Tasmania, the large island immediately south of Australia. At Tasmania the *Bounty* stopped briefly to plant the African trees and to pick up fuel wood. On October 24, after a full year's voyage, the ship arrived at Tahiti.

Bligh was able to persuade the chiefs of the tribes on Tahiti to present some of their breadfruit trees as a gift to King George. Nelson and his assistant proceeded to pot the young plants in a shelter on the shore. Bligh, aware of the scientific interest taken in his voyage, made precise notes about the trees he was collecting: "The natives reckon eight kinds of breadfruit trees, each of which they distinguish by a different name.... In the first, fourth and eighth class the leaf differs from the rest; the fourth is more sinuated; the eighth has a large broad leaf, not at all sinuated. The difference in the fruit is principally in the first and eighth class. In the first the fruit is rather large and more of an ob-

long form; in the eighth it is round and not above half the size of the others."

The visit was not a matter of all take and no give. Bligh had brought some plants for the Tahitians, and he looked around eagerly to see what they had done with gifts from earlier voyages. "I had the satisfaction," he wrote, "to see, brought to me, a fruit which they had not, till we introduced it. And among the articles which they brought off to the ship and offered for sale, were capsicums, pumpkins and two young goats." Among the new seeds he now gave them were melon, cucumber, salad greens, fruit stones and almonds. Also, "as they are very fond of sweet-smelling flowers with which the women delight to ornament themselves, I gave them some rose-seed." However, on the following day he "had the mortification to see that our garden-ground had been much trodden."

On January 31, 1789, getting ready for the return voyage, Bligh wrote in his diary: "This morning I ordered all the chests to be taken on shore, and the inside of the ship to be washed with boiling water to kill the cockroaches. We were constantly obliged to be at great pains to keep the ship clear of vermin. ... By the help of traps and good cats, we were freed from rats and mice." On March 31 Bligh noted: "Today all the plants are on board, being in 774 pots, 39 tubs and 24 boxes. The number of breadfruit plants was 1,015; besides which we had collected a number of other plants."

AT LENGTH on April 4, more than five months after its arrival at Tahiti, the *Bounty* was ready to sail for the West Indies. She set off westward for the Cape of Good Hope route. On April 27, after a brief stop at the Tonga

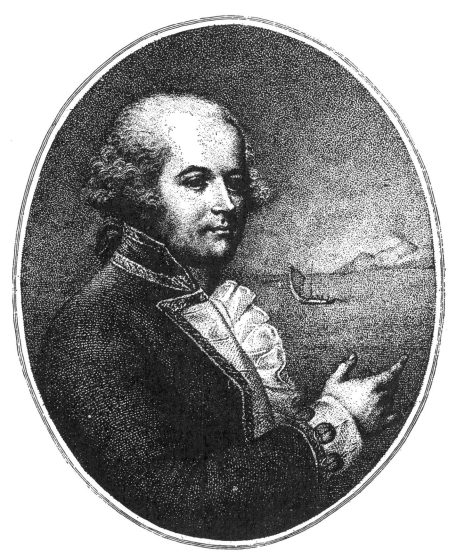

PORTRAIT OF BLIGH appears in his book *A Voyage to the South Sea.* In the background is the small boat in which he was set adrift by his crew.

island group, Bligh noted that "thus far, the voyage has advanced in a course of uninterrupted prosperity, and has been attended with many circumstances equally pleasing and satisfactory."

On the very next morning the famous mutiny broke out. The first thing Mr. Christian and his followers did after seizing the *Bounty* and putting off her captain was to throw the cargo overboard. Within a few hours the breadfruit were floating around in the Pacific.

Bligh's subsequent voyage of 3,600 miles in an open boat has become one of the epics of the sea. In October of 1789 he was in Batavia on his way home, and from there he wrote to Sir Joseph Banks:

"You will now, Sir, with all your generous endeavours for the public good, see an unfortunate end to the undertaking; and I feel very sensibly how you will receive the news. . . . To those, however, who may be disposed to blame, let them see I had in fact completed my undertaking. . . . I had most successfully got all my plants in a most flourishing and fine order. . . . I even rejected carrying stock for my own use, throwing away the hen-coops and every convenience. I roofed a place over the quarter-deck and filled it with plants, which I looked at with delight every day of my life."

Despite the disastrous end of the mission, Banks remained a staunch friend of Bligh. Shortly after the courts-martial of the mutineers in October, 1790, Banks began to appeal anew to the Ministry of the day, and in December, 1790, he gained approval for a second breadfruit voyage. Bligh was again picked for the job and this time given command of the *Providence*, a ship somewhat larger than the *Bounty*. She was to be accompanied by an armed brig, the *Assistance*. Two men from Kew Gardens, James Wiles and Christopher Smith, again went on the trip.

THE EXPEDITION sailed on August 3, 1791, and took the route around the Cape of Good Hope. Bligh reached Tasmania on February 8, 1792, and carried out some of his customary plantings. He found the date 1777 cut into trees by Cook and added the following inscription: "Near this tree Capt. William Bligh planted seven fruit trees in 1792: Messrs. S & W botanists." A few years later the French naturalist Jacques Labillardiere, seeing this inscription, was "scandalized by the despotism which condemned men of science to initials and gave a sea captain a monopoly of fame."

The *Providence* and the *Assistance* arrived at Tahiti on April 8, 1793. Their reception was pleasant. Arrangements were once more made to obtain breadfruit. Wiles and Smith built a shed on shore to shade the plants while they were being potted. After taking root, the plants were ferried out to the ship. At the end of three months Bligh noted with satisfaction· "All the plants are now in charming order, and spreading their leaves delightfully. I have completed nice airy spaces for them on the quarter-deck and galleries, and shall sail with every inch of space filled up." On July 18, as the ships were quitting Tahiti, the captain found time to report: "Upon a moderate calculation we suppose total of plants on board to number as follows: breadfruit 2,126, other plants 472, curiosity plants 36—total 2,634."

The expedition sailed west by way of the Fiji Islands and reached the coast of New Guinea on August 27. Ahead of them lay the dangerous passage through the Torres Strait between Australia and New Guinea. The commander of the *Assistance* wrote: "Every day now becomes more critical on account of the plants; a number of them have dropped off and our prospect of getting through becomes very uncertain. . . . It is absolutely necessary to shorten their allowance of water so that in case we are foiled in finding a passage there may be enough left to save the ship's company during the time of beating back. The want of water is all we dread."

The passage from the Pacific Ocean to the Indian Ocean took 19 days, and the vessels put in at the island of Timor on October 3. Bligh was becoming worried about his cargo. He wrote: "I can assign no reason, but the loss of our breadfruit at this time amounted to 224 pots." After taking on other varieties of plants at Timor, the ships set off on the long slow passage across the Indian

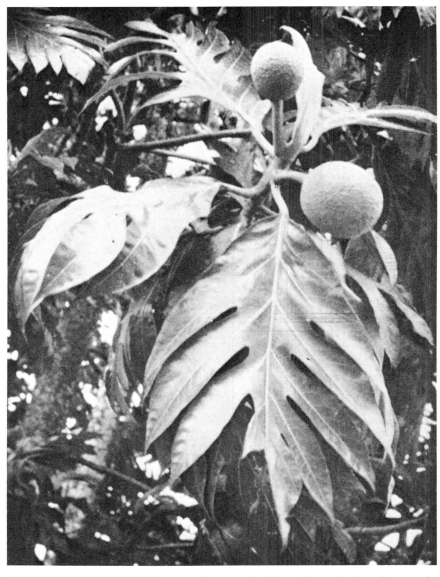

YOUNG BREADFRUITS were photographed in a botanical garden on the Caribbean island of St. Vincent, where Bligh left his first breadfruit plants.

Ocean. The season was now well into winter. Bligh had fair weather on his trip around the Cape of Good Hope but encountered severe gales on the northward leg of the voyage along the west coast of Africa. As he approached the island of St. Helena, where a selection of breadfruit was to be delivered, he remarked: "My plants have been shut up close these few days past; they are nevertheless doing well, but these adverse winds are much against them." On December 11, he counted survivors and discovered that he had only 830 plants left of the original 2,634.

Bligh informed the governor of St. Helena that he had orders to "give him into his care ten breadfruit plants, and one of every kind (of which I had five) as would secure to the islands a lasting supply of this valuable fruit which our most gracious King had ordered to be planted there." Before leaving St. Helena, Bligh received a letter from the governor and his council, expressing their gratitude to the king and stating that the sight of the *Providence* "had raised in them an inexpressible degree of wonder and delight to contemplate a floating garden transported in luxuriance from one extremity of the world to the other."

AFTER a rough passage across the South Atlantic, the *Providence* and her escort reached St. Vincent, their first port in the West Indies, on January 24, 1793. Arrangements were made for Negroes to carry the plants on their heads to the botanic garden two miles away. On the return trip they brought plants for Bligh to take to England.

Bligh was warmly received by the planters of St. Vincent. He reported: "A deputation from the Council and Assembly awaited on me the day after my arrival and presented me with a resolution and request to accept a piece of plate valued at 100 guineas as a mark of their approbation and esteem. They likewise did me the honor to give a public dinner to all my officers. . . . I left in all 544 plants at this place, and I received, for his Majesty's garden at Kew, 465 pots and 2 tubs containing botanic plants."

Bligh's party left St. Vincent on January 30, 1794, and arrived several days later at Port Royal, Jamaica. There the remaining breadfruit trees were delivered and Bligh again received the ceremonious thanks of the community.

Thus on the second try Bligh completed successfully one of the most difficult transplantation undertakings in the history of commercial horticulture. The French had brought in a few breadfruit before he finished his second voyage, but Bligh has always received credit for the successful introduction of the plant. With the help of Banks, he had shown how the transporting job could be done,

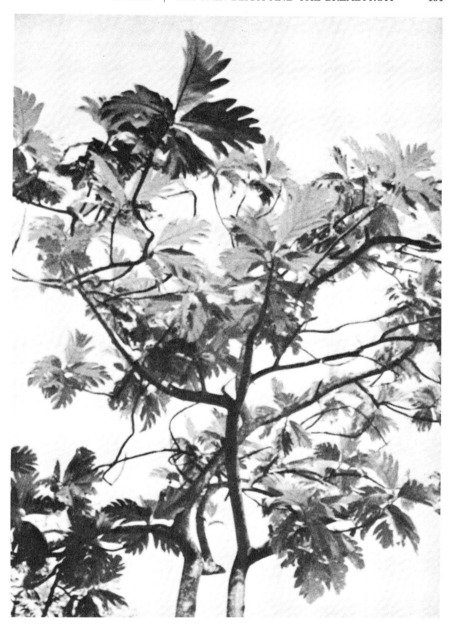

YOUNG BREADFRUIT TREE was photographed on Puerto Rico. The plant was brought to the West Indies to feed slaves, but they did not like it.

and it is probable that most of the trees growing in the West Indies today are the offspring of Bligh's stock.

After a few months' delay due to the outbreak of war with France, the *Providence* sailed for England on June 15, 1794. She carried from Jamaica specimens of the custard apple, avocado, cabbage tree, akee, wild mangosteen, naseberry and other plants. Altogether she brought 1,283 plants to Kew Gardens as the gleanings of her tropical voyage. On August 7 she dropped anchor at Deptford, her journey completed.

Little has been recorded of Bligh's reception in England. He was still disliked in many quarters for the *Bounty* epi-

sode, and his homecoming occasioned a renewal of hostile articles. But he apparently received a gold medal and in 1801 was elected a fellow of the Royal Society in consideration of his distinguished services to navigation and botany. Bligh remained in the Navy and was eventually promoted to the rank of vice-admiral. For a short time, 1806-1810, he was governor of the colony in New South Wales. He died in 1817 at the age of 64.

CONSIDERING the eagerness with which the West Indian planters had sought the breadfruit, the islands' reception of it was disappointing. Hinton

East, one of the proponents of the expedition and perhaps the leading planter and horticulturist in Jamaica at the time, had died shortly before the *Providence* arrived. The gardener Wiles, who stayed in the islands to superintend the cultivation of the new trees, wrote discouraged letters to Banks. Although the breadfruit trees eventually prospered in their new setting, they did not fulfill the planters' dreams. Apparently the Negro slaves did not care for the fruit. By 1850 breadfruit was being fed almost exclusively to pigs and poultry—with, however, excellent results.

More recently the breadfruit has staged a revival. Today West Indians, to whom the breadfruit is now a native tree, accept the fruit as a basic part of their diet. Although it has never become as important in the West Indies as it is in the South Seas, it is highly appreciated as an emergency food. It tides over a large part of the population during the periodic crop failures. Of 52 species of plants that Bligh brought to the West Indies, breadfruit has proved by far the most important.

III

SELECTION OF FOOD AND ITS INFLUENCE UPON HUMAN BEHAVIOR

SELECTION OF FOOD AND ITS INFLUENCE UPON HUMAN BEHAVIOR $\quad$ III

INTRODUCTION

Selection of foods is a complex process, and appears to be guided by color, odor, and taste. However, these are not simple, fixed qualities inherent in the food itself but are complex perceptions derived from interaction between physical stimuli emitted by the food and the sensory apparatus of the individual. Reactions to food on the basis of sensory perception are acquired and governed by cultural background and experience.

Man has a great ability to interpret food stimuli and attach specific meanings to them. Even the rat learns to avoid a food that has made it sick in the past; it can even determine which foods are poisonous by observing the feeding habits of other rats. The capacity of humans to attach meanings to foods is so great that psychological, social, and cultural factors often seem to play a greater role in the selection process than does the nutrient content or other physical qualities of the food in question.

Food technologists are concerned not only with preventing spoilage of foods but also with producing processed foods that preserve or imitate the qualities consumers find psychologically or socially desirable. One controversial aspect of this effort is described by G. O. Kermode in "Food Additives."

One of the important factors determining food preferences in adult humans is childhood experience with foods. Early and frequent exposure to particular foods may result in establishment of a pattern of likes and dislikes that persists throughout life. Although selection matures and changes as the individual becomes more sophisticated, such phrases as "home cooking" and "just like my mother cooked" reflect perceptions established early in life.

Another important factor in determining food preferences is the phenomenon of food taboos—social or religious sanctions against the consumption of certain foods. A food taboo may be absolute, as in the case of the Jewish and Islamic probibition against eating pork, or it may be applied only on particular occasions, as in the traditional Christian practice of giving up meat during Lent or the traditional Jewish practice of eating matzo (unleavened bread) during Passover. Some societies have food taboos that apply only to one sex or one age group. For example, a number of African tribes forbid women and girls to eat eggs.

It is not uncommon for individuals to develop a genuine aversion toward foods that are prohibited within their social groups. A classic example of this is the person born into a Jewish family who has long since broken with orthodox religious tenets but nonetheless recoils from the idea of eating pork. Various cultural groups around the world have instilled in their members a dislike of horsemeat, hippopotamus, worms, dog meat, and many other nutritionally sound and readily available foods that might serve as valuable sources of nutrients.

In contrast to the prohibited foods are the "superfoods" found in every society. These are foods held in such high esteem that they exert an influence on culture and social organization as well as on diet. Corn is a superfood for the Indians of Central America, while cassava plays the same role among certain West African peoples. The history of one superfood is discussed by Redcliffe Salaman in "The Social Influence of the Potato," a most important basic food to the Irish, and one upon which their economy and life was once dependent. The important nutrient salt has not only physiologic but also social bases for its selection. Its importance in the development of civilizations is well documented in "The Social Influence of Salt" by M. R. Bloch. The complex evolutionary pressures generated by the introduction of milk into the human diet about 10,000 years ago are discussed by Normal Kretchmer in "Lactose and Lactase." The gastrointestinal discomfort produced in people who are genetically unable to digest lactose in milk leads to their rejection of milk, despite conspicuous worldwide advertising.

Regardless of the factors responsible for the food choices discussed here, the ultimate composition of diet is determined by the availability of a food. Availability is often related to price. Thus, for many people, and particularly for the poor and for retired persons living on fixed incomes, price is an important determinant in selection of foods.

Food Additives

11

G. O. Kermode
March 1972

Perhaps as many as 2,500 substances are currently being added to foods for flavoring, coloring, preservation and other purposes. How are the necessity and safety of these substances determined?

Men have added nonfood substances to their food throughout recorded history, but in recent decades they have become concerned about such practices because of the large number of substances and motivations that have become involved. The questions at issue for any food additive are whether or not it is necessary and, if so, whether or not it is safe. For many years the United Nations (through the Food and Agriculture Organization and the World Health Organization) and many governments have kept watch on additives with these questions in view. The questions must be faced whenever a new additive is proposed; sometimes, as the recent case of cyclamate additives in the U.S. showed, they must be reconsidered when new evidence puts the safety of an old additive in doubt.

The distinction between food ingredients and food additives is somewhat imprecise. Sugar, being a natural product, is usually regarded as an ingredient, whereas saccharin, being an artificial sweetener, is likely to come under the heading of an additive. Perhaps the best method of classification is by function. Additives are employed for such purposes as enhancing flavor, improving color, extending shelf life and protecting the nutritional value of a food. They are, in short, valuable but not always essential items in the manufacture of food products.

Whatever one's views on additives may be, it is true that without additives many food products could not be offered for sale in their present form. This is exemplified in particular by the many convenience foods that have become popular in North America and in western Europe. Moreover, if food production is to increase enough to keep pace with population growth and the effort to improve nutrition generally in undernourished areas, chemicals that are not normally part of food will inevitably play an increasingly important role.

From the earliest times foods were preserved with incidental additives that resulted from cooking. Food was also preserved extensively in ancient times by heating, drying, salting, pickling, fermenting and smoking. Food colors were used in ancient Egypt. In China kerosene was burned to ripen bananas and peas; the reason the method succeeded, although the Chinese did not know it, was that the combustion produced the ripening agents ethylene and propylene. Flavoring and seasoning were arts in many ancient civilizations, with the result that spices and condiments were important items in commerce.

Additives have not invariably been employed with beneficial aims. The adulteration of food, in order to pass an inferior product off as a good one, is as old as trade. Expensive items such as tea, coffee, sugar, spices and essential oils were often adulterated. Common adulterants included coloring substances and burned or roasted vegetable material, which was mixed with flour. Bread, beer, and wine were widely adulterated.

Eventually such practices led the authorities of the time and place to try to suppress them. The earliest food laws were often designed to control the more obvious forms of adulteration and fraud. In addition to these efforts the merchant guilds tried to protect the genuineness and the reputation of their products. The means at hand for testing foods were limited; checking the appearance, taste and smell of a food was about all one could do. The basis of knowledge making possible the national food laws that are common today was not established until about the middle of the 19th century. In the latter part of the century pure-food laws were enacted in country after country to control the composition of food and regulate the use of additives.

These developments coincided with a number of discoveries, mainly in organic chemistry, that led to the production of several of the important food additives now in use. For example, discoveries that resulted in the development of aniline and the coal-tar dyes led eventually to many of the synthetic colors now added to food. The active principles of odor and flavor were isolated from vegetables and other organic materials, leading first to alcoholic solutions of those materials as flavors and later to synthetic flavors, some of which did not appear to be present in natural edible aromatic substances used to flavor foods and some of which proved to have more flavoring

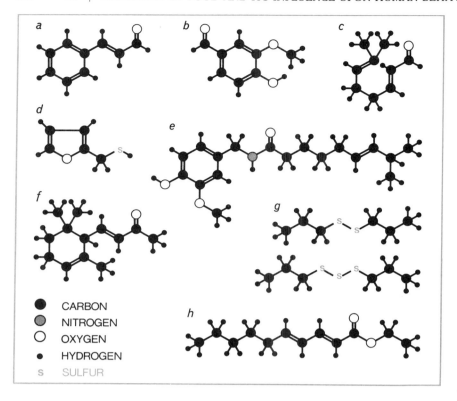

TYPICAL FLAVORING COMPOUNDS have chemical structures shown here. Cinnamaldehyde (*a*) supplies a cinnamon flavor; vanillin (*b*), a vanilla flavor; citral (*c*), lemon; furfuryl mercaptan (*d*), coffee; capsaicin (*e*), the pungent ingredient of red pepper; alphaionone (*f*), a principal component of strawberry and raspberry flavors; propyl disulfide (*g*), onion, and ethyl *trans*-2,*cis*-4-decadienoate (*h*), pear. Some 1,400 flavorings are in use.

cheaper or more effective than existing flavoring agents and flavor-enhancers. It is probably in this field that the greatest need for new additives will arise in the future, particularly for additives that can be put in simulated food products to imitate the complex flavor properties of traditional foods. At present the most widely sold simulated products are meat substitutes made from spun soybean proteins or proteins from other vegetables. With the addition of flavors, colors, vitamins, emulsifiers, acidifying agents and preservatives these proteins are sold as "vegetable steaks," "soya chicken breast" and "vegetable bacon" or are included in compounded products that normally have meat as a major ingredient. Other simulated foods are substitutes for dairy products. Flavored drinks, made so as to simulate the properties of genuine fruit juices, are also on the list. Because additive flavorings are expected to play such an expanding role in these products, they represent the field where ways of protecting the consumer's interest will need close attention, particularly with regard to designation and labeling of simulated foods.

Colors are put in food mainly to give it an appetizing appearance, on the tested assumption that the way food looks has an effect on its palatability. Foods are also colored to enhance the appreciation of flavor. Many people have become accustomed to the standardized color of a food product and would not accept the product if the color were substantially changed, even though nothing else had been done to the food. One need think only of blue or red butter to recognize the importance of accepted colors.

Much research has gone into food coloring. The colors most used in the food industry are synthetic dyestuffs. They are notably pure. Since they also have strong coloring power, little coloring is needed to achieve the desired result in a food product.

The manufacturer needs a color that not only produces the desired appearance but also will remain stable under certain conditions of manufacture, storage and cooking. Color put into candy, cakes and biscuits must be stable both to high temperature and to the action of carbon dioxide. Other colors must be able to withstand high processing temperatures and the action of acids.

Color regulation, like flavor regulation, varies from country to country. Many countries have fairly short lists of permitted food colors. The regulations specify purity and identity for the per-

power than the analogous natural flavors. By 1900 the flavorings in use were nearly all artificial and, except for vanilla, lemon, orange, peppermint and wintergreen, were being made with synthetic substances.

More than 40 functions now served by food additives can be listed. In this discussion, however, I shall group additives broadly in five categories: flavors, colors, preservatives, texture agents and a miscellaneous group.

Flavors constitute the largest class of food additives; estimates of the number of natural and synthetic flavors available range from 1,100 to 1,400. It is probably fair to say that flavors pose the largest regulatory task, not only because there are so many of them but also because of insufficient toxicological data, rapid changes in the field and many other factors. In general little is known about the toxicological aspects of flavors. Part of the problem is that many natural flavors have been used for centuries, and fully evaluating them all for safety would be an immense task. It is often argued that doing so would divert a large part of the effort that is needed to investigate the safety of more important and potentially more dangerous additives.

Over the past 30 years the use of flavorings has grown tremendously, paralleling the expansion in new types of food, new food-processing techniques and new methods of distribution. Governments have approached the question of controlling flavors from various directions. Some publish lists of permitted and prohibited flavors; some have a short list of prohibited flavors, many of which are natural, and others allow flavorings (both natural and synthetic) that are found only in the aromatic oils of edible plants.

Related to flavors are the additives known as flavor-enhancers. The commonest of them is monosodium glutamate (MSG), which is the monosodium salt of glutamic acid, one of the amino acids. A good deal of research is under way to find other flavor-enhancers, particularly in the group of substances known as the 5′-nucleotides. Similar work is being done on enhancers for fruit flavors. In recent years the use of maltol, which can intensify or modify the flavor of preserves, desserts, fruit, soft drinks and foods generally high in carbohydrates, has expanded greatly.

Manufacturers are also doing considerable research to find flavors that are

mitted colors and also restrict the number of foods to which color can be added. Since most of the lists are based on the toxicological evaluation of the dyes, one might expect a reasonable degree of uniformity among the lists. It is not so, however, and therefore one of the most trou-

blesome problems facing a food manufacturer who wants to export his products is the need to vary the color according to the different regulations of the importing countries.

The World Health Organization has evaluated more than 140 kinds of color-

ing matter, declaring a number to be unsafe and publishing a fairly short list of colors deemed to be safe. In some countries the food industry manages quite well with a choice of no more than a dozen dyes. Other countries allow more dyes. The difference is illustrated by a

CERTAIN COLORS employed as food additives are portrayed according to their chemical structure. The colors have both numerical and descriptive names: (a) red 2, amaranth; (b) red 3, erythrosine; (c) yellow 5, tartrazine; (d) yellow 6, sunset yellow; (e)

green 3, fast green; (f) violet 1, benzylviolet, and (g) blue 2, indigotine. The characteristic ring structure evident in the seven diagrams is more likely than an aliphatic, or open-chain, structure to produce color because of the way it absorbs and reflects light.

a   *b*   *c*

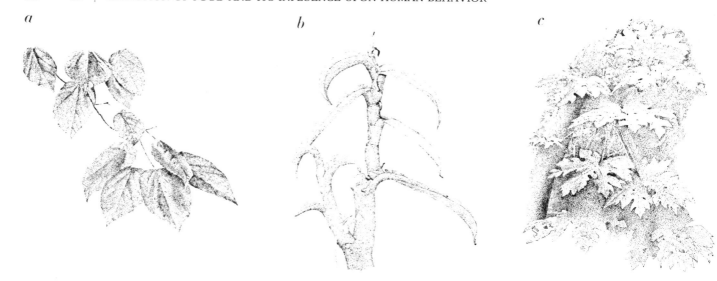

BOTANICAL SOURCES of four natural additives are depicted. The annatto (*a*) is a tropical tree, *Bixa orellana*, that produces a yellowish-red coloring agent made from the pulp around the seeds.

Natural vanilla extract comes from the pods of several species of orchid, chiefly *Vanilla planifolia* (*b*). Sap from the papaya tree (*c*), *Carica papaya*, is the source of the enzyme papain, which is

problem that the British will face when their country becomes a member of the European Economic Community: kippers will no longer be golden and sausages will no longer be "nicely pink" unless the Community's list of permitted colors is extended.

Preservative additives are one means of deterring food spoilage caused by microorganisms. The seriousness of spoilage is shown by the World Health Organization's estimate that about 20 percent of the world's food supply is lost in this way. Indeed, shortages of food in many parts of the world could be alleviated with the wider use of preservatives.

Spoilage can be prevented or retarded not only with additives but also with physical and biological processes such as heating, refrigeration, drying, freezing, souring, fermenting and curing. Some of these processes, however, achieve only partial preservation. Additives therefore have a role in prolonging a food's keeping qualities.

A number of different types of preservative have to be employed, depending on the kind of food, the method of manufacture, the way the food is packaged and stored and the nature of the microorganisms involved. Baked goods, for example, go stale rapidly. Once made, they are often exposed to mold spores that become active in warm weather or high humidity. In bread the spores produce a condition called "rope." Sodium diacetate, acetic acid, lactic acid, monocalcium phosphate, sodium propionate and calcium propionate are all effective in preventing rope. Sorbic

acid and its salts have many uses, such as preventing mold in cheese, syrup and confections containing fruit or sugar. Benzoic acid and sodium benzoate serve as preservatives in margarine, fruit-juice concentrates, juices and pickled vegetables. Sulfur dioxide is widely used to inhibit mold and discoloration in wine, fruit pulps, fruit-juice concentrates, fruit drinks requiring dilution and dried fruits and vegetables.

Sulfur dioxide is giving rise to concern in a number of countries where the average wine consumption is so high that the people who drink a good deal of wine are in danger of exceeding the acceptable average daily intake of sulfur dioxide. The acceptable daily level is 1.5 milligrams per kilogram of body weight, which means about 100 milligrams a day or a half-liter of wine containing 200 parts per million of sulfur dioxide. Studies on sulfite in the rat found that .1 percent in the diet inhibited the growth rate, probably because sulfite destroys vitamin B_1. The significance of this finding in man, whose diet does not consist exclusively of sulfited food as in the experiments with rats, is questionable; nonetheless, more work is needed to dispel the uncertainty about the toxicity of sulfur dioxide and sulfites.

As a result of such uncertainties serious attempts to find alternatives to preserving foods with chemicals are under way. Among the recent advances is the development of antibiotics as antimicrobial additives. Antibiotics commonly have a more transitory effect than the traditional preservatives and are more selective. These advantages are sig-

nificant when antibiotics are directed against known food pathogens and when their action is required only during the manufacturing stage. Antibiotics can be said to have a major disadvantage, however, in that by changing the normal spoilage pattern of certain foods they may result in unfamiliar forms of spoilage that consumers cannot recognize.

A number of countries have permitted such antibiotics as tetracyclines, nystatin, nisin and pimaricin as direct or indirect additives to chilled or raw fish, meat, poultry, cheese and bananas. The applications are strictly limited. Many other countries, although they recognize the efficacy of antibiotic additives, have taken the view that it would be unwise to approve them widely for food, since the antibiotics are important in medicine and their liberal use in food might produce resistant strains of pathogens that could affect humans.

Another development that has attracted interest as an alternative way of protecting food is the experimental work wherein ionizing radiation is employed to destroy the microorganisms and insects that cause food spoilage. An advantage of irradiation is that it produces little or no rise in the temperature of the food during treatment. A disadvantage at present is the possibility that irradiation will have an effect on the food and leave residues. For example, it is possible for the extranuclear structure of atoms to be excited under the influence of ionizing radiation. If the atoms are constituents of a molecule, the molecule as a whole may be excited, which may lead to rupture of one or more chemical

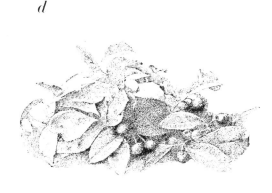

employed as a meat tenderizer. One source of wintergreen flavor is the leaves of the evergreen plant *Gaultheria procumbens* (d).

bonds, giving rise to free radicals. The free radicals may be capable of starting chemical chain reactions.

Nonetheless, work with irradiation has advanced to a point where in a small number of countries the sale of certain irradiated foodstuffs is now allowed. Irradiation raises the possibility that perishable foodstuffs could be more widely distributed in a fresh or nearly fresh condition. It is likely to take several years, however, for the irradiation of food to become a widespread practice because of the effort that must still be devoted to developing procedures for testing irradiated foods. The International Atomic Energy Agency, in conjunction with the Food and Agriculture Organization and the World Health Organization, has indicated a number of possible treatments by ionizing radiation to achieve long-term preservation, without refrigeration or chemical preservatives, of perishable foods and also to prevent food poisoning by destroying microorganisms such as salmonella.

Many traditional preservatives—notably salt, vinegar and sugar—still play an important role in homes and factories. It can be argued that recent improvements in food processing, coupled with improved standards of hygiene, should reduce the need for chemical preservatives. On the other hand, developments in making ready-to-use foods and the widespread resort to prepackaging have tended to increase the need for preservatives.

Related to preservatives are antioxidants, which are added to fatty foods primarily to prevent rancidity. Typical products containing these additives are margarine, cooking oils, biscuits, potato chips, cereals, salted nuts, soup mixes and precooked meals containing fish, poultry or meat. Certain foods, such as virgin olive oil, contain their own natural antioxidants in the form of tocopherols and therefore do not need the addition of antioxidants. If such foods are heated in a manufacturing process, however, they tend to lose their natural antioxidants, which should be restored if the product is to have a reasonable shelf life.

The most widely added antioxidants are butylated hydroxyanisole, butylated hydroxytoluene, propyl, octyl and dodecyl gallates and natural or synthetic tocopherols singly or in combination. Certain acids (ascorbic, citric and phosphoric) combined with antioxidants increase the antioxidant effect.

Preventing rancidity is not the only problem with a number of foods. The growing practice of using transparent wrapping for food presents its own problems by exposing the product to light and increasing the likelihood of discoloration. Ascorbic and isoascorbic acid have proved effective in preventing discoloration in certain fruit juices, soft drinks, canned vegetables, frozen fruits and cooked cured meat such as ham.

Often more than one antioxidant is put into a food, producing a synergistic action that allows more effective control of the product. Many countries authorize several antioxidants as food additives, but a number of others will allow only the so-called natural antioxidants, such as ascorbic acid (vitamin C) and the tocopherols (vitamin E). Much research is in progress to find compounds that are more potent than the present antioxidants. The search is particularly keen for antioxidants that are less likely than the present ones to impart odor, flavor or color to foods. Another quest is for antioxidants with a required solubility in both water and oil. With the development of simulated foods the search for antioxidants that are more effective in extending shelf life will gain further impetus.

In the class of texture agents I have included emulsifiers, stabilizers and thickening agents. In terms of quantity consumed they probably constitute the largest class of additives, being employed extensively in preparing bread, pastry, ice cream, frozen desserts, whipped products, margarine, candy and certain soft drinks and milk products. Many of the newer convenience foods have only become practicable as a result of the development of new and improved emulsifiers and stabilizers.

Among other things, the texture agents permit oil to be dispersed in water, produce a smooth and even texture and supply the desired body and consistency of many food products.

The first emulsifiers were few in number and were either natural substances such as gums, alginates and soaps or synthetic substances of fairly simple composition. Their action was often variable. Progress in chemical synthesis has now made available a large number of new texture agents with characteristics suitable for almost any requirement. Among the most common emulsifiers and stabilizers, aside from the natural ones, are stearyl tartrate, complete glycerol esters, partial glycerol esters, partial polyglycerol esters, propylene glycol esters, monostearin sodium sulfoacetate, sorbitan esters of fatty acids and their polyoxyethylene derivatives, cellulose ethers and sodium carboxymethyl cellulose. Thickeners include natural products such as agar, alginates, celluloses, starches, vegetable gums, dextrins and pectin; modified celluloses such as methyl cellulose, and starches modified by bleaching, oxidizing and phosphating.

The miscellaneous group of additives is so numerous that I can only indicate a few of the functions they serve. Acids, alkalis, buffers and neutralizing agents are added to many processed foods where the degree of acidity or alkalinity is important; manufacturers of baked goods, soft drinks, chocolate and processed cheese employ these additives extensively. The baking industry also makes heavy use of bleaching and maturing agents, which render flour whiter and bring it to maturity sooner. Sequestrants are added to food to bind trace metals and thus prevent any oxidative activity the metals in an ionized state might have on the food; in shortening, for example, unsequestered metals could catalyze processes leading to rancidity. Humectants, which are hygroscopic, offset changes in the humidity of the environment to which food is exposed, so that a desired level of moisture can be maintained in a food product such as shredded coconut. Anticaking agents keep many salts and powders free-flowing. Glazing agents make certain food surfaces shiny and in some cases protect the product from spoiling. Firming and crisping agents prevent flaccidity in processed fruits and vegetables and also aid the coagulation of certain cheeses. Release agents help food to separate from surfaces it touches during manufacture or transport. Foaming agents coupled with propellants make whipped

ANTICAKING AGENTS
Aluminum calcium silicate
Calcium silicate
Magnesium silicate
Sodium aluminosilicate
Sodium calcium aluminosilicate
Tricalcium silicate

CHEMICAL PRESERVATIVES
Ascorbic acid
Ascorbyl palmitate
Benzoic acid
Butylated hydroxyanisole
Butylated hydroxytoluene
Calcium ascorbate
Calcium propionate
Calcium sorbate
Caprylic acid
Dilauryl thiodipropionate
Erythorbic acid
Gum guaiac
Methylparaben
Potassium bisulfite
Potassium metabisulfite
Potassium sorbate
Propionic acid
Propyl gallate
Propylparaben
Sodium ascorbate
Sodium benzoate
Sodium bisulfite
Sodium metabisulfite
Sodium propionate
Sodium sorbate
Sodium sulfite
Sorbic acid
Stannous chloride
Sulfur dioxide
Thiodipropionic acid
Tocopherols

EMULSIFYING AGENTS
Cholic acid
Desoxycholic acid
Diacetyl tartaric acid esters
  of mono- and diglycerides
Glycocholic acid
Mono- and diglycerides
Monosodium phosphate
  derivatives of above
Propylene glycol
Ox bile extract
Taurocholic acid

NUTRIENTS AND DIETARY
SUPPLEMENTS
Alanine
Arginine
Ascorbic acid
Aspartic acid
Biotin
Calcium carbonate
Calcium citrate
Calcium glycerophosphate
Calcium oxide
Calcium pantothenate
Calcium phosphate
Calcium pyrophosphate
Calcium sulfate
Carotene
Choline bitartrate
Choline chloride
Copper gluconate
Cuprous iodide

Cysteine
Cystine
Ferric phosphate
Ferric pyrophosphate
Ferric sodium pyrophosphate
Ferrous gluconate
Ferrous lactate
Ferrous sulfate
Glycine
Histidine
Inositol
Iron, reduced
Isoleucine
Leucine
Linoleic acid
Lysine
Magnesium oxide
Magnesium phosphate
Magnesium sulfate
Manganese chloride
Manganese citrate
Manganese gluconate
Manganese glycerophosphate
Manganese hypophosphite
Manganese sulfate
Manganous oxide
Mannitol
Methionine
Methionine hydroxy analogue
Niacin
Niacinamide
D-pantothenyl alcohol
Phenylalanine
Potassium chloride
Potassium glycerophosphate
Potassium iodide
Proline
Pyridoxine hydrochloride
Riboflavin
Riboflavin-5-phosphate
Serine
Sodium pantothenate
Sodium phosphate
Sorbitol
Thiamine hydrochloride
Thiamine mononitrate
Threonine
Tocopherols
Tocopherol acetate
Tryptophane
Tyrosine
Valine
Vitamin A
Vitamin A acetate
Vitamin A palmitate
Vitamin B_{12}
Vitamin D_2
Vitamin D_3
Zinc sulfate
Zinc gluconate
Zinc chloride
Zinc oxide
Zinc stearate

SEQUESTRANTS
Calcium acetate
Calcium chloride
Calcium citrate
Calcium diacetate
Calcium gluconate
Calcium hexametaphosphate
Calcium phosphate, monobasic
Calcium phytate
Citric acid

Dipotassium phosphate
Disodium phosphate
Isopropyl citrate
Monoisopropyl citrate
Potassium citrate
Sodium acid phosphate
Sodium citrate
Sodium diacetate
Sodium gluconate
Sodium hexametaphosphate
Sodium metaphosphate
Sodium phosphate
Sodium potassium tartrate
Sodium pyrophosphate
Sodium pyrophosphate, tetra
Sodium tartrate
Sodium thiosulfate
Sodium tripolyphosphate
Stearyl citrate
Tartaric acid

STABILIZERS
Acacia (gum arabic)
Agar-agar
Ammonium alginate
Calcium alginate
Carob bean gum
Chondrus extract
Ghatti gum
Guar gum
Potassium alginate
Sodium alginate
Sterculia (or karaya) gum
Tragacanth

MISCELLANEOUS ADDITIVES
Acetic acid
Adipic acid
Aluminum ammonium sulfate
Aluminum potassium sulfate
Aluminum sodium sulfate
Aluminum sulfate
Ammonium bicarbonate
Ammonium carbonate
Ammonium hydroxide
Ammonium phosphate
Ammonium sulfate
Beeswax
Bentonite
Butane
Caffeine
Calcium carbonate
Calcium chloride
Calcium citrate
Calcium gluconate
Calcium hydroxide
Calcium lactate
Calcium oxide
Calcium phosphate
Caramel
Carbon dioxide
Carnauba wax
Citric acid
Dextrans
Ethyl formate
Glutamic acid
Glutamic acid hydrochloride
Glycerin
Glyceryl monostearate
Helium
Hydrochloric acid
Hydrogen peroxide
Lactic acid
Lecithin

Magnesium carbonate
Magnesium hydroxide
Magnesium oxide
Magnesium stearate
Malic acid
Methylcellulose
Monoammonium glutamate
Monopotassium glutamate
Nitrogen
Nitrous oxide
Papain
Phosphoric acid
Potassium acid tartrate
Potassium bicarbonate
Potassium carbonate
Potassium citrate
Potassium hydroxide
Potassium sulfate
Propane
Propylene glycol
Rennet
Silica aerogel
Sodium acetate
Sodium acid pyrophosphate
Sodium aluminum phosphate
Sodium bicarbonate
Sodium carbonate
Sodium citrate
Sodium carboxy-
  methylcellulose
Sodium caseinate
Sodium citrate
Sodium hydroxide
Sodium pectinate
Sodium phosphate
Sodium potassium tartrate
Sodium sesquicarbonate
Sodium tripolyphosphate
Succinic acid
Sulfuric acid
Tartaric acid
Triacetin
Triethyl citrate

SYNTHETIC FLAVORING
SUBSTANCES
Acetaldehyde
Acetoin
Aconitic acid
Anethole
Benzaldehyde
N-butyric acid
d- or l-carvone
Cinnamaldehyde
Citral
Decanal
Diacetyl
Ethyl acetate
Ethyl butyrate
Ethyl vanillin
Eugenol
Geraniol
Geranyl acetate
Glycerol tributyrate
Limonene
Linalool
Linalyl acetate
1-malic acid
Methyl anthranilate
3-Methyl-3-phenyl
  glycidic acid ethyl ester
Piperonal
Vanillin

GROUP OF ADDITIVES included in the U.S. Food and Drug Administration's list of additives "generally recognized as safe" is given, except for large groups of natural flavors and oils. To be on this list an additive must have been in use before 1958 and have met certain specifications of safety. Additives brought into use since 1958 must be approved individually. Occasionally substances are removed from the list by the FDA in the light of new evidence; recent examples include the cyclamate sweeteners and saccharin.

toppings come out of their containers as a foam, whereas foam inhibitors have an opposite role, where a tendency to foam, as with pineapple juice, makes filling a container difficult. Clarifying agents remove small particles of minerals from liquids such as vinegar, which might otherwise turn cloudy. Solvents serve as carriers for flavors, colors and other additives, and solvent extraction is the method whereby oil is obtained from oilseeds, coffee is decaffeinated and a number of instant beverages are prepared.

Additives have become a public issue because of recurrent episodes bringing into question the safety of certain additives that have been used for some time. Cyclamates were tested extensively in the U.S. before they were put on the market as artificial sweeteners, but in 1969 it was reported that large doses had caused bladder cancer in rats. The U.S. Government ordered cyclamates off the market. Subsequently it was reported that rats fed with cyclamate and saccharin at a sixth of the dose that led to the original ban also developed bladder cancer. As a result saccharin is now being critically reviewed in the U.S. and other countries. Sodium nitrite, which fixes a red color in frankfurters, sausages and hams, is currently under review in many countries because of the possibility that it may form a cancer-producing agent during digestion and storage. Laboratory evidence has linked monosodium glutamate with the "Chinese restaurant syndrome" (more precisely Kwok's disease), a tightening of the muscles of the face and neck, occasionally accompanied by headache, nausea and giddiness, experienced by some people who have eaten in restaurants where monosodium glutamate has been used in large amounts. Many countries have therefore restricted the use of monosodium glutamate or required its presence in food to be prominently stated on the label.

Food additives, unlike the chemicals put in pesticide preparations, are not designed to be toxic, and most of them would have to be ingested in large single doses to produce acute toxic symptoms. Many additives by nature are of extremely low potential toxicity. It is therefore difficult to determine their possible hazards to man, even after exhaustive testing. It is probably true to say that there will always be an area of doubt concerning the possible effects of ingesting small amounts of additives over the course of a lifetime. One cannot be fully sure of the safety of an additive until it has been consumed by people of all ages in specified amounts over a long period

of time and has been shown conclusively, by careful toxicological examination, to have no harmful effects.

Since humans cannot be used for testing by exposing them to unknown chemicals for a substantial period of time, tests are made on rats and other animals such as mice and dogs. Test animals are fed quantities of the additive that far exceed the amount likely to be found in food. Tests are made both for short periods and over the animal's lifetime and are often continued into succeeding generations. Any change in growth, body function, tissue and reproduction is reported, as is the incidence of tumors.

The largest dose that appears to produce no effects in animals is taken, and a safety factor reducing that dose by about 100 is applied in most countries in order to arrive at an acceptable dose for humans. The "acceptable daily intake" thus calculated is the daily intake that for an entire lifetime appears to be without appreciable risk on the basis of all known facts at the time. It is expressed in terms of milligrams of the additive per kilogram of body weight. One must then calculate how much of the additive a person might be expected to ingest in a day from all dietary sources and compare this figure with the acceptable daily intake in order to decide whether the applications of the additive should be permitted and whether the specific tolerances or maximum limits required for it by good manufacturing practices in individual foods are safe to the health of the consumer.

Many national authorities publish information on the tests they require for proposed additives. International guidelines have been published by the Joint Expert Committee on Food Additives of the Food and Agriculture Organization and the World Health Organization. They require a comprehensive series of tests on laboratory animals, including short- and long-term studies covering acute toxicity, metabolism of the additive and carcinogenic effects, among others.

Assessing safety on the basis of toxicological tests calls for expert judgment of all the evidence available. The judgment may have to be modified in the light of further experiments and experience with the additive in food for humans. The tests required to obtain approval of an additive can cost upward of $100,000.

It is therefore the hope of the government and the food industry in many countries that the work of such international bodies as the Codex Alimentarius Commission of the Food and Agriculture

Organization and the World Health Organization will lead to a greater exchange of toxicological data and to the evaluation of the safety of more additives as soon as possible. The commission has published a list of six general principles on the use of food additives. The first is that the use of an additive is justified only when it has the purpose of maintaining a food's nutritional quality, enhancing its keeping quality or stability, making the food attractive, providing aid in processing, packing, transporting or storing food or providing essential components for foods for special diets, and that an additive is not justified if the proposed level of use constitutes a hazard to the consumer's health, if the additive causes a substantial reduction in the nutritive value of a food, if it disguises faulty quality or the use of processing and handling techniques that are not allowed, if it deceives the customer or if the desired effect can be obtained by other manufacturing processes that are economically and technologically satisfactory.

The second principle is that the amount of additive should not exceed the level reasonably required to achieve the desired effect under good manufacturing practice. The third principle calls for additives to conform with an approved standard of purity; the fourth holds that all additives, in use or proposed, should be subjected to adequate toxicological evaluation and that permitted additives should be kept under observation for possible deleterious effects; the fifth states that approval of an additive should be limited to specific foods for specific purposes and under specific conditions, and the sixth relates to the use of additives in foods consumed mainly by special groups in the community. In this case the intake of the food by the group should be taken into account before authorizing the use of the additive.

Food additives have become part of everyday life and undoubtedly will play an increasing role with advances in food technology. The prospect is not necessarily bad, because properly used additives can bring the consumer significant benefits. Moreover, provided that in each case sound justification for the additive is demonstrated, that government and manufacturers exercise the utmost care to ensure that the additive entails no appreciable risks to health and that clear labeling informs the consumer of the nature and composition of the product he is buying, consumers should be reasonably assured as to the safety of officially authorized food additives.

The Social Influence of the Potato

by Redcliffe N. Salaman
December 1952

*The humble tuber has shaped many cultures, notably
the Peruvian and the Irish. For some peoples the
richness of its food content and the ease of its
cultivation have ironically been a disaster*

THE potato has had much to do with shaping human society. Two cultures in particular, each in its own way, offer striking examples of its influence. One is Ireland, whose history has been bound up with the potato for more than 300 years. The other is ancient Peru, where for some 2,000 years the potato was not only the staple of life but a spiritual symbol as well. It was from Peru, in fact, that the tuber came to Europe; investigations in recent years have left little doubt that the first European potatoes were of the Peruvian species *Solanum andigenum*. The potato did not arrive in Europe until near the end of the 16th century. It has since been enormously improved. The tuber of today is a triumph of breeding and selection; it differs from its Peruvian ancestor as much as does the race horse from its wild progenitor.

The birthplace of this Peruvian potato, and the place where it was first cultivated, was in the uplands of the Andes between the altitudes of 6,000 and 14,000 feet. In these lofty valleys and plateaus the potato's nutritive value, its bountiful bearing and its good keeping qualities, in an environment where the failure of crops was all too common, made it the pre-eminently suitable food. The pre-Inca Indians who cultivated it were probably the first farmers in history to make a practice of reversing the sod. They worked in teams of at least four persons—two diggers dragging plows to cut the turf, and two others, generally women, following them to turn it over. The Peruvians were also pioneers in the art of preserving food. After harvesting the potatoes they dehydrated part of the crop to keep it for later use. They spread the tubers on the ground and exposed them to the night frosts, then trod them with bare feet during the heat of the day to press out the moisture. After several days of this treatment the

potatoes were dried and stored. The product, hard and chalk-white inside and still covered with its brown skin, was known as *chuño*. There was also a refinement of the process in which the potatoes, after the freezing, thawing and treading, were kept in running water for two months. This product, called *tunta*, was snow-white except for the eyes.

THE esteem in which the potato was held by the Peruvians is shown by the fact that they often buried bowls

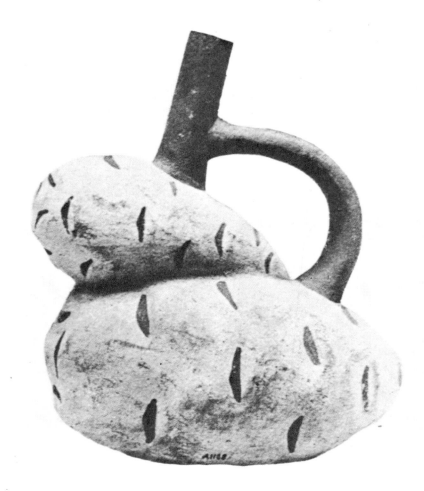

PERUVIAN VESSEL was made to look like the *tunta*. Most of the Peruvian potato vessels, however, also look like people (*see photograph on page 118*).

of *chuño*, doubtless as food for the departed, in their tombs, and that in much of their pottery the potato is the motif of the design. I have collected photographs of 70 such Peruvian pots from the museums of the world. Some of them date back to about the time of the beginning of the Christian Era, and the evidence indicates the potato must have been cultivated in pre-Inca Peru as early as 500 B.C.

The potato design on these pots is generally anthropomorphic. It almost always represents a human being, or at least a human head. The design is so cleverly made that it is equally convincing as a representation of a human figure or of a potato tuber. In one pot several tubers are combined to form a head, trunk and arms. All of the figures bear on the head and body many deeply incised tuber "eyes."

Now a peculiar feature of these sculptures is that the human figures are generally mutilated. Of the 27 pots of out-spoken anthropomorphic design, 22 exhibit mutilations of the mouth or nose or of both. Sometimes the end of the nose is sliced off; sometimes one or both lips are cut out, so that the teeth appear to sprout from the exposed gums. What explanation is to be ascribed to this curious syndrome—potato tuber, human figure, facial mutilation?

We start with the assumption that the pots depict a sacrificial mutilation designed as a fertility rite to further the productivity of the plant. The germinal foci of the potato tuber lie in the "eyes," and it is a common tradition that a well developed "eye" and a strong bud issuing from it are favorable omens for a bountiful crop. Let us now suppose that the Peruvians regarded these foci not as "eyes" but as "mouths." For this there is morphological support. The "eye" of the more commonly grown S. *andigenum* varieties is very deep, and it is bordered above and below by bolster-like swellings which might be described as lips. From between these lips project the buds, which we must now regard as teeth.

Accepting this symbolization, it follows that the bigger the mouth and more prominent the teeth, the better the prospects for a good crop.

The Peruvian was a confirmed animist. The spirit of the potato, *Papa mama*, needed not only invocation but guidance and strength to carry out its task. A common symbol of strength-giving in primitive rites is the outpouring of blood, and in this case it would have followed the mutilations.

It may be objected that this explanation is an armchair theory lacking factual support. Happily such criticism can be met. We have evidence on the point from the early Spanish soldier Cieza de Léon. In 1545 he witnessed in Inca Peru an elaborate ritual in which the blood of a llama was poured over the seed potatoes before planting. Later visitors to Peru described scenes in

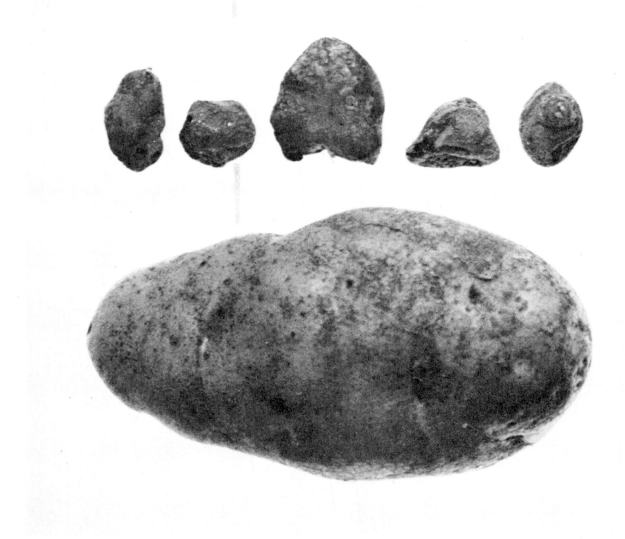

OLD AND NEW POTATOES are compared in their actual size. At the bottom is a modern specimen. At the top are ancient Peruvian *chuños* in the American Museum of Natural History. They were dried by freezing.

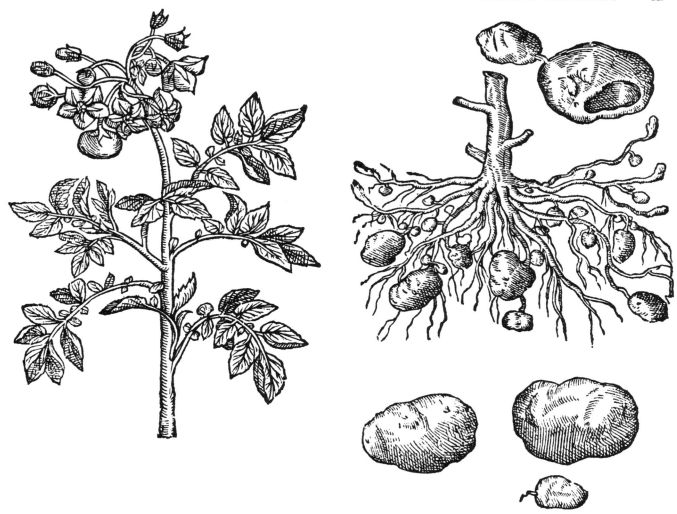

FIRST SCIENTIFIC DESCRIPTION of the potato was published in 1601 by the famous French botanist Caro-lus Clusius, or Charles de l'Escluse. This woodcut is reproduced from his book *Rariorum Plantarum Historia*.

which the womenfolk collected the blood of warriors and carried it off to pour on the potato fields, or soaked *chuño* in the blood and ate it. Potatoes of a blood-red color were, and still are, highly prized in the Peru-Bolivia region. Travelers have told me of seeing a curi-ous ceremony: upon finding a blood-red tuber in the field, a farm man or woman rushes to the nearest person of the op-posite sex and hits or touches him in the face with it.

The pots themselves give further sup-port to the fertility-symbolism theory. One of them shows not only several mutilated heads of human beings (formed from tubers) but also a large jaguar's head, with mouth open and teeth displayed, as if reinforcing the symbolism suggested by the mutilated heads. Finally, there is an early Mochica pot which seems to sum up the whole story: we see a man built up from a po-tato tuber, with his lips and the end of

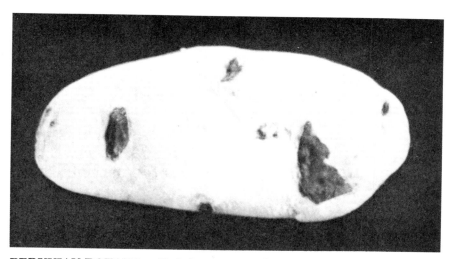

PERUVIAN POTATO called the *tunta* is white except for the eyes. It was made from the already dried *chuño* by long immersion in running water.

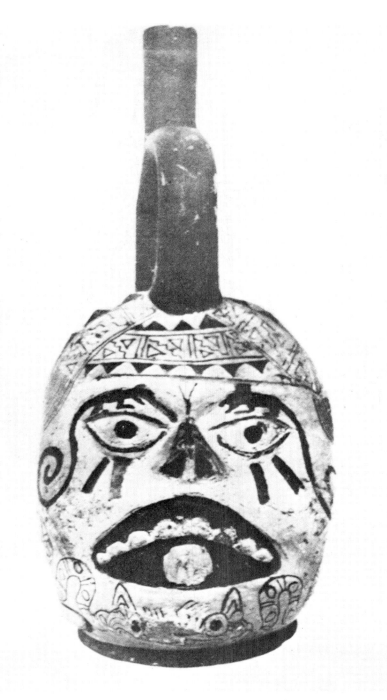

MUTILATED HEAD is worked into the potato design of another Peruvian vessel. The mutilations may have suggested bleeding, symbol of strength.

his nose cut off and his body bestrewn with "eyes" from which extrude well developed buds. In the man's hand is the digging-stick with which he will plant the tuber seed.

WHEN the potato arrived in Europe, it soon acquired a semi-religious aura there too, but in reverse—the people regarded it as a sinister creation. The Highlanders of Scotland, objecting violently to the tuber as a food, noted significantly that the potato was not mentioned in the Bible. In Russia a century later the introduction of the potato met with open revolt. The Church of the Old Believers wove a nexus of myth around the tuber which, by a miracle of inductive logic, led them to alter the Ukrainian name for a potato, *bulba*, into *gulba*, which connoted something sexually perverse and unclean. England's John Ruskin, in his *The Queen of the Air*, called the potato "the scarcely innocent underground stem of one of a tribe set aside for evil." Throughout the 17th and the 18th centuries there was a widespread and persistent belief that the potato induced leprosy. When that fell disease no longer aroused popular fear, the potato was accused of being the cause of scrofula.

But the tuber was eventually accepted everywhere. It is in Ireland, the classic land of the potato, that one finds the clearest evidence of the influence which a cheap, nutritious foodstuff can exercise on a society. The potato reached Ireland around 1588. The Desmond Revolt at that time and the Cromwellian storm in the mid-17th century uprooted the Irish peasantry and destroyed their herds, their homes and their crops. But by the end of the 17th century the potato had helped them to recover. In Munster and Connaught it had become the basic food of nine tenths of the population. In 1672 John Beale recorded that "potatoes were a relief to Ireland in their last famine; they yield meat and drink"— a signpost on the road along which the Irish economy was traveling. As we journey through the next two centuries, how often we hear the potato spoken of as the lifeline of the people, the trusted bulwark against ever-recurring failures of the cereal crop!

The Irish potato economy has been held partly responsible, and I think rightly, for the rise in population which, setting in early in the 18th century, was to assume alarming proportions toward its end. It is not true, as was once thought, that the potato has aphrodisiac powers, but it may fairly be said that the potato did a great deal to make large families possible. It provided a maximum of sustenance with a minimum of labor. When the potatoes had been earthed up in early June, there was nothing to do until October, and even then tubers were often left in the ground to be lifted as required—a custom which proved of great value in times of "trouble." The output of an Irish acre was sufficient to supply a married couple and four children with all they needed in the way of potatoes and still leave enough for the pigs and hens, notwithstanding that the average man consumed 12 pounds, the wife 10 pounds, and each child 5 pounds per day.

If food was no limiting factor, neither was clothing; no one wore shoes, and the children ran naked, at least in summer. Housing was of the simplest: it was commonly allowed that a singlechambered black hut could be erected for £3, and a partitioned dwelling for £5. Of furniture there was little more than the three-legged iron cauldron, a few rough stools and perhaps a table. Beds, as such, were a luxury; a straw mattress on the raised part of the floor sufficed. The cow, the pig and the poultry lived under the same roof, providing welcome heat in the winter months. Why, then, should the poor delay marriage, seeing that they couldn't be poorer and might well be happier?

TOWARD the middle of the 18th century a disturbing sign appeared: here and there the potato crop began to fail. Sometimes the cause was excessive rainfall, sometimes drought. And then in 1809 a virus disease struck the crop. By 1817 the disease had brought famine and typhus to the people. The government began to spend large sums for organized relief. In 1833 virus diseases of the potato caused a spurt of emigration to the U. S.

These failures of the potato crop led many to warn the government and the people against undue reliance on the potato. It was too late; the potato had not only fashioned the pattern of the people's lives but also widened the gulf dividing the Protestant ruling caste from the Catholic workers and farmers. The impoverished and subject population felt that its refuge and protection was the potato economy. The relations between the working classes, the small bourgeoisie and the Protestant ascendancy had become so stereotyped, so firmly embedded in an economic nexus in which the potato was the least common denominator, that the people were held in bondage to it.

Then in 1845 and 1846 came the total destruction of the potato crop by the previously unknown fungus *Phytophthora infestans*. The tale of this fatal mold and of the Great Famine that followed has been told too often to need repetition here. Notwithstanding a sustained effort by the government and the people of England to meet the emergency, death and emigration reduced the population of Ireland from 9 million to 6.5 million within six years, and in a couple of decades it had fallen to 4 million.

The common idea that Ireland attained its economic and political independence by political action and revolution is, I believe, but half the truth. Ireland could never have been really independent until it freed itself from its economic thralldom to the potato. That was not effected by legislation, violence or famine. The old economy was defeated by a newer economy, by free trade and by the importation of cheap American food.

IRELAND is the extreme example of the impact of the potato on social organization. In most of England its effect was blunted by the sturdy independence of the people; in truth the potato there was for a long time a luxury food, and was accepted by the industrial workers only reluctantly after wheat prices skyrocketed during the Napoleonic Wars. The English working man had long regarded the Irishman as a man enslaved by his potato diet, and he struggled to ward off a similar subjection.

The danger the English worker recognized more than 150 years ago has not disappeared. Before World War II a potato economy was being created in rural Poland, and today one exists along part of the Chilean coast of South America and west of it on the Pacific island of Chiloé. As in Ireland just over a hundred years ago, the Chilean crops were destroyed in 1950 suddenly and unexpectedly—and by the same agent.

A cheap, abundant and easily raised food still has its dangers!

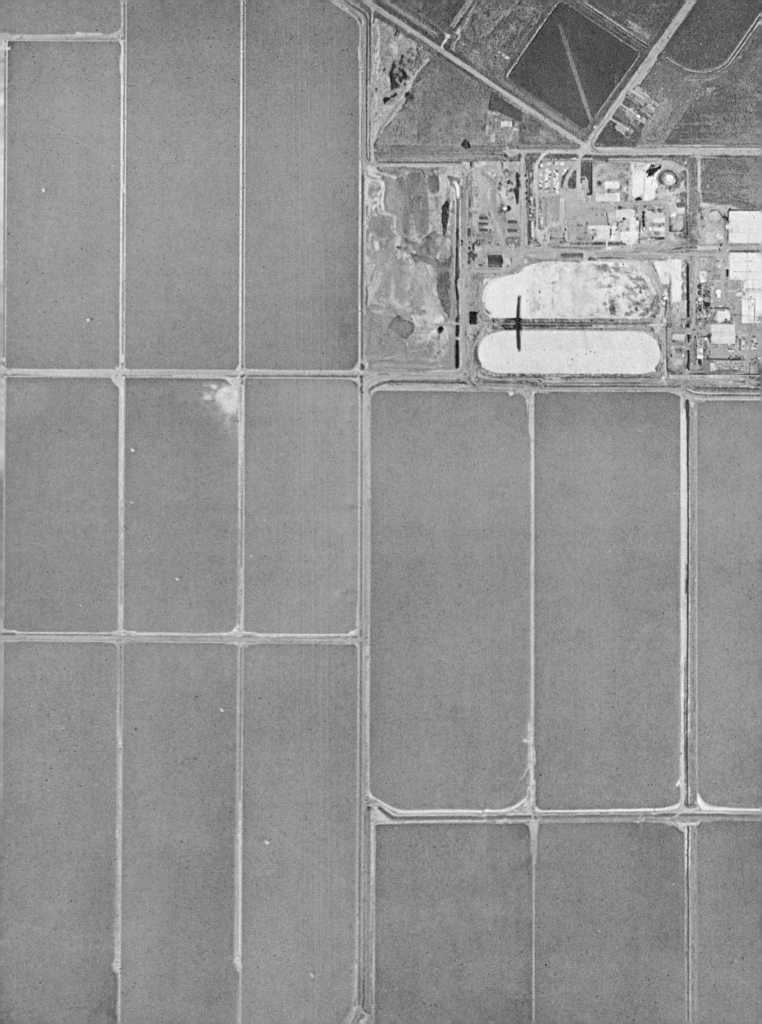

The Social Influence of Salt

by M. R. Bloch
July 1963

Salt is a necessity of human life, and many people are addicted to using more of it than they need. Its sources are surprisingly limited, a fact that has shaped history in many curious respects

The Bible assigns a high value to salt ("Ye are the salt of the earth"). The great importance of salt to man was noted by a number of ancient writers (Plutarch, for example); indeed, "salt hunger" has a folklore all of its own. Typical is a pathetic story recounted in 1708 by a French cleric named J. Bion:

"In France...there are some poor peasants and their whole families who, for want of salt, eat no soup sometimes in a whole week; though it be their common nourishment. A man in that case, grieved to see his wife and children in a starving, languishing condition, ventures to go abroad, to buy salt in the Provinces where it is three parts in four cheaper. If discovered, he is certainly sent to the galleys. It is a very melancholy sight to see a wife and children lament their father, whom they see laden with chains and irrevocably lost; and that for no other crime but endeavoring to procure subsistence for those to whom he gave birth."

For want of salt men have risked their lives and endured the most disagreeable circumstances. Over large areas of Africa, lacking other sources, people used to drink the urine of animals for its salt. We are not likely to think of salt as one of the major necessities of life, but in fact it is as essential as water, and for precisely the same reason.

The chemical requirements of the human body demand that the salt concentration in the blood be kept constant. If the body does not get enough salt, a hormonal mechanism compensates by reducing the excretion of salt in the urine and sweat. But it cannot reduce this output to zero. On a completely saltless diet the body steadily loses small amounts of salt via the kidneys and sweat glands. It then attempts to adjust to this by accelerating its secretion of water, so that the blood's salt concentration can be maintained at the vital level. The result is a gradual desiccation of the body and finally death. The organism literally dies of thirst.

In the case of lack of water to drink, the crucial factor—the salt concentration in the blood—is the same but the hormonal mechanism works in the opposite direction. It operates to reduce the secretion of water and increase the salt secretion, in order to maintain the correct salt level; nonetheless, the inevitable, irreducible water losses lead to death. In short, the body's normal craving for salt and for water are both aspects of the same vital need: a saline internal fluid.

In regions of the world where the population lives mainly on meat or fish the year round salt is no great problem—the meat or fish provide enough. (Curiously, however, salt is habit-forming: people who live on a high salt intake become addicted to it. Obviously they must also secrete it at a higher rate.) Salt deprivation is a predicament of the vast areas where meat is scarce and men depend primarily on a vegetarian diet. On such a diet a human being needs a minimum of two to five grams of additional salt per day in mineral form. In many regions no mineral source is available. This was the case in parts of precolonial Africa. Its people survived only by drinking the blood and urine of cattle and wild animals, which roamed over wide areas collecting and concentrating the salt in their systems by feeding on plants. As a result inner Africa was able to support only a thin human population.

Aside from serving as a staple of the diet, salt is a necessity in civilized communities for storing meat and fish. It performs its function as a preservative by extracting water from the animal tissues; the dehydrated meat is then immune from attack by bacteria. There are, of course, other methods of preserving meat, but salt is still the most important one around the world.

It was the availability of mineral salt that enabled dense populations to arise and flourish in the valleys of the Jordan, the Nile, the Tigris-Euphrates, the Yellow River of China and the Salt River of Arizona. The same is almost certainly true of the valleys of Mexico and Peru, and of many in the far-flung Roman Empire.

Today the world population of three billion consumes an estimated 80 million tons of salt a year. But the per capita consumption varies widely. Some populations live on the edge of necessity, averaging two grams per day. Other countries enjoy the luxury of using salt for the production of such chemicals as sodium bicarbonate and polyvinyl chloride. In the U.S. the per capita use of salt is 280 grams a day, four times the world average. A salt shortage in the U.S. would result in some pinch of living standards; in Bengal, where the average daily consumption is five grams, it would mean famine and wholesale death.

In view of all this, it is interesting to investigate the history of the salt econ-

MODERN SALT PANS of the Leslie Salt Company in California get their color from reddish microorganisms in the brine with which the pans are filled. When solar evaporation concentrates the brine, the salt is deposited in layers, which can then be harvested. The buildings of the salt-processing plant appear at lower left. The two white oblong areas are mounds of harvested salt. The approximate scale of distance in this aerial photograph is one inch to 1,800 feet.

omy and its influence on civilization. In a very literal sense, as we shall see, salt has represented tides in the affairs of mankind. The investigation must depend largely on indirect evidence, because written history, oddly enough, does not furnish much information on the subject. There is much eloquent evidence, however, in the archaeological record.

In such an inquiry we cannot do better than to begin by hunting for the sources of possible supply. Where and how did man find salt-rich sites for his early civilizations?

We think at once, of course, of the Dead Sea, the world's saltiest body of water. Near the shores of the sea is a hill of salt known as Jebel Usdum (Mount Sodom). There salt has been quarried since early times, going back before the Bronze Age, and it is no coincidence that some of the earliest known agricultural settlements arose in

this area, at Jericho and near the mouth of the Jordan at the north end of the Dead Sea. There were other places in the ancient world where salt could be had merely by digging it out of the ground. Herodotus mentioned salt quarries in North Africa; it is known that the Phoenicians quarried salt in Spain; and prehistoric salt quarries containing stone axes have been found in Asia Minor (Armenia), South America and at pre-Columbian sites in Arizona.

Quarrying led to attempts to mine salt in deeper levels. Remains of such mines have been found at Hallstatt in the Austrian Alps and in several other places [see map on pages 124 and 125]. The tools were primitive and the yields low. Nevertheless, salt mining made Hallstatt an important center of ancient middle Europe. A salt mine at Camp Verde in Arizona made possible the Salt River valley civilization of pre-Columbian times.

Easier than quarrying and mining was the production of salt from concentrated brines. All one had to do was to wall the natural brine in a shallow enclosure, let the sun evaporate the water and then harvest the deposited layers of salt. At the edges of the Dead Sea there are remains of rectangular "solar pans" that were diked in by ancient salt-makers. In China, in a salt-water swamp at the great bend of the Yellow River, ancient solar pans are still in operation [see illustration below]. They were described in 1882 by the German geologist and explorer Baron Ferdinand von Richthofen as follows:

"The floor of the valley is drained by 150 corporations; each corporation has a strip 600 feet wide running across the length of the valley down to the lake.... Every winter holes are made in the soil, 20 feet deep and 50 feet wide.... There the concentrated brine collects. Around these holes, flat fields with low dividing

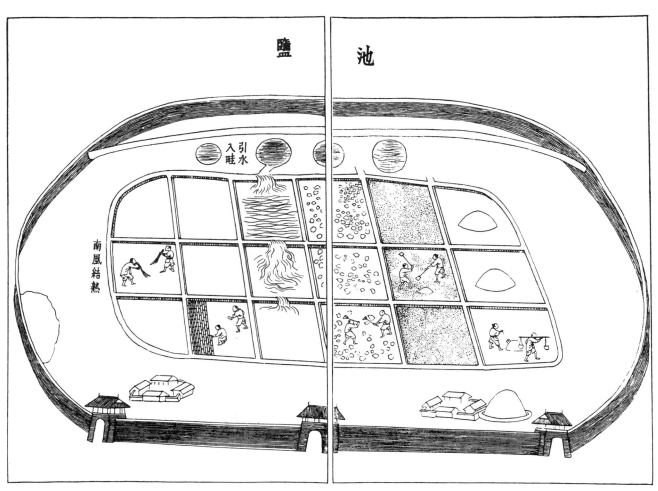

CHINESE SALT PAN described in the text has been used from earliest times to the present. It is located in a salt-water swamp at the great bend of the Yellow River in China. Circles at top represent large holes in which brine collects. The drawings on these two pages first appeared in 1637 in the book *Tien Kung Khai Wu* ("The Exploitation of the Worlds of Nature") by Sung Ying-Hsing.

walls are constructed. The summer's task is to lift the brine from the holes into these fields. This is done with a swinging bucket."

There were salt swamps in Persia, the deserts of Egypt and the Sahara. Early man came to recognize the oases of the mineral by their red color. The redness is due to the fact that in briny, shallow ponds reddish microorganisms multiply. Usually the redder the brine, the higher its salt content. The similarity of the red brine to blood, in taste as well as color, must have made a profound impression on primitive folk.

Indeed, the Bible indicates this, as we read in the Second Book of Kings: "And they rose up early in the morning, and the sun shone upon the water, and the Moabites saw the water on the other side as red as blood. And they said, This is blood...." The passage probably refers to salt pans at Sodom. The name Sodom itself very likely came from the Hebrew words *sade* ("field") and *adom* ("red"). In a cave near the Dead Sea archaeologists have found a piece of reddish salt, made by careful crystallization around a wooden stick, along with remains that are dated from the time of the Bar-Kochba Jewish uprising against Rome about A.D. 130.

In contrast to the salt from solar pans, salt quarried from the ground is gray; it usually contains gypsum and has less savor because it does not dissolve completely. A map made around A.D. 450 shows two ships sailing on the Dead Sea, one loaded with reddish salt from the solar ponds and the other with gray salt from a quarry at Mount Sodom.

Rare are the places in the world where salt can be obtained so easily. Inland peoples in most regions of the earth had to search for salt and work hard to extract it. In China some ingenious engineer about A.D. 400 conceived the idea of drilling deep into mountains to salt deposits and bringing up the brine via pipes made of bamboo; some of these salt holes are as deep as 3,000 feet. The brine was then evaporated over fires fueled by coal, wood or natural gas.

Elsewhere early settlements grew up around salty springs, which hunting tribes located by following animals to them. It was difficult to concentrate salt from these dilute sources, but the hunters kept wood fires going and boiled away the water. These salt-boiling civilizations go back to Neolithic times. Among the centers were the Tirol region of the Alps, the Moselle and Franche-Comté areas in France, the Saale and Lüneburg areas in Germany and Droitwich in England. Whole forests were burned up in this industry, and the saltmakers had to haul their wood from farther and farther away, often on river rafts from distant places.

The most abundant and ubiquitous

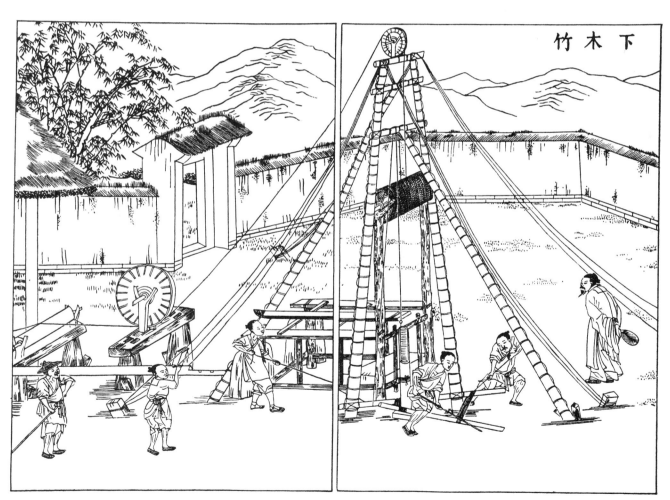

CHINESE SALT DRILLS were first used about A.D. 400 to reach salt deposits as much as 3,000 feet below the surface. The brines were pumped to the surface through bamboo pipes. These drawings of the pan and drill were photographed from a reprinted edition of *Tien Kung Khai Wu*. The reprinted edition, published in 1930, is in the collection of the East Asian Library of Columbia University.

source of salt on our planet is of course the ocean. Its content of salts is low—only about 3 per cent, compared with close to 30 per cent in the Dead Sea. The ocean nonetheless was and still is the main source that has sustained the earth's human populations. Of the 80 million tons of salt produced today, some 30 million are extracted from ocean water by means of solar energy according to a system that apparently goes back at least to Mycenaean times some 3,500 years ago and possibly to the early Minoan civilization about 5,000 years ago.

This system is useful only in regions of abundant sunshine. The peoples of rainy northern Europe—Britain, the Netherlands, Scandinavia—were blessed, however, with stored solar energy in the form of peat. Along the coastal areas of the North Sea they dug out immense quantities of peat that had been soaked with sea water at low tide. This they dried and burned; then they extracted the salt from the ashes with sea water, filtered the extract and evaporated the water in caldrons—using peat for the fires. The remaining concentrate (more than 90 per cent salt) was dried beside the fire in small clay vessels. The final salt loaves represented money in prehistoric times, and they still do in parts of Africa. This use of salt as money is embedded in language; the word "salary" is one example.

In the span of northern European history from Neolithic times until the peat began to give out about 400 years ago, millions of tons of peat were harvested for salt. It was a cheap, convenient method and it made the civilization of northern Europe possible.

Sunshine, however, is cheaper, and it is inexhaustible. It is gratifying to note in this day of talk of harnessing solar energy that solar energy is already harnessed on a considerable scale to provide man with one of the chief necessities of life. Huge areas of the earth's sunny zones are devoted to solar saltmaking. Ocean water is pumped into flat, low-lying, diked compounds connected by canals; there the water evaporates under the sun and leaves a harvest of salt. It takes 50,000 cubic yards of sea water, spread over 100,000 square yards of flatland, to produce 1,000 tons of salt per year. This is enough to support the salt needs of a population of 100,000 comfortably.

Until a few years ago the techniques employed for producing and harvesting the salt were exactly the same as those invented thousands of years ago. New methods of treating the brine and more efficient pumping and harvesting are now improving the yields. Saltmaking, which includes fractional harvesting of the various salts of different solubility, is a high art.

Of all the basic necessities of life, salt is unique in that it is confined to certain limited locations. Men can make a living by hunting, fishing, raising animals and cultivating land over vast areas of the earth, but salt can come only from the comparatively few places where it is

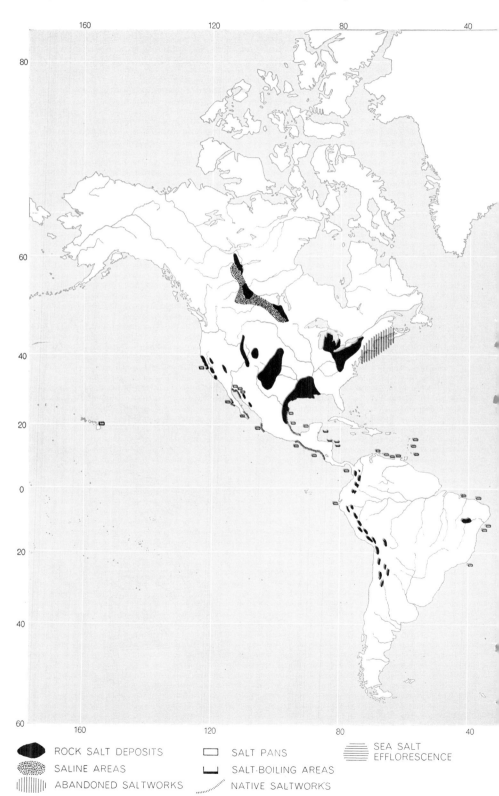

ROCK SALT DEPOSITS   SALT PANS   SEA SALT EFFLORESCENCE
SALINE AREAS   SALT-BOILING AREAS
ABANDONED SALTWORKS   NATIVE SALTWORKS

readily obtainable from salt lakes, mines, springs, or the ocean shores and means are at hand for extracting it. This fact, from the very beginning of civilization, has operated to make transport one of the cardinal necessities of civilized life.

To perceive this we need only look at the maps of the ancient civilizations. In Palestine agriculture spread up the Jordan River from the Dead Sea, and places such as Magdala on the Sea of Galilee became fishing and salting centers. In Egypt early farming depended

on boats bringing salt up the Nile from the salt swamps at the river mouth and on caravans bringing it in from the salt lakes in the deserts. In France the hinterland was nourished by salt carried up the Rhone from pans near Marseilles. The same pattern is visible in Mesopotamia,

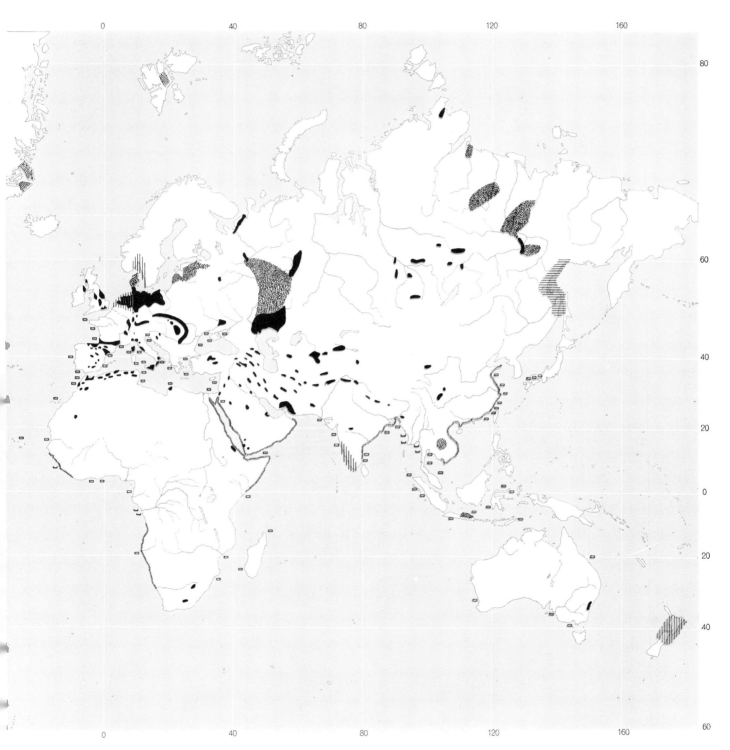

SALT IN ANCIENT TIMES was usually obtained from the types of source (*keyed at left*) indicated in the map on these two pages. Rock salt was generally dug directly out of the ground. "Saline areas" provided salt through soil compounds and salt springs. In "Salt-boiling areas" sea water or brine was boiled to produce salt. "Sea salt efflorescence" resulted from the freezing of sea water.

Persia, India, China and pre-Columbian Mexico.

River transportation was obviously the easiest. For so precious a commodity, however, every possible means was pressed into service. Caravans of camels, horses, donkeys and llamas carried salt across deserts and over mountains to salt-hungry populations. (A camel can carry some 300 pounds.) Up to a few

years ago a great caravan brought salt twice a year to Timbuktu in Mali from the Taodeni salt swamp in the Sahara Desert. To maintain Timbuktu, with its celebrated market, a caravan of 2,000 camels left the town semiannually on a 450-mile journey to the swamp for the single purpose of bringing back 300 tons of salt.

Salt was also an important item of

ocean-going commerce. Hundreds of ships plied the Atlantic and northern European waters to bring salt to the Netherlands, Britain, Scandinavia and Russia. Spain and Portugal traded salt to Africa, India and the Americas, and Britain later joined in this trade, shipping salt from Cheshire, where it was produced with the help of coal. In the time of the Hanseatic League, France sent salt by

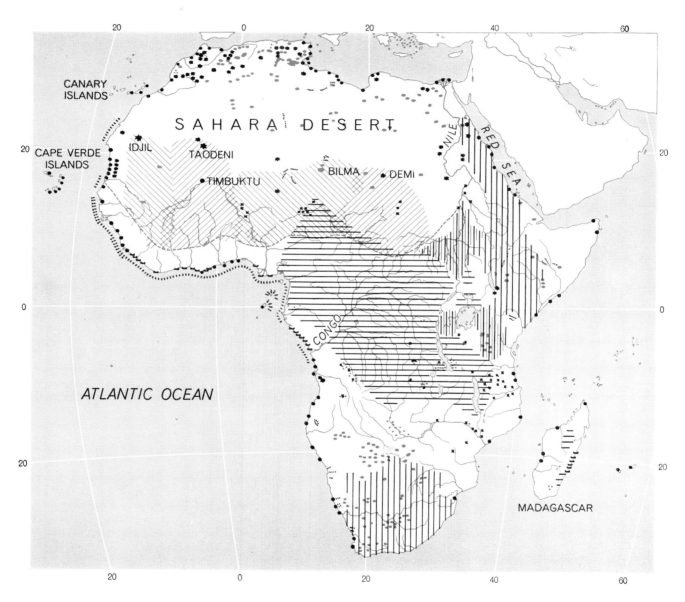

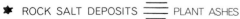 ROCK SALT DEPOSITS ═══ PLANT ASHES

✕ SALIFEROUS SOILS ‖‖‖ SALT FROM CONSUMPTION OF ANIMAL BLOOD

▒ SALT EFFLORESCENCE ‖‖‖ SALT FROM CONSUMPTION OF CATTLE URINE

⬮ SALT LAKES ⌇⌇⌇ SALT IMPORTS FROM EUROPE BEFORE 1800

· SALT SPRINGS ⌇⌇⌇ SALT IMPORTS FROM EUROPE AFTER 1800

▃ SALT-BOILING OPERATIONS

● NATURAL FORMATIONS OF SEA SALT OR SALIFEROUS BEACH DEPOSITS

⸼⸼ SOUTHERN LIMIT OF THE SALT TRADE SOUTH FROM THE SAHARA

SALT IN PRECOLONIAL AFRICA was sufficiently scarce to require the importation of salt as well as the exploitation of various native sources. The imports and different sources are keyed at left. The ashes of burned plants were used as condiments and as a substitute for normal salt. The hatched areas associated with Idjil, Taodeni, Bilma and Demi represent the areas in which salt from each of these sources was distributed.

the thousands of tons to the Baltic countries (the Baltic waters being relatively low in salt content). A single ship could carry more than 150 tons—as much as a caravan of 1,000 camels.

The salt trade, particularly the overland traffic, inevitably had military, social and political consequences. The caravans and ships, and the depots to which they delivered their salt, had to be protected against bandits and marauders. It became necessary to provide them with convoys and to fortify way stations, shipping ports and trading posts. In short, the system of "protection" came into existence. As the most valuable single commodity in commerce, salt required the services of powerful protectors.

A certain political pattern seems to emerge: where salt was plentiful, the society tended to be free, independent and democratic; where it was scarce, he who controlled the salt controlled the people.

In the very early settlement of Jericho the farmers pursued an independent existence and needed no fortifications to defend their abundant source of salt. (The town's famous walls were built later.) Along the shores of the Mediterranean and the North Sea, farmers and fishermen also nourished free societies. We know that the economy of the Athenians depended in considerable part on the salting of meat and hides, for which they sacrificed hundreds of cattle daily on the Acropolis. Salted fish was a staple of the diet throughout the Hellenistic world, thanks to the salty Mediterranean. Later the empire of the Caesars, utilizing the seacoasts and ocean coasts along its borders, was able to produce about a million tons of salt a year for the population of the empire, which is estimated to have totaled some 100 million.

In northern Europe the abundance of fish, peat and tidally shallow, salty seacoast allowed the Dutch, the English and the French to be more than self-sufficient. They were able to maintain small, independent communities that not only supported themselves but also sold their salted fish to markets as far away as the Mediterranean. In the Middle Ages the Dutch shipped salted herring to half of Europe. When peat and wood gave out, the English turned to coal as a fuel for saltmaking, and this use of coal made Britain the world's foremost salt producer during the 18th and 19th centuries.

In contrast, areas of the world that had to import most of their salt or

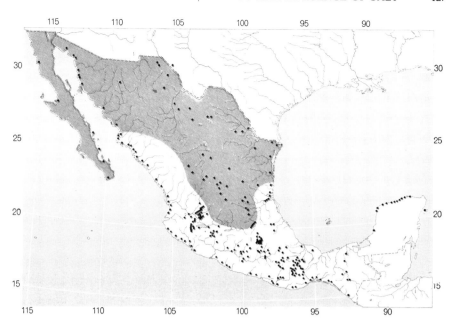

SALT IN PRE-COLUMBIAN MEXICO influenced the distribution of agricultural populations. This map shows available salt sources before (*dots*) and after the Spanish Conquest in 1519 (*crosses*). Most of the indigenous populations occupied southern Mexico (*unshaded*).

obtain it from small, isolated sources show a more autocratic pattern—a history of frequent conflict, monopoly and all-powerful rulers. In the ancient river-valley civilizations of the Nile, Babylon, India, China, Mexico and Peru the kings and priests maintained their rule and obtained their income through their monopoly of salt, on which the population was helplessly dependent. By their control of the military forces that guarded the stores of salt these rulers exercised a power of life and death over their people.

In middle Europe during Roman times salt was a focus of instability. Unlike the salt-rich Dutch, English and French, the German tribes fought wars over their meager salt sources, so Tacitus tells us, and small dukedoms consolidated around the centers of production located at Halle, Hallstatt, Seille and Lüneburg.

In Africa the scarcity of salt made it more precious than human freedom; it was, in fact, a most powerful factor in the slave trade. Families in the African interior sold children into slavery for a handful of salt. As recently as 1882 a traveler in British East Africa reported that he was offered a young girl for four loaves of salt.

Students of recent history will also recall that the salt monopoly and salt tax (*gabelle*) in France was one of the main causes of the French Revolution, and that Mahatma Gandhi climaxed his crusade for emancipation of the Indian

people by leading them in the famous salt march.

What is most startling in the whole salt story is that geological history has played a crucial but unappreciated role in the world's salt supply. Bear in mind that a large share of the salt (more than a third) is obtained from low-lying flat lands at the ocean's edge; that is, from natural or diked pans of sea water, which can be evaporated by the sun or by the use of fuel. What happens when the ocean rises because of melting of the glaciers?

We know that within the history of human civilization the sea level has risen and fallen periodically in what is called eustatic ebb and flow. From tracing old shore lines, from carbon-14 dating of plant and animal remains and from historical records, we can make a rough chart of these oscillations [*see illustration on page 98*]. It appears that after the last continental glaciation the average sea level rose some 20 feet and then settled down to a cycle of minor rises and falls.

At the height of the ancient Greek and Phoenician civilizations the sea level was more than three feet lower than it is today. For 1,000 years or so saltmaking in solar pans and in peat marshes flourished in the Mediterranean, the Atlantic and the North Sea. But the sea was rising. By A.D. 500 it had risen more than six feet (about three feet higher than it is now). This may seem a rather minor change. It was enough, however, to inundate most of the sea salt ponds all over the world!

The solar pans of Athlit in Palestine sank below sea level. So did those at Marseilles and Narbonne in France and at other places around the Mediterranean; only at the mouth of the Po River and a few other places did the salt pans survive. In northern Europe the marshes were similarly flooded and salt-making all but stopped. Only a few North Sea islands and Duurstede in the Netherlands provided any salt.

The effects on Europe were nearly catastrophic. The Belgian historian Henri Pirenne observes that Europe fell into an economic dark age. The salt traffic virtually disappeared; the coasts of Britain and France were deserted; the northern part of the continent became an "underdeveloped" area, and people began to

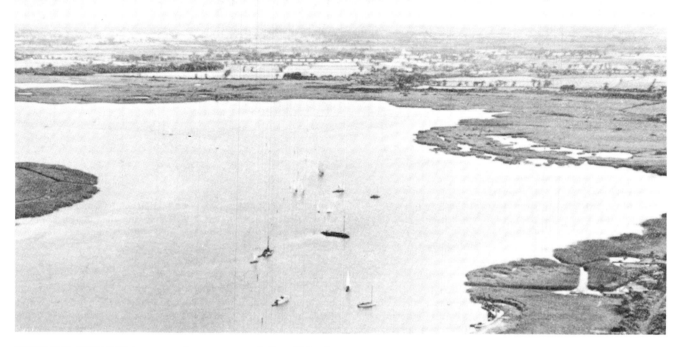

HICKLING "BROAD" is among the numerous shallow "lakes" and inlets on the east coast of England that were created by the removal of immense quantities of peat. The peat, soaked in sea water, was dried and burned for salt. This practice was prevalent from about the ninth until the 16th century, when the rising sea level flooded the areas and rendered them useless as sources of salt.

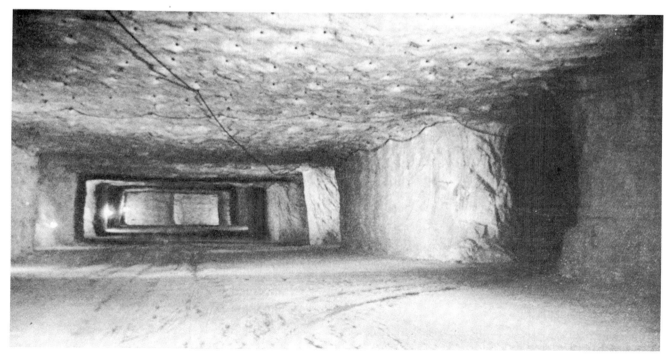

HUGE ROCK SALT DEPOSIT at the Fairport Harbor Mine of the Morton Salt Company near Cleveland is mined at a level 2,000 feet below the surface. "Room and pillar" mining has left pillars of rock salt to support the ceiling, which is about 18 feet high.

migrate to the more arid areas of the Mediterranean in quest of lifesaving salt.

The salt mines, the desert salt lakes and the Dead Sea became the saving sources for European civilization. This explains the otherwise senseless determination of the Roman emperors Vespasian and Titus to conquer the deserts around the Dead Sea. In the sixth century A.D. the ports and other towns of Palestine became great trade centers and grew to cities of 100,000 or more. For the salt and salted food they provided to the collapsing West they received gold, marble and other luxuries.

The sea receded, and Europe came back. By the 10th century the English, French and Dutch were again making salt in their peat bogs. Essex, according to the *Domesday Book* of the time of William the Conqueror, was operating hundreds of salt pans; the island of Yarmouth had revived as the center of Britain's fish-salting industry; and salt production was in full swing in Normandy, on the west coast of France, at the mouth of the Rhone, in Sicily and the Crimea.

The revival of European saltmaking brought invaders; Europe's population vacuum began to fill up violently. From the north the Norsemen took over the British and French salt centers; from the east the Arabs invaded France and clashed with the Norman conquerors in Provence.

In the 16th century the oscillating sea level again flooded saltmaking centers along the European coasts and made lakes of the peat excavations—now known as the "broads" of eastern England, the "meers" of the Netherlands and the "claires" of France. The rising

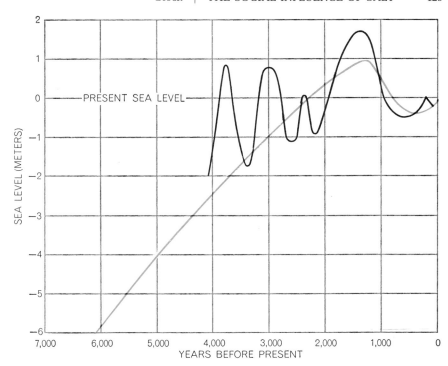

EUSTATIC CHANGES OF SEA LEVEL over the past 6,000 years have greatly affected the production of salt, as discussed in the text. In the past 4,000 years there have been small but important oscillations (*black curve*) in the over-all rise of sea level (*colored curve*).

tides covered part of the "red hills" in Essex and elsewhere on the shores of the North Sea; these hills were formed by the piling up of hundreds of thousands of tons of broken clay forms in which peat salt was cast over the centuries from Neolithic times on.

Recent rises in sea level have not gone as catastrophically high as during Europe's dark age. Industrialization has largely removed the danger of salt famine from the Western world. In the U.S., for example, large quantities of salt are produced from natural salt lakes, from rock salt and by drilling into deep underground salt deposits where water is pumped in and the brine pumped out —as well as from solar pans on the California coast.

Yet some 30 per cent of the world's salt is still obtained from seacoast solar ponds, which are vulnerable to a rise in sea level. Thus the small eustatic fluctuations of the ocean level may produce profound effects on human civilization in the future as they have in the past.

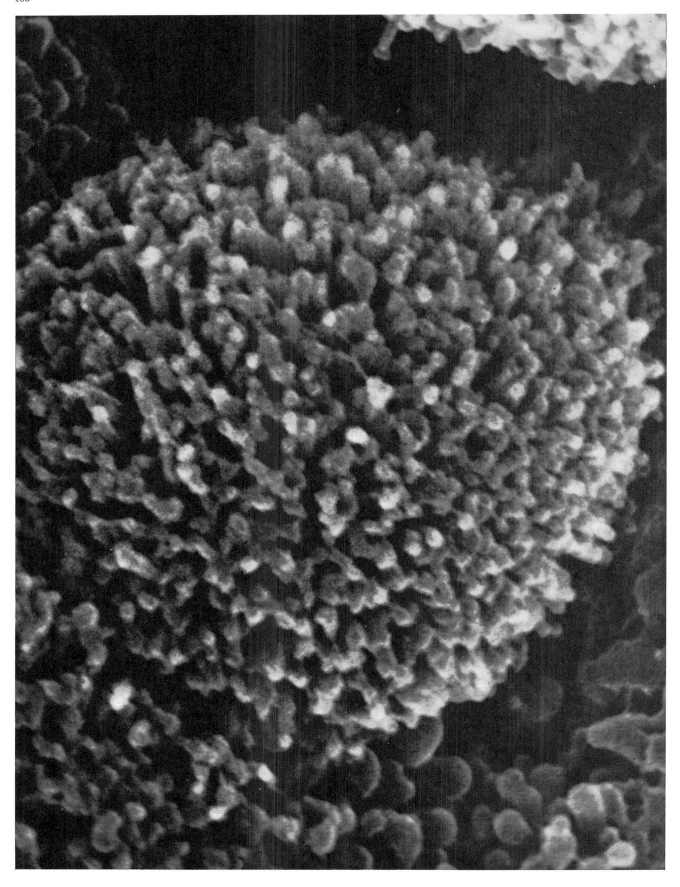

LACTOSE IS DIGESTED BY LACTASE in the intestine, a single epithelial cell of which is enlarged 37,500 diameters in this scanning electron micrograph made by Jeanne M. Riddle of the Wayne State University School of Medicine. The cell, on the surface of one of the finger-like villi that stud the lining of the intestine, is in turn covered by innumerable fine processes called microvilli.

Lactose and Lactase

14

by Norman Kretchmer
October 1972

Lactose is milk sugar; the enzyme lactase breaks it down. For want of lactase most adults cannot digest milk. In populations that drink milk the adults have more lactase, perhaps through natural selection

Milk is the universal food of newborn mammals, but some human infants cannot digest it because they lack sufficient quantities of lactase, the enzyme that breaks down lactose, or milk sugar. Adults of all animal species other than man also lack the enzyme—and so, it is now clear, do most human beings after between two and four years of age. That this general adult deficiency in lactase has come as a surprise to physiologists and nutritionists can perhaps be attributed to a kind of ethnic chauvinism, since the few human populations in which tolerance of lactose has been found to exceed intolerance include most northern European and white American ethnic groups.

Milk is a nearly complete human food, and in powdered form it can be conveniently stored and shipped long distances. Hence it is a popular source of protein and other nutrients in many programs of aid to nutritionally impoverished children, including American blacks. The discovery that many of these children are physiologically intolerant to lactose is therefore a matter of concern and its implications are currently being examined by such agencies as the U.S. Office of Child Development and the Protein Advisory Group of the United Nations System.

Lactose is one of the three major solid components of milk and its only carbohydrate; the other components are fats and proteins. Lactose is a disaccharide composed of the monosaccharides glucose and galactose. It is synthesized only by the cells of the lactating mammary gland, through the reaction of glucose with the compound uridine diphosphate galactose [*see illustrations on next page*]. One of the proteins found in milk, alpha-lactalbumin, is required for the synthesis of lactose. This protein apparently does not actually enter into the reaction; what it does is "specify" the action of the enzyme galactosyl transferase, modifying the enzyme so that in the presence of alpha-lactalbumin and glucose it catalyzes the synthesis of lactose.

In the nonlactating mammary gland, where alpha-lactalbumin is not present, the enzyme synthesizes instead of lactose a more complicated carbohydrate, N-acetyl lactosamine. Test-tube studies have shown that alpha-lactalbumin is manufactured only in the presence of certain hormones: insulin, cortisone, estrogen and prolactin; its synthesis is inhibited by the hormone progesterone. It is when progesterone levels decrease late in pregnancy that the manufacture of alpha-lactalbumin, and thus of lactose, is initiated [see "Milk," by Stuart Patton; SCIENTIFIC AMERICAN Offprint 1147].

The concentration of lactose in milk from different sources varies considerably. Human milk is the sweetest, with 7.5 grams of lactose per 100 milliliters of milk. Cow's milk has 4.5 grams per 100 milliliters. The only mammals that do not have any lactose—or any other carbohydrate—in their milk are certain of the Pinnipedia: the seals, sea lions and walruses of the Pacific basin. If these animals are given lactose in any form, they become sick. (In 1933 there was a report of a baby walrus that was fed cow's milk while being shipped from Alaska to California. The animal suffered from severe diarrhea throughout the voyage and was very sick by the time it arrived in San Diego.) Of these pinnipeds the California sea lion has been the most intensively studied. No alpha-lactalbumin is synthesized by its mammary gland. When alpha-lactalbumin from either rat's milk or cow's milk is added to a preparation of sea lion mammary gland in a test tube, however, the glandular tissue does manufacture lactose.

In general, low concentrations of lactose are associated with high concentrations of milk fat (which is particularly useful to marine mammals). The Pacific pinnipeds have more than 35 grams of fat per 100 milliliters of milk, compared with less than four grams in the cow. In the whale and the bear (an ancient ancestor of which may also be an ancestor of the Pacific pinnipeds) the lactose in milk is low and the fat content is high.

Lactase, the enzyme that breaks down lactose ingested in milk or a milk product, is a specific intestinal beta-galactosidase that acts only on lactose, primarily in the jejunum, the second of the small intestine's three main segments. The functional units of the wall of the small intestine are the villus (composed of metabolically active, differentiated, nondividing cells) and the crypt (a set of dividing cells from which those of the villus are derived). Lactase is not present in the dividing cells. It appears in the differentiated cells, specifically within the brush border of the cells at the surface of the villus [*see illustrations on page 134*]. Lactase splits the disaccharide lactose into its two component monosaccharides, glucose and galactose. Some of the released glucose can be utilized directly by the cells of the villus; the remainder, along with the galactose, enters the bloodstream, and both sugars are metabolized by the liver. Neither Gary Gray of the Stanford University School of Medicine nor other investigators have been able to distinguish any qualitative biochemical or physical difference among the lactases isolated from the intestine of infants, tolerant adults and intolerant adults. The difference appears to be

LACTOSE, a disaccharide composed of the monosaccharides glucose and galactose, is the carbohydrate of milk, the other major components of which are fats, proteins and water.

merely quantitative; there is simply very little lactase in the intestine of a lactose-intolerant person. In the intestine of Pacific pinnipeds, Philip Sunshine of the Stanford School of Medicine found, there is no lactase at all, even in infancy.

Lactase is not present in the intestine of the embryo or the fetus until the middle of the last stage of gestation. Its activity attains a maximum immediately after birth. Thereafter it decreases, reaching a low level, for example, immediately after weaning in the rat and after one and a half to three years in most children. The exact mechanism involved in the appearance and disappearance of the lactase is not known, but such a pattern of waxing and waning activity is common in the course of development; in general terms, one can say that it results from differential action of the gene or genes concerned.

Soon after the turn of the century the distinguished American pediatrician Abraham Jacobi pointed out that diarrhea in babies could be associated with the ingestion of carbohydrates. In 1921 another pediatrician, John Howland, said that "there is with many patients an abnormal response on the part of the intestinal tract to carbohydrates, which expresses itself in the form of diarrhea and excessive fermentation." He suggested as the cause a deficiency in the hydrolysis, or enzymatic breakdown, of lactose.

The physiology is now well established. If the amount of lactose presented to the intestinal cells exceeds the hydrolytic capacity of the available lactase (whether because the lactase level is low or because an unusually large amount of lactose is ingested), a portion of the lactose remains undigested. Some of it passes into the blood and is eventually excreted in the urine. The remainder moves on into the large intestine, where two processes ensue. One is physical: the lactose molecules increase the particle content of the intestinal fluid compared with the fluid in cells outside the intestine and therefore by osmotic action draw water out of the tissues into the intestine. The other is biochemical: the glucose is fermented by the bacteria in the colon. Organic acids and carbon dioxide are generated and the symptoms can be those of any fermentative diarrhea, including a bloated feeling, flatulence, belching, cramps and a watery, explosive diarrhea.

At the end of the 1950's Paolo Durand of the University of Genoa and Aaron Holzel and his colleagues at the University of Manchester reported detailed studies of infants who were unable to digest lactose and who reacted to milk sugar with severe diarrhea, malnutrition and even death. This work stimulated a revival of interest in lactose and lactase, and there followed a period of active investigation of lactose intolerance. Many cases were reported, including some in which lactase inactivity could be demonstrated in tissue taken from the patient's intestine by biopsy. It became clear that intolerance in infants could be a congenital condition (as in Holzel's two patients, who were siblings) or, more frequently, could be secondary to various diseases and other stresses: cystic fibrosis, celiac disease, malnutrition, the ingestion of certain drugs, surgery and even non-

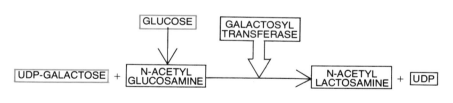

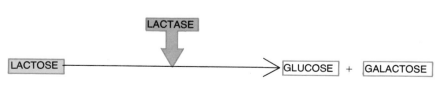

SYNTHESIS OF LACTOSE in the mammary gland begins late in pregnancy when specific hormones and the protein alpha-lactalbumin are present. The latter modifies the enzyme galactosyl transferase, "specifying" it so that it catalyzes the synthesis of lactose from glucose and galactose (top). In the nonlactating gland the glucose takes part in a different reaction (middle). In intestine lactase breaks down lactose to glucose and galactose (bottom).

specific diarrhea. During this period of investigation, it should be noted, intolerance to lactose was generally assumed to be the unusual condition and the condition worthy of study.

In 1965 Pedro Cuatrecasas and his colleagues and Theodore M. Bayless and Norton S. Rosensweig, all of whom were then at the Johns Hopkins School of Medicine, administered lactose to American blacks and whites, none of whom had had gastrointestinal complaints, and reported some startling findings. Whereas only from 6 to 15 percent of the whites showed clinical symptoms of intolerance, about 70 percent of the blacks were intolerant. This immediately suggested that many human adults might be unable to digest lactose and, more specifically, that there might be significant differences among ethnic groups. The possibility was soon confirmed: G. C. Cook and S. Kajubi of Makerere University College examined two different tribes in Uganda. They found that only 20 percent of the adults of the cattle-herding Tussi tribe were intolerant to lactose but that 80 percent of the nonpastoral Ganda were intolerant. Soon one paper after another reported a general intolerance to lactose among many ethnic groups, including Japanese, other Orientals, Jews in Israel, Eskimos and South American Indians.

In these studies various measures of intolerance were applied. One was the appearance of clinical symptoms—flatulence and diarrhea—after the ingestion of a dose of lactose, which was generally standardized at two grams of lactose per kilogram (2.2 pounds) of body weight, up to a maximum of either 50 or 100 grams. Another measure was a finding of low lactase activity (less than two units per gram of wet weight of tissue) determined through an intestinal biopsy after ingestion of the same dose of lactose. A third was an elevation of blood glucose of less than 20 milligrams per 100 milliliters of blood after ingestion of the lactose. Since clinical symptoms are variable and the biopsy method is inconvenient for the subject being tested, the blood glucose method is preferable. It is a direct measure of lactose breakdown, and false-negative results are rare if the glucose is measured 15 minutes after lactose is administered.

By 1970 enough data had been accumulated to indicate that many more groups all over the world are intolerant to lactose than are tolerant. As a matter of fact, real adult tolerance to lactose has so far been observed only in northern Europeans, approximately 90 percent of whom tolerate lactose, and in the

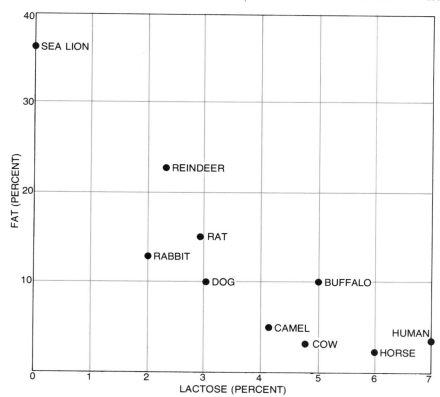

CONCENTRATION OF LACTOSE varies with the source of the milk. In general the less lactose, the more fat, which can also be utilized by the newborn animal as an energy source.

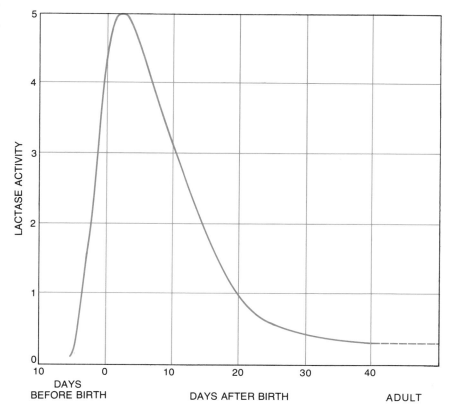

LACTASE is present in mammals other than man, and in most humans, in the fetus before birth and in infancy. The general shape of the curve of enzyme activity, shown here for the rat, is about the same in all species. Enzyme activity, given here in relative units, is determined by measuring glucose release from intestinal tissue in the presence of lactose.

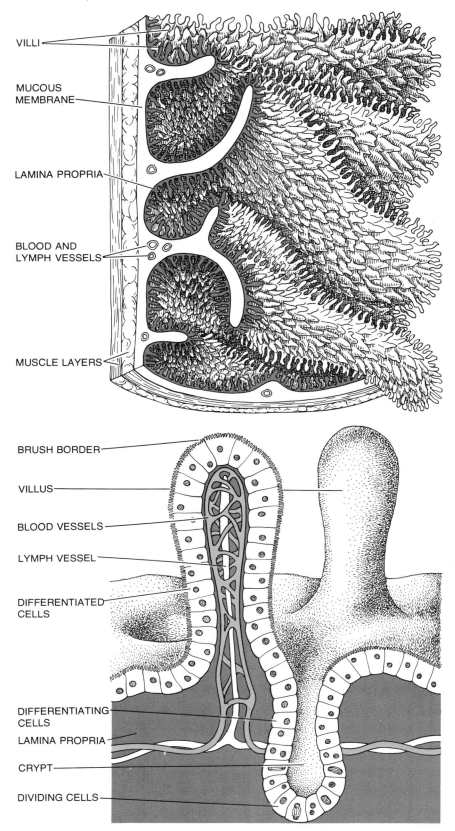

VILLI

MUCOUS MEMBRANE

LAMINA PROPRIA

BLOOD AND LYMPH VESSELS

MUSCLE LAYERS

BRUSH BORDER

VILLUS

BLOOD VESSELS

LYMPH VESSEL

DIFFERENTIATED CELLS

DIFFERENTIATING CELLS

LAMINA PROPRIA

CRYPT

DIVIDING CELLS

WALL OF SMALL INTESTINE, seen in longitudinal section (*top*), has outer muscle layers, a submucosa layer and an inner mucous membrane. The mucous membrane (*bottom*) has a connective-tissue layer (lamina propria), which contains blood and lymph capillaries, and an inner surface of epithelial cells. The cells multiply and differentiate in the crypts and migrate to the villi. At what stage the lactase is manufactured is not known; it is found primarily in the microvilli, which constitute the brush border of the differentiated cells.

members of two nomadic pastoral tribes in Africa, of whom about 80 percent are tolerant. Although many other generally tolerant groups will be found, they will always belong to a minority of the human species. In this situation it is clearly more interesting and potentially more fruitful to focus the investigation on tolerant people in an effort to explain adult tolerance, a characteristic in which man differs from all other mammals.

There are two kinds of explanation of adult tolerance to lactose. The first, and perhaps the most immediately apparent, originates with the fact that most people who tolerate lactose have a history of drinking milk. Maybe the mere presence of milk in the diet suffices to stimulate lactase activity in the individual, perhaps by "turning on" genes that encode the synthesis of the enzyme. Individual enzymatic adaptation to an environmental stimulus is well known, but it is not transferable genetically. The other explanation of tolerance is based on the concept of evolution through natural selection. If in particular populations it became biologically advantageous to be able to digest milk, then the survival of individuals with a genetic mutation that led to higher intestinal lactase activity in adulthood would have been favored. An individual who derived his ability to digest lactose from this classical form of Darwinian adaptation would be expected to be able to transfer the trait genetically.

These two points of view have become the subject of considerable controversy. I suspect that each of the explanations is valid for some of the adult tolerance being observed, and I should like to examine both of them.

The possibility of individual adaptation to lactose has been considered since the beginning of the century, usually through attempts to relate lactase activity to the concentration of milk in the diet of animals. Almost without exception the studies showed that although there was a slight increase in lactase activity when a constant diet of milk or milk products was consumed, there was no significant change in the characteristic curve reflecting the developmental rise and fall of enzymatic activity. Recently there have been reports pointing toward adaptation, however. Some studies, with human subjects as well as rats, indicated that continued intensive feeding of milk or lactose not only made it possible for the individual to tolerate the sugar but also resulted in a measurable increase in lactase activity. The discrepancy among the findings could be partly attributable to improvement in methods for assaying the enzyme activity.

On balance it would appear that individual adaptation may be able to explain at least some cases of adult tolerance. I shall cite two recent studies. John Godell, working in Lagos, selected six Nigerian medical students who were absolutely intolerant to lactose and who showed no physiological evidence of lactose hydrolysis. He fed them increasing amounts of the sugar for six months. Godell found that although the students did develop tolerance for the lactose, there was nevertheless no evidence of an increase of glucose in the blood—and thus of enzymatic adaptation—following test doses of the sugar. The conjecture is that the diet brought about a change in the bacterial flora in the intestine, and that the ingested lactose was being metabolized by the new bacteria.

In our laboratory at the Stanford School of Medicine Emanuel Lebenthal and Sunshine found that in rats given lactose the usual pattern of a developmental decrease in lactase activity is maintained but the activity level is somewhat higher at the end of the experiment. The rise in activity does not appear to be the result of an actual increase in lactase synthesis, however. We treated the rats with actinomycin, which prevents the synthesis of new protein from newly activated genes. The actinomycin had no effect on the slight increase in lactase activity, indicating that the mechanism leading to the increase was not gene activation. It appears, rather, that the presence of additional amounts of the enzyme's substrate, lactose, somehow "protects" the lactase from degradation. Such a process has been noted in many other enzyme-substrate systems. The additional lactase activity that results from this protection is sufficient to improve the rat's tolerance of lactose, but that additional activity is dependent on the continued presence of the lactose.

Testing the second hypothesis—that adult lactose tolerance is primarily the result of a long-term process of genetic selection—is more complicated. It involves data and reasoning from such disparate areas as history, anthropology, nutrition, genetics and sociology as well as biochemistry.

As I have noted, the work of Cuatrecasas, of Bayless and Rosensweig and of Cook and Kajubi in the mid-1960's pointed to the likelihood of significant differences in adult lactose tolerance among ethnic groups. It also suggested that one ought to study in particular black Americans and their ancestral pop-

ulations in Africa. The west coast of Africa was the primary source of slaves for the New World. With the objective of studying lactose tolerance in Nigeria, we developed a joint project with a group from the University of Lagos Teaching Hospital headed by Olikoye Ransome-Kuti.

The four largest ethnic groups in Nigeria are the Yoruba in western Nigeria, the Ibo in the east and the Fulani and Hausa in the north. These groups have different origins and primary occupations. The Yoruba and the Ibo differ somewhat anthropometrically, but both are Negro ethnic groups that probably came originally from the Congo Basin; they were hunters and gatherers who became farmers. They eventually settled south of the Niger and Benue rivers in an area infested with the tsetse fly, so that they never acquired cattle (or any other beast of burden). Hence it was not until recent times that milk appeared in their diet beyond the age of weaning. After the colonization of their part of Nigeria by the British late in the 19th century, a number of Yoruba and Ibo, motivated by their intense desire for education, migrated to England and northern Europe; they acquired Western dietary habits and in some cases Western spouses, and many eventually returned to Nigeria.

The Fulani are Hamites who have been pastoral people for thousands of years, originally perhaps in western Asia and more recently in northwestern Africa. Wherever they went, they took their cattle with them, and many of the Fulani are still nomads who herd their cattle from one grazing ground to another. About 300 years ago the Fulani appeared in what is now Nigeria and waged war on the Hausa. (The Fulani also tried to invade Yorubaland but were defeated by the tsetse fly.) After the invasion of the Hausa region some of the Fulani moved into villages and towns.

As a result of intermarriage between the Fulani and the Hausa there appeared a new group known as the town-Fulani or the Hausa-Fulani, whose members no longer raise cattle and whose ingestion of lactose is quite different from that of the pastoral Fulani. The pastoral Fulani do their milking in the early morning and drink some fresh milk. The milk reaches the market in the villages and towns only in a fermented form, however, as a kind of yogurt called *nono*. As the *nono* stands in the morning sun it becomes a completely fermented, watery preparation, which is then thickened with millet or some other cereal. The final product is almost completely

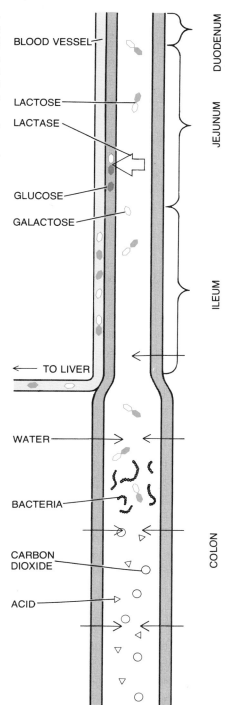

DIGESTION OF LACTOSE is accomplished primarily in the jejunum, where lactase splits it into glucose and galactose. Some glucose is utilized locally; the rest enters the bloodstream with the galactose and both are utilized in the liver. In the absence of enough lactase some undigested lactose enters the bloodstream; most goes on into the ileum and the colon, where it draws water from the tissues into the intestine by osmotic action. The undigested lactose is also fermented by bacteria in the colon, giving rise to various acids and carbon dioxide gas.

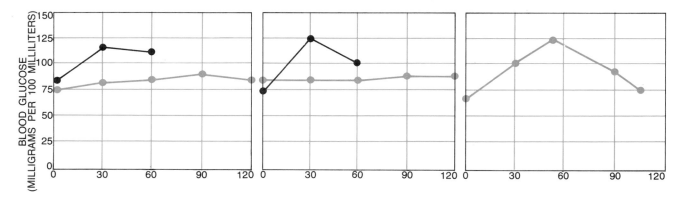

LACTOSE INTOLERANCE is determined by measuring blood glucose after ingestion of lactose. The absence of a significant rise in blood glucose after lactose ingestion (*color*) as contrasted with a rise in blood glucose after ingestion of sucrose, another sugar (*black*), indicates that a Yoruba male (*left*) and an American Jewish male (*middle*) are lactose-intolerant. On the other hand, the definite rise in blood glucose after ingestion of lactose in a Fulani male (*right*) shows that the Fulani is tolerant to lactose.

free of lactose and can be ingested without trouble even by a person who cannot digest lactose.

We tested members of each of these Nigerian populations. Of all the Yorubas above the age of four who were tested, we found only one person in whom the blood glucose rose to more than 20 milligrams per 100 milliliters following administration of the test dose of lactose. She was a nurse who had spent six years in the United Kingdom and had grown accustomed to a British diet that included milk. At first, she said, the milk disagreed with her, but later she could tolerate it with no adverse side effects. None of the Ibos who were studied showed an elevation of glucose in blood greater than 20 milligrams per 100 milliliters. (The major problem in all these studies is determining ethnic purity. All the Yorubas and Ibos who participated in this portion of the study indicated that there had been no intermarriages in their families.) Most of the Hausa and Hausa-Fulani

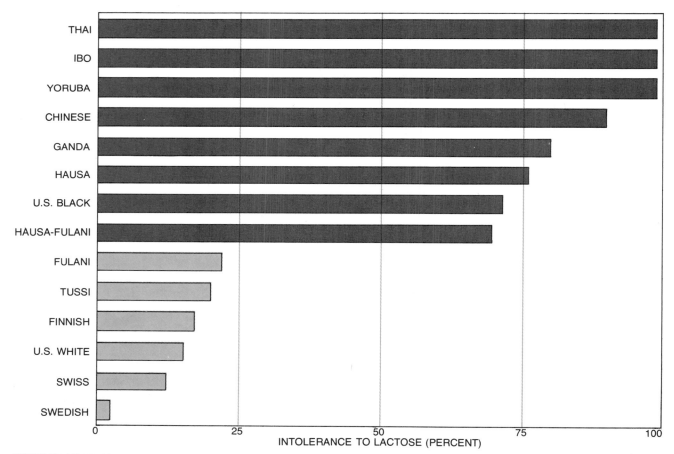

INTOLERANCE VARIES WIDELY among populations. The bars are based on tests conducted by a number of investigators by different methods; they may not be strictly comparable or accurately reflect the situation in entire populations. Among the groups studied to date lactose intolerance is prevalent except among northern Europeans (and their descendants) and herders in Africa.

(70 to 80 percent) were intolerant to lactose. In contrast most of the nomadic Fulani (78 percent) were tolerant to it. In their ability to hydrolyze lactose they resembled the pastoral Tussi of Uganda and northern Europeans more than they resembled their nearest neighbors.

Once the distribution of lactose intolerance and tolerance was determined in the major Nigerian populations, we went on to study the genetics of the situation by determining the results of mixed marriages. One of the common marriages in western Nigeria is between a Yoruba male and a British or other northern European female; the reverse situation is less common. Our tests showed that when a tolerant northern European marries a lactose-intolerant Yoruba, the offspring are most likely to be lactose-tolerant. If a tolerant child resulting from such a marriage marries a pure Yoruba, then the children are also predominantly tolerant. There is no sex linkage of the genes involved: in the few cases in which a Yoruba female had married a northern European male, the children were predominantly tolerant.

On the basis of these findings one can say that lactose tolerance is transmitted genetically and is dominant, that is, genes for tolerance from one of the parents are sufficient to make the child tolerant. On the other hand, the children of two pure Yorubas are always intolerant to lactose, as are the children of a lactose-intolerant European female and a Yoruba male. In other words, intolerance is also transmitted genetically and is probably a recessive trait, that is, both parents must be lactose-intolerant to produce an intolerant child. When the town-dwelling royal line of the Fulani was investigated, its members were all found to be unable to digest lactose—except for the children of one wife, a pastoral Fulani, who were tolerant.

Among the children of Yoruba-European marriages the genetic cross occurred one generation ago or at the most two generations. Among the Hausa-Fulani it may have been as much as 15 generations ago. This should explain the general intolerance of the Hausa-Fulani. Presumably the initial offspring of the lactose-tolerant Fulani and the lactose-intolerant Hausa were predominantly tolerant. As the generations passed, however, intolerance again became more prevalent. The genes for lactase can therefore be considered incompletely dominant.

The blacks brought to America were primarily Yoruba or Ibo or similar West African peoples who were originally

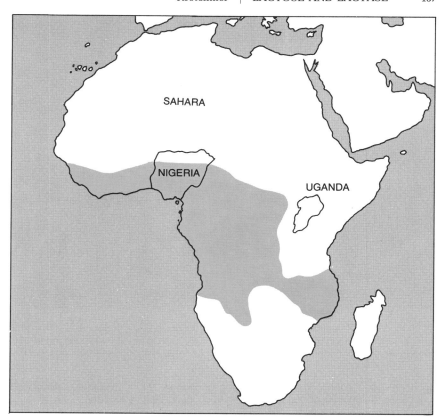

GEOGRAPHICAL EXTENT of dairying coincides roughly with areas of general lactose tolerance. According to Frederick J. Simoons of the University of California at Davis, there is a broad belt (color) across Africa in which dairying is not traditional. Migrations affect the tolerance pattern, however. For example, the Ganda, a lactose-intolerant group living in Uganda, came to that milk-drinking region from the nonmilking central Congo.

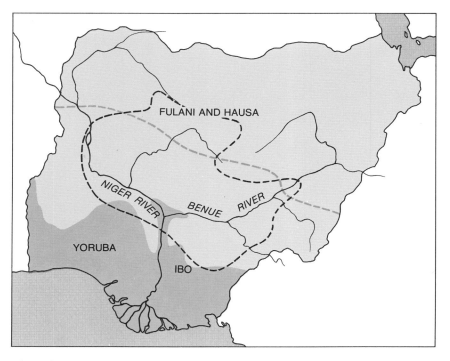

LARGEST ETHNIC GROUPS in Nigeria are the Ibo in the east, the Yoruba in the west and the Hausa and Fulani in the north. Map shows regions of mangrove swamp or forest (dark color) and grassland or desert (light color). Southern livestock limit (broken colored line) is set by climate, vegetation and tsetse fly infestation (broken black line).

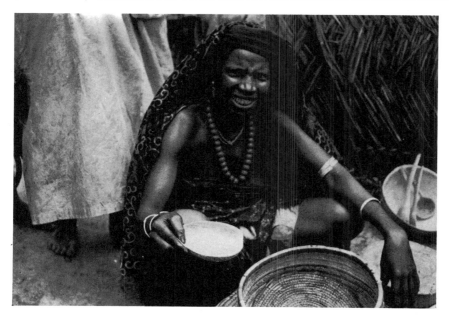

FULANI WOMAN offers *nono*, a yogurt-like milk drink, for sale in the marketplace of a town in northern Nigeria. The pastoral Fulani drink fresh milk. The partially fermented *nono*, with reduced lactose content, is tolerated by villagers who could not digest milk.

intolerant to lactose. American blacks have been in this country for between 10 and 15 generations, in the course of which a certain complement of white northern European genes has entered the black population. Presumably as a result lactose intolerance among American blacks has been reduced to approximately 70 percent. One can speculate that if this gene flow eventually stopped, lactose intolerance would approach 100 percent among American blacks.

What events in human cultural history might have influenced the development of tolerance to lactose in the adults of some groups? Frederick J. Si-moons of the University of California at Davis has proposed a hypothesis based on the development of dairying. It would appear that the milking of cattle, sheep, goats or reindeer did not begin until about 10,000 years ago, some 100 million years after the origin of mammals and therefore long after the mammalian developmental pattern of lactase activity had been well established. Man presumably shared that pattern, and so adults were intolerant to lactose. When some small groups of humans began to milk animals, a selective advantage was conferred on individuals who, because of a chance mutation, had high enough lactase activity to digest lactose. A person who could not digest lactose might have difficulty in a society that ingested nonfermented milk or milk products, but the lactose-tolerant individual was more adaptable: he could survive perfectly well in either a milk-drinking or a non-milk-drinking society.

The genetic mutation resulting in the capability to digest lactose probably occurred at least 10,000 years ago. People tivity could be members of a dairying culture, utilize their own product for food (as the Fulani do today) and then sell it in the form of a yogurt (as the Fulani do) or cheese to the general, lactose-intolerant population. These statements are presumptions, not facts, but they are based soundly on the idea that tolerance to lactose is a mutation that endowed the individual with a nutritional genetic advantage and on the basic assumption, which is supported by fact, that lactose intolerance is the normal genetic state of adult man and that lactose tolerance is in a sense abnormal.

What are the implications of all of this for nutrition policy? It should be pointed out that many people who are intolerant to lactose are nevertheless able to drink some milk or eat some milk products; the relation of clinical symptoms to lactose ingestion is quantitative. For most people, even after the age of four, drinking moderate amounts of milk has no adverse effects and is actually nutritionally beneficial. It may well be, however, that programs of indiscriminate, large-scale distribution of milk powder to intolerant populations should be modified, or that current moves toward supplying lactose-free milk powder should be encouraged.

IV

NUTRIENTS REQUIRED BY MAN AND THEIR UTILIZATION

IV

NUTRIENTS
REQUIRED BY MAN
AND THEIR UTILIZATION

INTRODUCTION

The fundamental processes of all living matter—energy transfer, development of structure, growth, and reproduction—are determined by simple and complex molecules present in all species. This underlying similarity of life processes is reflected in the elemental composition of living forms. In all species, carbon, oxygen, hydrogen, nitrogen, phosphorous, and sulfur are present in similar proportions and account for over 99 percent of an organism's mass. Irrespective of this basic uniformity of life processes, millions of species of animals and plants have evolved, each different from the others. And although of the thousands of different compounds that make up an organism the basic ones are the same in all species, many of the more complex molecules are unique to the species; some are even specific to individuals within a species.

If one were to compare the structures of the thousands of chemical compounds contained in foods with the chemicals that make up a human body, it would become obvious that the only way molecules that make up the organism can be synthesized from food is for the food to be broken down into small simple molecules. These small molecules are used for energy and for the synthesis of molecules characteristic of human protoplasm. Together with other compounds that the organism takes in and cannot synthesize for itself, these small molecules are the essential nutrients.

The outstanding achievement of nutritional science has been the isolation, and determination of structure, of the approximately 50 nutrients essential for man. The molecular role of many of these nutrients in metabolic processes has been elucidated. Diseases associated with lack of an essential nutrient have been identified and are consequently now curable or preventable.

By the end of the nineteenth century those nutrients needed most had been identified. Carbohydrates and fats were recognized as needed sources of energy. Protein (but not the individual amino acids) and an ill-defined group of minerals were known to be essential. In 1903 F. Gowland Hopkins recognized the need for accessory, organic growth factors, now known as vitamins. Subsequently, 16 different vitamins, 9 amino acids, and a group of highly unsaturated fatty acids were identified as essential for man. The list of essential organic nutrients was probably completed by mid-century, with the discovery of vitamin B-12. The article "Biotin" by John D. Woodward relates the story of one of the last vitamins to be discovered.

The discovery of inorganic nutrients has proceeded along with that of the vitamins. We now recognize as essential at least 18 elements that may be supplied as inorganic compounds. Additional elements may be needed, but in such small quantities that they are present in adequate quantities in all but the most highly purified diets. In "The Chemical Elements of Life" Earl Frieden tells of the search to identify other essential trace elements.

It is as important to know how much of each nutrient is required as to know which nutrients are essential in diet. Because we are each unique in structure, function, activity, stage of development, and reaction to environment, determination of individual requirements has proven quite difficult. Requirements determined for experimental animals can only serve as gross approximations of requirements for human beings. Nevertheless, even with incomplete data, it is desirable to make practical recommendations. Nevin Scrimshaw and Vernon Young describe the factors affecting recommended dietary allowances in "Human Nutritional Requirements."

Knowledge of the essential nutrients and the approximate amounts required by man has permitted the development of chemically defined diets, using synthetic or purified chemicals. These diets have been used in experimental or therapeutic situations. On synthetic diets adults have remained well and active and children have grown normally for several years. A further development of this principle has been the ability to develop feeding mixtures that completely bypass the intestine. These diets are particularly useful in patients with diseases of the alimentary tract. Stanley Dudrick and Jonathan Rhoads discuss this technique in "Total Intravenous Feeding." Since the publication of this article in 1972, techniques have been developed for emulsifying unsaturated fatty acids in a form suitable for intravenous feeding, so that it is now possible to supply a completely adequate diet parenterally.

The polyunsaturated fatty acids were shown to be essential nutrients 40 years ago. The exact function of these compounds remained unknown until recently, despite considerable research. In "Prostaglandins" John Pike describes how an apparently unrelated observation in reproductive biology led to the elucidation of how polyunsaturated fatty acids are chemically modified by the body to become potent regulators of metabolic processes.

15   Biotin

John D. Woodward
June 1961

*This little known but remarkably potent member of
the family of B vitamins has been a biochemical
puzzle for three decades. The details of its functions
are only now beginning to emerge*

Hardly anyone who is not a biologist or a biochemist will have heard of biotin. The name of this vitamin does not appear on the labels of tonics and vitamin pills; dietitians do not compile lists of foods that contain it. Perhaps there has never been a case of natural biotin deficiency. Yet anyone deprived of the minute traces of the substance that are required by probably every cell of the body would surely die.

The requirement is extremely small, and biotin is widely distributed. From the point of view of nutrition it can safely be ignored. Nevertheless the amazingly potent vitamin has fascinated biochemists for many years. Since the turn of the century different workers have "discovered" it at least three times and given it half a dozen names. About 20 years ago the diverse lines of research were finally brought together, and the names were shown to apply to a single substance. The chemical structure of biotin was worked out soon afterward. But the job of discovering its essential function, or functions, in the chemistry of living cells has barely begun.

The story goes back to 1901 and some experiments of the Belgian microbiologist E. Wildiers on the culture of yeast cells. His simple medium contained all the nutrients then thought to be essential, but the cells often grew poorly. He found he could obtain normal growth by adding small amounts of brewer's wort (an extract of ground malt) or extracts of dead yeast cells. The extracts evidently contained an unknown nutrient; Wildiers named it "Bios."

It was many years before Wildiers's observations gained general acceptance. Eventually it became clear that his hypothetical material represented not one but a number of distinct growth factors—water-soluble B vitamins including the now familiar thiamin (B_1), riboflavin (B_2), pyridoxine (B_6) and nicotinic acid (pellagra-preventive factor). One of the Bios fractions, unlike the others, was readily adsorbed by charcoal and so could be separated, at least partially, from the rest of the complex.

In the early 1930's this fraction, designated II*b*, attracted the attention of Fritz Kögl, an organic chemist at the University of Utrecht. Up to that time all the known sources of Bios II*b* contained it in exceedingly tiny amounts, so Kögl began by looking for a richer raw material. Egg yolk was one of the best sources he could find. By 1936 Kögl and B. Tönnis succeeded in isolating about a milligram (less than .00004 ounce) of "beautiful crystals" that strongly promoted the growth of yeast. This scarcely visible quantity they had extracted, in a series of 16 different and tedious steps, from 550 pounds of dried duck-egg yolks. With so small a sample they could do little more than determine the melting point of the crystals. The great biological activity of the substance in yeast cultures, however, convinced the chemists that they had found the active principle of Bios II*b*. They called the elusive compound biotin.

At about the time that Kögl was beginning his research, Franklin E. Allison and his colleagues in the Bureau of Chemistry and Soils of the U. S. Department of Agriculture embarked on a study of another microorganism, the nitrogen-fixing bacterium *Rhizobium trifolii*. They found that the growth and respiration of this organism were stimulated by extracts from various organic sources. Because they believed that an unknown factor in the extracts acted in conjunction with an enzyme, they called the factor coenzyme R (for "respiration"). Philip M. West and P. W. Wilson at the University of Wisconsin noted a similarity between the growth-promoting effects of coenzyme R and of biotin. This suggested that they might be the same substance hiding behind different names. By then Kögl had improved his extraction methods and had a larger supply of crystalline biotin. A test of the material on a culture of *Rhizobium* was made by R. Nilsson, G. Bjälfe and D. Burström of the University of Uppsala in Sweden; they found it to have exactly the same stimulating effects as coenzyme R. In this respect, at least, the two were identical.

The next chapter of the story is drawn from the field of animal nutrition. It opens with a flashback to 1916, when W. G. Bateman of Yale University made the casual observation that raw egg white in the diet of animals had a toxic effect. Nothing came of this until 11 years later, when Margaret A. Boas at the Lister Institute of Preventive Medicine in London happened on the same phenomenon. She was using raw egg white as a source of protein in the diet of rats. After a few weeks the animals developed dermatitis and hemorrhages of the skin; their hair fell out; their limbs became paralyzed; they lost considerable weight and eventually they died. Only raw or cold-dried egg white produced the symptoms. Cooking made it harmless. Subsequent investigation showed that the effects of raw egg white could be alleviated or prevented by any one of a variety of foodstuffs. The action was thought to be due to a substance, common to all these foods, that was dubbed protective factor X.

The search for the protective factor was taken up by Paul György, originally at the University of Heidelberg and later at the University of Cambridge and

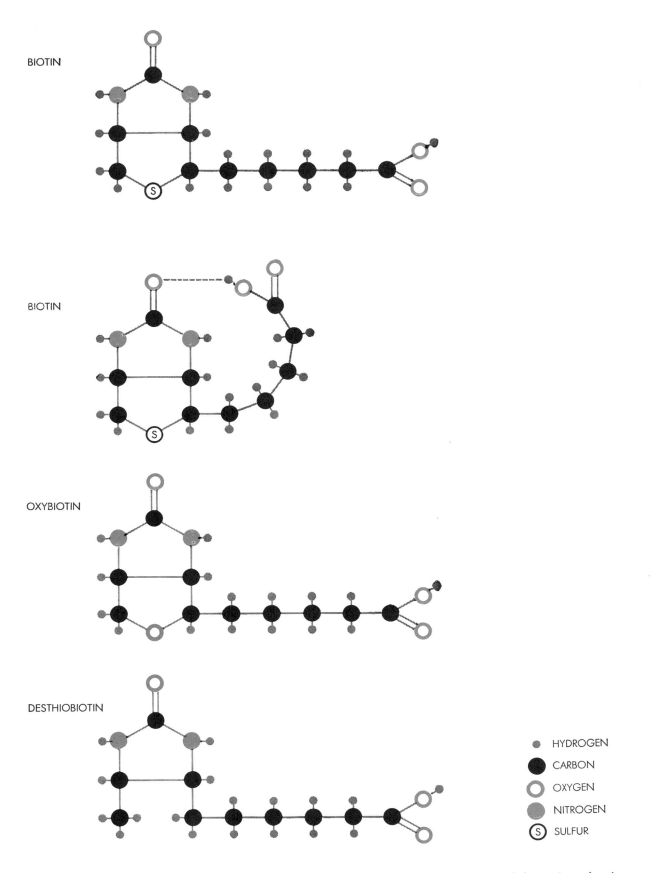

BIOTIN

BIOTIN

OXYBIOTIN

DESTHIOBIOTIN

- HYDROGEN
- CARBON
- OXYGEN
- NITROGEN
- (S) SULFUR

BIOTIN AND RELATED COMPOUNDS are depicted in these structural diagrams. The second biotin molecule is hypothetical; it shows side chain twisted so that a hydrogen bond (*broken line*) forms between oxygen and hydrogen. This might change the con- figuration of the molecule and thus activate the nitrogen atoms. Oxybiotin resembles biotin in biological activity; its molecule con- tains an oxygen atom instead of a sulfur atom. Desthiobiotin lacks the sulfur atom; it is probably the immediate precursor of biotin.

Western Reserve University. He learned that liver is a good source of the protective factor, which he had named "vitamin H." Concentrates prepared from liver had more than 3,000 times the power of liver itself to protect rats on an egg-white diet.

By that time preliminary work on the chemical and physical properties of biotin had turned up some provocative similarities between biotin and concentrates of vitamin H. On the other hand, it should be remembered that there was

no evidence of a physiological connection between the two. Biotin was a growth factor for microorganisms; vitamin H prevented egg-white injury in animals. György now suspected a connection, however, and asked Kögl for a sample of his crystalline biotin. Tested on animals, it showed the same protective action against egg-white injury that vitamin H did. In fact, the pure biotin was immensely more potent than the rather crude liver extracts of vitamin H. Would vitamin H concentrates in turn support

the growth of biotin-requiring microorganisms? They did. Moreover, the addition of raw egg white to an otherwise adequate culture medium prevented the growth of these organisms. More biotin or vitamin H overcame the toxic effect and growth resumed.

In 1940 György and Vincent du Vigneaud and his colleagues at the Cornell University Medical College independently isolated crystalline vitamin H from highly active liver concentrates and showed that it matched Kögl's biotin in

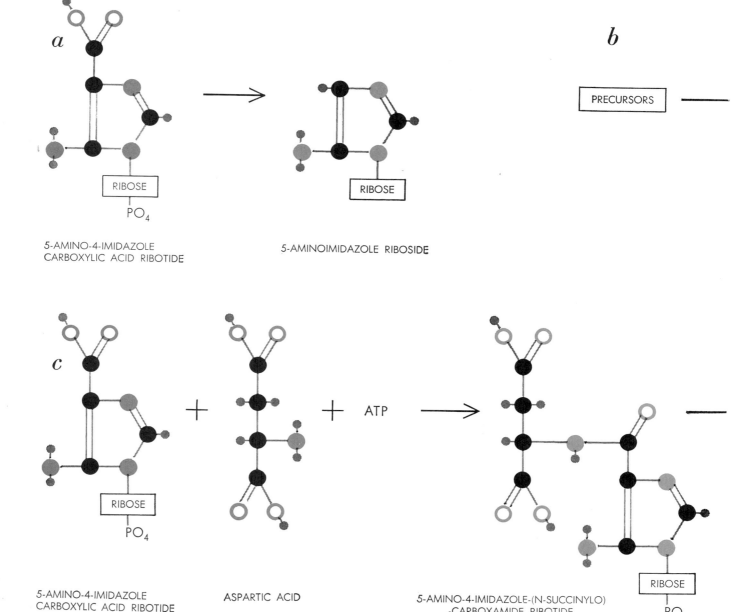

a

5-AMINO-4-IMIDAZOLE
CARBOXYLIC ACID RIBOTIDE

5-AMINOIMIDAZOLE RIBOSIDE

b

PRECURSORS

c

5-AMINO-4-IMIDAZOLE
CARBOXYLIC ACID RIBOTIDE

ASPARTIC ACID

ATP

5-AMINO-4-IMIDAZOLE-(N-SUCCINYLO)
-CARBOXAMIDE RIBOTIDE

SYNTHESIS OF PURINES depends on biotin. When yeast is deprived of biotin, the synthesis stops with the intermediate shown at left in a. This, in turn, breaks down spontaneously to 5-ami-noimidazole riboside, which accumulates in the culture medium. The stoppage is caused by a lack of aspartic acid, which is made with the aid of biotin (b). When biotin, or aspartic acid, is fed to

physiological and physical properties. It also yielded the same breakdown products on chemical analysis. There was no longer any doubt that the two compounds were one and the same.

Shortly afterward, biotin was isolated from milk. With so plentiful a source it was now possible to accumulate enough of the vitamin for a concerted attack on its chemical structure. Du Vigneaud and others proceeded to dissect the molecule and by 1942 were able to write its complete structural formula [see illustration on page 143]. The next year Stanton A. Harris and his colleagues at the research laboratory of Merck & Co., Inc., clinched this part of the problem when they synthesized a substance with the proposed structure. It was identical with natural biotin, both chemically and in its physiological action.

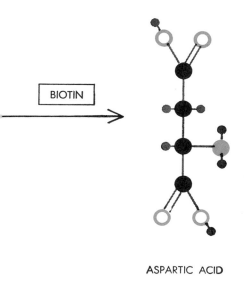

BIOTIN →

ASPARTIC ACID

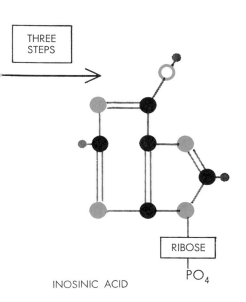

THREE STEPS →

INOSINIC ACID

RIBOSE

PO$_4$

the yeast, the assembly line resumes. Inosinic acid, which is one of the purines, is the end product of this particular process.

So closed a most satisfying chapter in biological research. Bios IIb, coenzyme R, protective factor X, vitamin H and biotin had been shown to be the same substance—an essential preliminary to any attempt to understand its biochemical function.

Today biotin is known to be very widely distributed. In fact, it is probably an essential constituent of all living cells, both plant and animal. Yet its potency is so great that no cell contains more than a trace of it. Liver, one of the richest sources, contains less than one part of biotin per million. Kögl spent five years accumulating 70 milligrams of the crystalline material. He estimated that he would have needed 360 tons of yeast or about $175,000 worth of eggs (1937 prices) to extract one gram.

Kögl's refined material was not free biotin but its methyl ester, in which the final hydroxyl (OH) of the carboxyl group (COOH) is replaced by a methyl group (CH$_3$). In tissues biotin is also often found in combination with other compounds rather than free. Proteins are a common partner, and the compounds the two substances form have been named bioto-proteins. The toxic material in egg white is the protein avidin. It combines with biotin in a complex that the digestive enzymes of higher animals cannot split apart and that is not absorbed from the alimentary canal. Thus raw egg white exerts its toxic action by inducing a deficiency of biotin. Cooking or any heat treatment denatures avidin, destroying its power to combine with biotin. Moreover, the avidin-biotin complex readily breaks down when it is heated.

Under normal circumstances human beings and other mammals do not suffer biotin deficiency even when the vitamin is eliminated from the diet. The intestines contain bacteria that synthesize biotin for themselves and incidentally for their host. Therefore the deficiency can be induced in test animals only by feeding them avidin or by eliminating the intestinal flora with antibacterial drugs. Using these techniques various workers have studied biotin deficiency in many species of higher animal, including rats, mice, hamsters, dogs,

cattle, pigs, monkeys and even man. A biotin-free diet alone can induce deficiency symptoms in chickens, presumably because of the low bacterial content of their alimentary tract.

The precise symptoms of biotin deficiency vary from species to species, but skin lesions, dermatitis, loss of hair and nervous disorders usually characterize the disease. Human volunteers at the University of Georgia School of Medicine, put on a diet containing about half a pound of dried egg white a day, developed a scaling dermatitis and a peculiar gray pallor. Lassitude, mental depression and muscle pains accompanied these symptoms. Administration of biotin promptly relieved the condition.

Of course, the observation of such gross effects cannot by itself elucidate the biochemical role of biotin. Experiments now under way in many laboratories, on a wide variety of cells and tissues, are directed at two fundamental problems: the precise function of biotin in the cell and the way in which it is synthesized by the organisms that manufacture it.

One difficulty in understanding how biotin works is that it seems to play a number of different roles. Almost all the other B vitamins, which are "cousins" of biotin, have been shown to have unique and specific functions at the cellular level. Biotin participates in many different biochemical reactions and transformations: it helps convert carbon dioxide to carbohydrates; it acts in removing amino (NH$_2$) groups from certain amino acids and the carboxyl group from certain other organic acids that are key intermediates in the breakdown of carbohydrates; it plays an essential part in the synthesis of aspartic acid and of fatty acids; there is evidence that it is involved in glucose oxidation and the metabolism of pyruvic acid. The list shows that biotin participates in the metabolism of the three principal constituents of living organisms: carbohydrates, fats and proteins. This apparent diversity of function suggests that biochemists have been unable to see the forest for the trees. The role of biotin may be more subtle than has been supposed. Perhaps the vitamin acts to synthesize specific enzymes rather than to assist in their chemical function, serving as a toolmaker rather than as a tool.

Some evidence for a fundamental role of this sort has come out of experiments in our laboratory at the University of Birmingham in England. In the course of investigation of biotin deficiency in

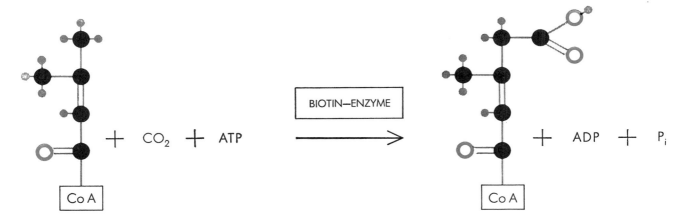

BETA- METHYL-CROTONYL-Co A   BETA- METHYL-GLUTACONYL-CoA

CARBON DIOXIDE TRANSFER is effected by an enzyme that contains biotin. Adenosine triphosphate (ATP) supplies energy for many cellular reactions. The biotin-enzyme directs the union of carbon dioxide and beta-methyl-crotonyl-CoA to give beta-methyl-glutaconyl-CoA, adenosine diphosphate (ADP) and inorganic phosphate (P_i). Proposed details of this reaction are shown below.

yeast D. Peter Lones, Cyril Rainbow and I found an unexpected compound accumulating in the culture medium. It was a material now known to be an intermediate in the synthesis of purines by cells. The purines, essential components of nucleic acids and other cell constituents, are compounds having a common double-ring framework of carbon and nitrogen atoms [see illustration on pages 144 and 145]. Largely through the elegant studies of John M. Buchanan at the Massachusetts Institute of Technology and G. Robert Greenberg, then at Western Reserve University, each step in the biosynthesis of purines has been delineated.

About halfway along this cellular assembly line aspartic acid is incorporated into the growing framework of the molecule. Biotin-deficient yeast is unable to manufacture enough aspartic acid to keep pace with the purine assembly process. This results in a pile-up of the unfinished purine intermediate, which eventually spills out of the cells into the surrounding medium. If aspartic acid itself is included in the medium, the bottleneck is broken, the assembly line starts moving again and the intermediate compound no longer accumulates. Other recent work indicates that biotin can also function as a coenzyme, as Allison originally supposed. Whereas some of

the enzymes for which biotin was once thought to be a cofactor have now been shown to be active without it, Salih J. Wakil at the University of Wisconsin has obtained an enzyme, involved in the synthesis of fatty acids, that does require the vitamin. The activity of the enzyme preparation is proportional to its biotin content. Moreover, the activity disappears with the addition of avidin and reappears when more biotin is added. A similar biotin-containing enzyme has been described by Feodor Lynen of the Max Planck Institute for Cell Chemistry in Munich. Both this enzyme and Wakil's seem to effect the uptake of carbon dioxide through the intermediate forma-

| BIOTIN—ENZYME | + ATP ⟶ ADP— | BIOTIN—ENZYME | + P_i |

| ADP— | BIOTIN—ENZYME | + CO_2 ⟶ CO_2— | BIOTIN—ENZYME | + ADP |

| CO_2— | BIOTIN—ENZYME | + BETA-METHYL-CROTONYL-CoA ⟶ | BIOTIN—ENZYME | + BETA-METHYL-GLUTACONYL-CoA |

PROPOSED SEQUENCE OF REACTIONS to account for the transfer of carbon dioxide is diagramed. In the first step ATP reacts with the biotin-enzyme. In the second step carbon dioxide com- bines with the biotin-enzyme. The carbon dioxide is transferred to beta-methyl-crotonyl-CoA in the third step, producing beta-methyl-glutaconyl-CoA. CoA is an abbreviation for coenzyme A.

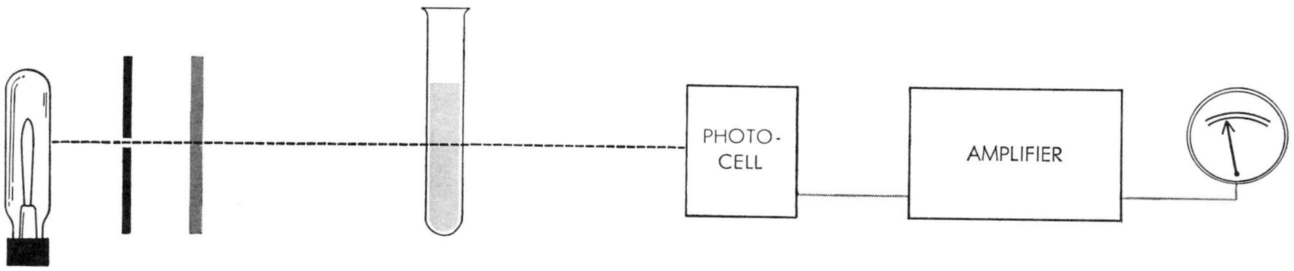

MICROBIOLOGICAL ASSAY OF BIOTIN employs cultures of yeast cells. It can detect a biotin concentration of only one part in 500,000 million. More yeast cells appear in a culture as the concentration of biotin rises, making the suspension more turbid. A light (*left*) shines through a diaphragm, a filter and the culture in the test tube until it hits a photocell, which detects changes in light intensity. The amount of light transmitted by the culture registers on the ammeter at right, giving the measure of the concentration of biotin. With a compound as active as biotin such a method of quantative measurement is essential to the understanding of its functions.

tion of an active "carboxylated" biotin. Lynen has provisionally identified such an intermediate, in which carbon dioxide is attached at one of the nitrogen atoms of the biotin molecule. He suggests that there are many biotin-containing enzymes that transfer carbon dioxide in different reactions.

W. Traub of the University of London has suggested a mechanism by which the nitrogen atoms in the biotin molecule may be enabled to participate in these reactions. Examining the spatial arrangement of the molecule, he found that under certain conditions the keto (C-O) oxygen of the ring and one oxygen of the carboxyl group in the side chain may come close enough to each other for a special kind of intramolecular bond—the hydrogen bond—to form between them. This would distort the molecule in such a way that it would increase the chemical reactivity of the nitrogen atoms in the ring.

As for the synthesis of biotin by living cells, the process has not yet been traced very far. The immediate precursor of the vitamin is probably desthiobiotin, which lacks only the sulfur atom of the biotin molecule [*see illustration on page 143*]. Part of the carbon skeleton is thought to be supplied by pimelic acid, a seven-carbon compound. In fact, pimelic acid acts like biotin in certain microorganisms and stimulates the production of biotin in others.

Here matters stand as these lines are written. The story, which nicely illustrates the trend in modern biology, began with the recognition of an undefined principle in brewer's wort and it closes with the consideration of individual atoms in a precisely known molecular structure. There is still a lot to learn, and biotin is very much a "hot" topic today. By the time this article is published the chances are that someone will have made a further important contribution to the understanding of this unfamiliar but vital substance.

16

The Chemical Elements of Life

by Earl Frieden
July 1972

Until recently it was believed that living matter incorporated 20 of the natural elements. Now it has been shown that a role is played by four others: fluorine, silicon, tin and vanadium

How many of the 90 naturally occurring elements are essential to life? After more than a century of increasingly refined investigation, the question still cannot be answered with certainty. Only a year or so ago the best answer would have been 20. Since then four more elements have been shown to be essential for the growth of young animals: fluorine, silicon, tin and vanadium. Nickel may soon be added to the list. In many cases the exact role played by these and other trace elements remains unknown or unclear. These gaps in knowledge could be critical during a period when the biosphere is being increasingly contaminated by synthetic chemicals and subjected to a potentially harmful redistribution of salts and metal ions. In addition, new and exotic chemical forms of metals (such as methyl mercury) are being discovered, and a complex series of competitive and synergistic relations among mineral salts has been encountered. We are led to the realization that we are ignorant of many basic facts about how our chemical milieu affects our biological fate.

Biologists and chemists have long been fascinated by the way evolution has selected certain elements as the building blocks of living organisms and has ignored others. The composition of the earth and its atmosphere obviously sets a limit on what elements are available. The earth itself is hardly a chip off the universe. The solar system, like the universe, seems to be 99 percent hydrogen and helium. In the earth's crust helium is essentially nonexistent (except in a few rare deposits) and hydrogen atoms constitute only about .22 percent of the total. Eight elements provide more than 98 percent of the atoms in the earth's crust: oxygen (47 percent), silicon (28 percent), aluminum (7.9 percent), iron

(4.5 percent), calcium (3.5 percent), sodium (2.5 percent), potassium (2.5 percent) and magnesium (2.2 percent). Of these eight elements only five are among the 11 that account for more than 99.9 percent of the atoms in the human body. Not surprisingly nine of the 11 are also the nine most abundant elements in seawater [*See illustration on page 150*].

Two elements, hydrogen and oxygen, account for 88.5 percent of the atoms in the human body; hydrogen supplies 63 percent of the total and oxygen 25.5 percent. Carbon accounts for another 9.5 percent and nitrogen 1.4 percent. The remaining 20 elements now thought to be essential for mammalian life account for less than .7 percent of the body's atoms.

The Background of Selection

Three characteristics of the biosphere or of the elements themselves appear to have played a major part in directing the chemistry of living forms. First and foremost there is the ubiquity of water, the solvent base of all life on the earth. Water is a unique compound; its stability and boiling point are both unusually high for a molecule of its simple composition. Many of the other compounds essential for life derive their usefulness from their response to water: whether they are soluble or insoluble, whether or not (if they are soluble) they carry an electric charge in solution and, not least, what effect they have on the viscosity of water.

The second directing force involves the chemical properties of carbon, which evolution selected over silicon as the central building block for constructing giant molecules. Silicon is 146 times more plentiful than carbon in the earth's crust and exhibits many of the same

properties. Silicon is directly below carbon in the periodic table of the elements; like carbon, it has the capacity to gain four electrons and form four covalent bonds.

The crucial difference that led to the preference for carbon compounds over silicon compounds seems traceable to two chemical features: the unusual sta-

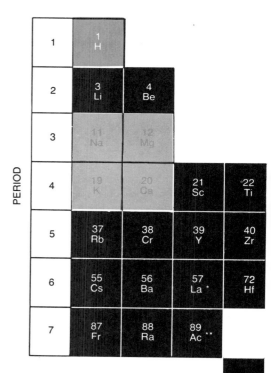

ESSENTIAL LIFE ELEMENTS, 24 by the latest count, are clustered in the upper half of the periodic table. The elements are ar-

bility of carbon dioxide, which is readily soluble in water and always monomeric (it remains a single molecule), and the almost unique ability of carbon to form long chains and stable rings with five or six members. This versatility of the carbon atom is responsible for the millions of organic compounds found on the earth.

Silicon, in contrast, is insoluble in water and forms only relatively short chains with itself. It can enter into longer chains, however, by forming alternating bonds with oxygen, creating the compounds known as silicones (–Si–O–Si–O–Si–). Carbon-to-carbon bonds are more stable than silicon-to-silicon bonds, but not so stable as to be virtually immutable, as the silicon-oxygen polymers are. Nevertheless, silicon has recently been shown to be essential in a way as yet unknown for normal bone development and full growth in chicks.

The third force influencing the evolutionary selection of the elements essential for life is related to an atom's size and charge density. Obviously the heavy synthetic elements from neptunium (atomic number 93) to lawrencium (No. 103), along with two lighter synthetic elements, technetium (No. 43) and promethium (No. 61), were never available in nature. (The atomic number expresses the number of protons in the nucleus of an atom or the number of electrons around the nucleus.) The eight heavy elements in another group (Nos. 84 and 85 and Nos. 87 through 92) are too radioactive to be useful in living structures. Six more elements are inert gases with virtually no useful chemical reactivities: helium, neon, argon, krypton, xenon and radon. On various plausible grounds one can exclude another 24 elements, or a total of 38 natural elements, as being clearly unsatisfactory for incorporation in living organisms because of their relative unavailability (particularly the elements in the lanthanide and actinide series) or their high toxicity (for example mercury and lead). This leaves 52 of the 90 natural elements as being potentially useful.

Only three of the 24 elements known to be essential for animal life have an atomic number above 34. All three are needed only in trace amounts: molybdenum (No. 42), tin (No. 50) and iodine (No. 53). The four most abundant atoms in living organisms—hydrogen, carbon, oxygen and nitrogen—have atomic numbers of 1, 6, 7 and 8. Their preponderance seems attributable to their being the smallest and lightest elements that can achieve stable electronic configurations by adding one to four electrons. The ability to add electrons by sharing them with other atoms is the first step in forming chemical bonds leading to stable molecules. The seven next most abundant elements in living organisms all have atomic numbers below 21. In the order of their abundance in mammals they are calcium (No. 20), phosphorus (No. 15), potassium (No. 19), sulfur (No. 16), sodium (No. 11), magnesium (No. 12) and chlorine (No. 17). The remaining 10 elements known to be present in either plants or animals are needed only in traces. With the exception of fluorine (No. 9) and silicon (No. 14), the remaining eight occupy positions between No. 23 and No. 34 in the periodic table [see illustration below]. It is inter-

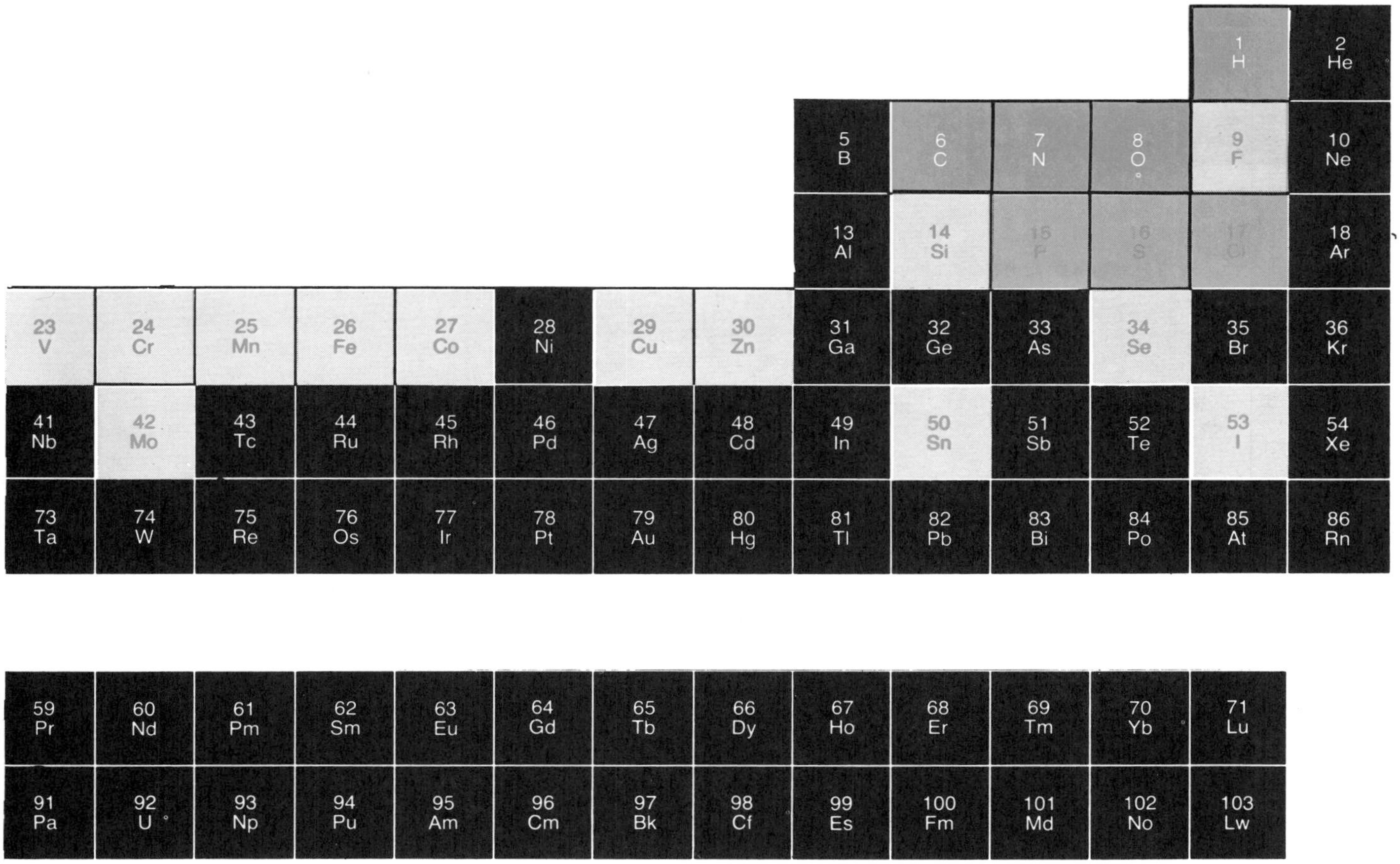

ranged according to their atomic number, which is equivalent to the number of protons in the atom's nucleus. The four most abundant elements that are found in living organisms (hydrogen, oxygen, carbon and nitrogen) are indicated by dark color. The seven next most common elements are in lighter color. The 13 elements that are shown in lightest color are needed only in traces.

esting that this interval embraces three elements for which evolution has evidently found no role: gallium, germanium and arsenic. None of the metals with properties similar to those of gallium (such as aluminum and indium) has proved to be useful to living organisms. On the other hand, since silicon and tin, two elements with chemical activities similar to those of germanium, have just joined the list of essential elements, it seems possible that germanium too, in spite of its rarity, will turn out to have an essential role. Arsenic, of course, is a well-known poison.

Functions of Essential Elements

Some useful generalizations can be made about the role of the various elements. Six elements—carbon, nitrogen, hydrogen, oxygen, phosphorus and sulfur—make up the molecular building blocks of living matter: amino acids, sugars, fatty acids, purines, pyrimidines and nucleotides. These molecules not only have independent biochemical roles but also are the respective constituents of the following large molecules: proteins, glycogen, starch, lipids and nucleic acids. Several of the 20 amino acids contain sulfur in addition to carbon, hydrogen and oxygen. Phosphorus plays an important role in the nucleotides such as adenosine triphosphate (ATP), which is central to the energetics of the cell. ATP includes components that are also one of the four nucleotides needed to form the double helix of deoxyribonucleic acid (DNA), which incorporates the genetic blueprint of all plants and animals. Both sulfur and phosphorus are present in many of the small accessory molecules called coenzymes. In bony animals phosphorus and calcium help to create strong supporting structures.

The electrochemical properties of living matter depend critically on elements or combinations of elements that either gain or lose electrons when they are dissolved in water, thus forming ions. The principal cations (electron-deficient, or positively charged, ions) are provided by four metals: sodium, potassium, calcium and magnesium. The principal anions (ions with a negative charge because they have surplus electrons) are provided by the chloride ion and by sulfur and phosphorus in the form of sulfate ions and phosphate ions. These seven ions maintain the electrical neutrality of body fluids and cells and also play a part in maintaining the proper liquid volume of the blood and other fluid systems. Whereas the cell membrane serves as a physical barrier to the exchange of large molecules, it allows small molecules to pass freely. The electrochemical functions of the anions and cations serve to maintain the appropriate relation of osmotic pressure and charge distribution on the two sides of the cell membrane.

One of the striking features of the ion distribution is the specificity of these different ions. Cells are rich in potassium and magnesium, and the surrounding plasma is rich in sodium and calcium. It seems likely that the distribution of ions in the plasma of higher animals reflects the oceanic origin of their evolutionary antecedents. One would like to know how primitive cells learned to exclude the sodium and calcium ions in which they were bathed and to develop an internal milieu enriched in potassium and magnesium.

The third and last group of essential elements consists of the trace elements. The fact that they are required in extremely minute quantities in no way diminishes their great importance. In this sense they are comparable to the vitamins. We now know that the great majority of the trace elements, represented by metallic ions, serve chiefly as key components of essential enzyme systems or of proteins with vital functions (such as hemoglobin and myoglobin, which respectively transports oxygen in the blood and stores oxygen in muscle). The heaviest essential element, iodine, is an essential constituent of the thyroid hormones thyroxine and triiodothyronine, although its precise role in hormonal activity is still not understood.

COMPOSITION OF UNIVERSE		COMPOSITION OF EARTH'S CRUST		COMPOSITION OF SEAWATER		COMPOSITION OF HUMAN BODY	
PERCENT OF TOTAL NUMBER OF ATOMS							
H	91	O	47	H	66	H	63
He	9.1	Si	28	O	33	O	25.5
O	.057	Al	7.9	Cl	.33	C	9.5
N	.042	Fe	4.5	Na	.28	N	1.4
C	.021	Ca	3.5	Mg	.033	Ca	.31
Si	.003	Na	2.5	S	.017	P	.22
Ne	.003	K	2.5	Ca	.006	Cl	.03
Mg	.002	Mg	2.2	K	.006	K	.06
Fe	.002	Ti	.46	C	.0014	S	.05
S	.001	H	.22	Br	.0005	Na	.03
		C	.19			Mg	.01
ALL OTHERS<.01		ALL OTHERS<.1		ALL OTHERS<.1		ALL OTHERS<.01	

Al	ALUMINUM	C	CARBON	Fe	IRON	O	OXYGEN	S	SULFUR
B	BORON	Cl	CHLORINE	Mg	MAGNESIUM	K	POTASSIUM	Ti	TITANIUM
Br	BROMINE	He	HELIUM	Ne	NEON	Si	SILICON		
Ca	CALCIUM	H	HYDROGEN	N	NITROGEN	Na	SODIUM		

CHEMICAL SELECTIVITY OF EVOLUTION can be demonstrated by comparing the composition of the human body with the approximate composition of seawater, the earth's crust and the universe at large. The percentages are based on the total number of atoms in each case; because of rounding the totals do not exactly equal 100. Elements in the colored boxes in the last column appear in one or more columns at the left. Thus one sees that phosphorus, the sixth most plentiful element in the body, is a rare element in inanimate nature. Carbon, the third most plentiful element, is also very scarce elsewhere.

The Trace Elements

To demonstrate that a particular element is essential to life becomes increasingly difficult as one lowers the threshold of the amount of a substance recognizable as a "trace." It has been known for more than 100 years, for example, that iron and iodine are essential to man. In a rapidly developing period of biochemistry between 1928 and 1935 four more elements, all metals, were shown to be

ELEMENT	SYMBOL	ATOMIC NUMBER	COMMENTS
HYDROGEN	H	1	Required for water and organic compounds.
HELIUM	He	2	Inert and unused.
LITHIUM	Li	3	Probably unused.
BERYLLIUM	Be	4	Probably unused; toxic.
BORON	B	5	Essential in some plants; function unknown.
CARBON	C	6	Required for organic compounds.
NITROGEN	N	7	Required for many organic compounds.
OXYGEN	O	8	Required for water and organic compounds.
FLUORINE	F	9	Growth factor in rats; possible constituent of teeth and bone.
NEON	Ne	10	Inert and unused.
SODIUM	Na	11	Principal extracellular cation.
MAGNESIUM	Mg	12	Required for activity of many enzymes; in chlorophyll.
ALUMINUM	Al	13	Essentiality under study.
SILICON	Si	14	Possible structural unit of diatoms; recently shown to be essential in chicks.
PHOSPHORUS	P	15	Essential for biochemical synthesis and energy transfer.
SULFUR	S	16	Required for proteins and other biological compounds.
CHLORINE	Cl	17	Principal cellular and extracellular anion.
ARGON	A	18	Inert and unused.
POTASSIUM	K	19	Principal cellular cation.
CALCIUM	Ca	20	Major component of bone; required for some enzymes.
SCANDIUM	Sc	21	Probably unused.
TITANIUM	Ti	22	Probably unused.
VANADIUM	V	23	Essential in lower plants, certain marine animals and rats.
CHROMIUM	Cr	24	Essential in higher animals; related to action of insulin.
MANGANESE	Mn	25	Required for activity of several enzymes.
IRON	Fe	26	Most important transition metal ion; essential for hemoglobin and many enzymes.
COBALT	Co	27	Required for activity of several enzymes; in vitamin B_{12}.
NICKEL	Ni	28	Essentiality under study.
COPPER	Cu	29	Essential in oxidative and other enzymes and hemocyanin.
ZINC	Zn	30	Required for activity of many enzymes.
GALLIUM	Ga	31	Probably unused.
GERMANIUM	Ge	32	Probably unused.
ARSENIC	As	33	Probably unused; toxic.
SELENIUM	Se	34	Essential for liver function.
MOLYBDENUM	Mo	42	Required for activity of several enzymes.
TIN	Sn	50	Essential in rats; function unknown.
IODINE	I	53	Essential constituent of the thyroid hormones.

SOME TWO-THIRDS OF LIGHTEST ELEMENTS, or 21 out of the first 34 elements in the periodic table, are now known to be essential for animal life. These 21 plus molybdenum (No. 42), tin (No. 50) and iodine (No. 53) constitute the total list of the 24 essential elements, which are here enclosed in colored boxes. It is possible that still other light elements will turn out to be essential. The most likely candidates are aluminum, nickel and germanium. The element boron already appears to be essential for some plants.

essential: copper, manganese, zinc and cobalt. The demonstration can be credited chiefly to a group of investigators at the University of Wisconsin led by C. A. Elvehjem, E. B. Hart and W. R. Todd. At that time it seemed that these four metals might be the last of the essential trace elements. In the next 30 years, however, three more elements were shown to be essential: chromium, selenium and molybdenum. Fluorine, silicon, tin and vanadium have been added since 1970.

The essentiality of five of these last seven elements was discovered through

the careful, painstaking efforts of Klaus Schwarz and his associates, initially located at the National Institutes of Health and now based at the Veterans Administration Hospital in Long Beach, Calif. For the past 15 years Schwarz's group has made a systematic study of the trace-element requirements of rats and other small animals. The animals are maintained from birth in a completely isolated sterile environment [*see illustration on page 154*].

The apparatus is constructed entirely of plastics to eliminate the stray contaminants contained in metal, glass and

rubber. Although even plastics may contain some trace elements, they are so tightly bound in the structural lattice of the material that they cannot be leached out or be picked up by an animal even through contact. A typical isolator system houses 32 animals in individual acrylic cages. Highly efficient air filters remove all trace substances that might be present in the dust in the air. Thus the animals' only access to essential nutrients is through their diet. They receive chemically pure amino acids instead of natural proteins, and all other dietary ingredients are screened for metal contaminants.

Since the standards of purity employed in these experiments far exceed those for reagents normally regarded as analytically pure, Schwarz and his coworkers have had to develop many new analytical chemical methods. The most difficult problem turned out to be the purification of salt mixtures. Even the purest commercial reagents were contaminated with traces of metal ions. It was also found that trace elements could be passed from mothers to their offspring. To minimize this source of contamination animals are weaned as quickly as possible, usually from 18 to 20 days after birth.

With these precautions Schwarz and his colleagues have within the past several years been able to produce a new deficiency disease in rats. The animals grow poorly, lose hair and muscle tone, develop shaggy fur and exhibit other detrimental changes [*see illustration on page 155*]. When standard laboratory food is given these animals, they regain their normal appearance. At first it was thought that all the symptoms were caused by the lack of one particular trace element. Eventually four different elements had to be supplied to complete the highly purified diets the animals had been receiving. The four elements proved to be fluorine, silicon, tin and vanadium. A convenient source of these elements is yeast ash or liver preparations from a healthy animal. The animals on the deficiency diet grew less than half as fast as those on a normal or supplemented diet. Growth alone, however, may not tell the entire story. There is some evidence that even the addition of the four elements may not reverse the loss of hair and skin changes resulting from the deficiency diet.

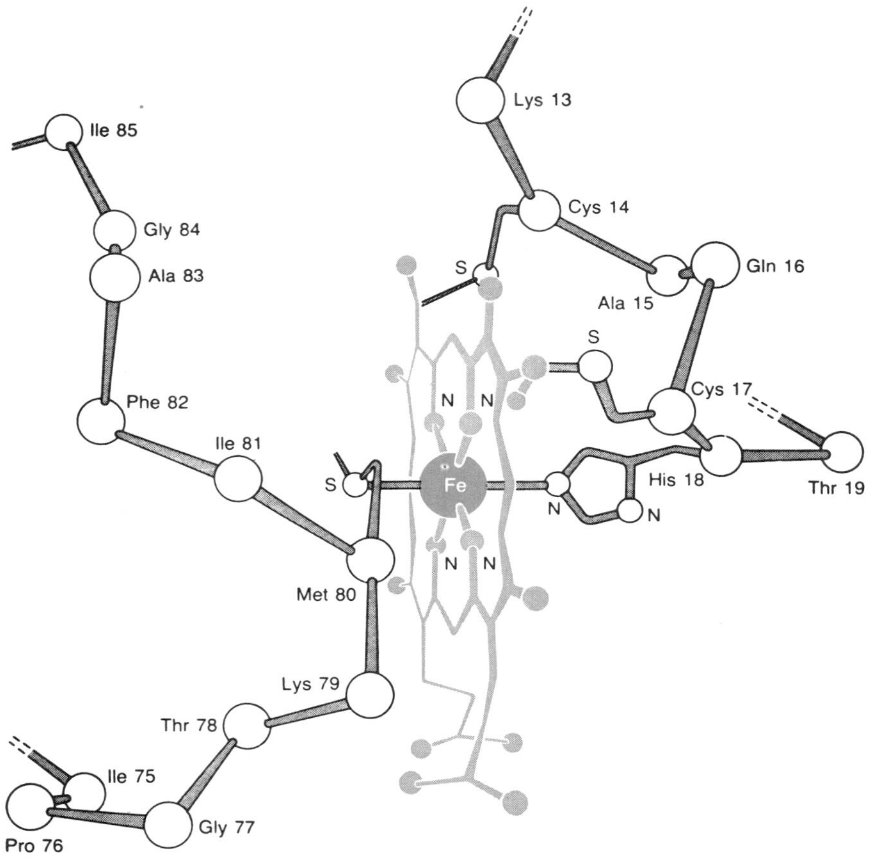

Functions of Trace Elements

The addition of tin and vanadium to the list of essential trace metals brings

Ala	ALANINE	His	HISTIDINE	Phe	PHENYLALANINE
Cys	CYSTEINE	Ile	ISOLEUCINE	Pro	PROLINE
Gln	GLUTAMINE	Lys	LYSINE	Thr	THREONINE
Gly	GLYCINE	Met	METHIONINE		

THE METALLOENZYME CYTOCHROME *c* is typical of metal-protein complexes in which trace metals play a crucial role. Cytochrome *c* belongs to a family of enzymes that extract energy from food molecules. It consists of a protein chain of 104 amino acid units attached to a heme group (*color*), a rosette of atoms with an atom of iron at the center. This simplified molecular diagram shows only the heme group and several of the amino acid units closest to it. The iron atom has six coordination sites enabling it to form six bonds with neighboring atoms. Four bonds connect to nitrogen atoms in the heme group itself, and the remaining two bonds link up with amino acid units in the protein chain (histidine at site No. 18 and methionine at site No. 80). The illustration is based on the work of Richard E. Dickerson of the California Institute of Technology, in whose laboratory the complete structure of horse-heart cytochrome *c* was recently determined.

to 10 the total number of trace metals needed by animals and plants. What role do these metals play? For six of the eight trace metals recognized from earlier studies (that is, for iron, zinc, copper, cobalt, manganese and molybdenum) we are reasonably sure of the answer. The six are constituents of a wide range of enzymes that participate in a variety of metabolic processes [see illustration at right].

In addition to its role in hemoglobin and myoglobin, iron appears in succinate dehydrogenase, one of the enzymes needed for the utilization of energy from sugars and starches. Enzymes incorporating zinc help to control the formation of carbon dioxide and the digestion of proteins. Copper is present in more than a dozen enzymes, whose roles range from the utilization of iron to the pigmentation of the skin. Cobalt appears in enzymes involved in the synthesis of DNA and the metabolism of amino acids. Enzymes incorporating manganese are involved in the formation of urea and the metabolism of pyruvate. Enzymes incorporating molybdenum participate in purine metabolism and the utilization of nitrogen.

These six metals belong to a group known as transition elements. They owe their uniqueness to their ability to form strong complexes with ligands, or molecular groups, of the type present in the side chains of proteins. Enzymes in which transition metals are tightly incorporated are called metalloenzymes, since the metal is usually embedded deep inside the structure of the protein. If the metal atom is removed, the protein usually loses its capacity to function as an enzyme. There is also a group of enzymes in which the metal ion is more loosely associated with the protein but is nonetheless essential for the enzyme's activity. Enzymes in this group are known as metal-ion-activated enzymes. In either group the role of the metal ion may be to maintain the proper conformation of the protein, to bind the substrate (the molecule acted on) to the protein or to donate or accept electrons in reactions where the substrate is reduced or oxidized.

In 1968 the complete three-dimensional structure of the first metalloenzyme, cytochrome c, was published [see "The Structure and History of an Ancient Protein," by Richard E. Dickerson; SCIENTIFIC AMERICAN Offprint 1245]. Cytochrome c, a red enzyme containing iron, is universally present in plants and animals. It is one of a series of enzymes, all called cytochromes, that extract en-

METAL	ENZYME	BIOLOGICAL FUNCTION
IRON	FERREDOXIN	Photosynthesis
	SUCCINATE DEHYDROGENASE	Aerobic oxidation of carbohydrates
IRON IN HEME	ALDEHYDE OXIDASE	Aldehyde oxidation
	CYTOCHROMES	Electron transfer
	CATALASE	Protection against hydrogen peroxide
	[HEMOGLOBIN]	Oxygen transport
COPPER	CERULOPLASMIN	Iron utilization
	CYTOCHROME OXIDASE	Principal terminal oxidase
	LYSINE OXIDASE	Elasticity of aortic walls
	TYROSINASE	Skin pigmentation
	PLASTOCYANIN	Photosynthesis
	[HEMOCYANIN]	Oxygen transport in invertebrates
ZINC	CARBONIC ANHYDRASE	CO_2 formation; regulation of acidity
	CARBOXYPEPTIDASE	Protein digestion
	ALCOHOL DEHYDROGENASE	Alcohol metabolism
MANGANESE	ARGINASE	Urea formation
	PYRUVATE CARBOXYLASE	Pyruvate metabolism
COBALT	RIBONUCLEOTIDE REDUCTASE	DNA biosynthesis
	GLUTAMATE MUTASE	Amino acid metabolism
MOLYBDENUM	XANTHINE OXIDASE	Purine metabolism
	NITRATE REDUCTASE	Nitrate utilization
CALCIUM	LIPASES	Lipid digestion
MAGNESIUM	HEXOKINASE	Phosphate transfer

WIDE VARIETY OF METALLOENZYMES is required for the successful functioning of living organisms. Some of the most important are given in this list. The giant oxygen-transporting molecules hemoglobin and hemocyanin are included in the list (in brackets) even though they are not strictly enzymes, that is, they do not act as biological catalysts.

ergy from food molecules by the stepwise addition of oxygen.

The complete amino acid sequence of cytochrome c obtained from the human heart was determined some 10 years ago by a group led by Emil L. Smith of the University of California at Los Angeles and by Emanuel Margoliash of Northwestern University. The iron atom is partially complexed with an intricate organic molecule, protoporphyrin, to form a heme group similar to that in hemoglobin. Of the iron atom's six coordination sites, four are attached to the heme group through nitrogen atoms. The other two sites form bonds with the protein chain; one bond is through a nitrogen atom in the side chain of a histidine unit at site No. 18 in the protein sequence and the other bond is through a sulfur atom in the side chain of a methionine unit at site No. 80 [see illustration on opposite page].

Although the cytochrome c molecule is complicated, it is one of the simplest of the metalloenzymes. Cytochrome oxidase, probably the single most important enzyme in most cells, since it is responsible for transferring electrons to oxygen to form water, is far more complicated. Each molecule contains about 12 times as many atoms as cytochrome c, including two copper atoms and two heme groups, both of which participate in transferring the electrons.

More complicated yet is cysteamine oxygenase, which catalyzes the addition of oxygen to a molecule of cysteamine; it contains one atom each of three different metals: iron, copper and zinc. There are many other combinations of metal ions and unique molecular assemblies. An extreme example is xanthine oxidase, which contains eight iron atoms, two molybdenum atoms and two molecules incorporating riboflavin (one of the B vitamins) in a giant molecule more than 25 times the size of cytochrome c.

The metal-containing proteins of another group, the metalloproteins, closely resemble the metalloenzymes except that they lack an obvious catalytic function. Hemoglobin itself is an example. Others are hemocyanin, the copper-containing blue protein that carries oxygen in many invertebrates, metallothionein, a protein involved in the absorption and storage of zinc, and transferrin, a protein that transports iron in the bloodstream. There may be many more such compounds still unrecognized because their function has escaped detection.

The Newest Essential Elements

Much remains to be learned about the specific biochemical role of the most recently discovered essential elements. In 1957 Schwarz and Calvin M. Foltz, working at the National Institutes of Health, showed that selenium helped to prevent several serious deficiency diseases in different animals, including liver necrosis and muscular dystrophy. Rats were protected against death from liver necrosis by a diet containing one-tenth of a part per million of selenium. Comparably low doses reversed the white muscle disease observed in cattle and sheep that happen to graze in areas where selenium is scarce.

In April a group at the University of Wisconsin under J. T. Rotruck reported a direct biochemical role for selenium.

Oxidative damage to red blood cells was detected in rats kept on a selenium-deficient diet. This damage was related to reduced activity of an enzyme, glutathione peroxidase, that helps to protect hemoglobin against the injurious oxidative effects of hydrogen peroxide. The enzyme uses hydrogen peroxide to catalyze the oxidation of glutathione, thus keeping hydrogen peroxide from oxidizing the reduced state of iron in hemoglobin. Oxidized glutathione can readily be converted to reduced glutathione by a variety of intracellular mechanisms. There is some reason to believe glutathione peroxidase may even contain some form of selenium acting as an integral part of the functional enzyme molecule.

The physiological importance of chromium was established in 1959 by Schwarz and Walter Mertz. They found that chromium deficiency is characterized by impaired growth and reduced life-span, corneal lesions and a defect in sugar metabolism. When the diet is deficient in chromium, glucose is removed from the bloodstream only half as fast as it is normally. In rats the deficiency is relieved by a single administration of 20 micrograms of certain trivalent chromic salts. It now appears that the chromium ion works in conjunction with insulin, and that in at least some cases

diabetes may reflect faulty chromium metabolism.

After developing the all-plastic trace-element isolator described above, Schwarz, David B. Milne and Elizabeth Vineyard discovered that tin, not previously suspected as being essential, was necessary for normal growth. Without one or two parts per million of tin in their diet, rats grow at only about two-thirds the normal rate.

The next element shown to be essential in mammals by the Schwarz group was vanadium, an element that had been detected earlier in certain marine invertebrates but whose essentiality had not been demonstrated. On a diet in which vanadium is totally excluded rats suffer a retardation of about 30 percent in growth rate. Schwarz and Milne found that normal growth is restored by adding one-tenth of a part per million of vanadium to the diet. At higher concentrations vanadium is known to have several biological effects, but its essential role in trace amounts remains to be established. A high dose of vanadium blocks the synthesis of cholesterol and reduces the amount of phospholipid and cholesterol in the blood. Vanadium also promotes the mineralization of teeth and is effective as a catalyst in the oxidation of many biological substances.

The third element most recently iden-

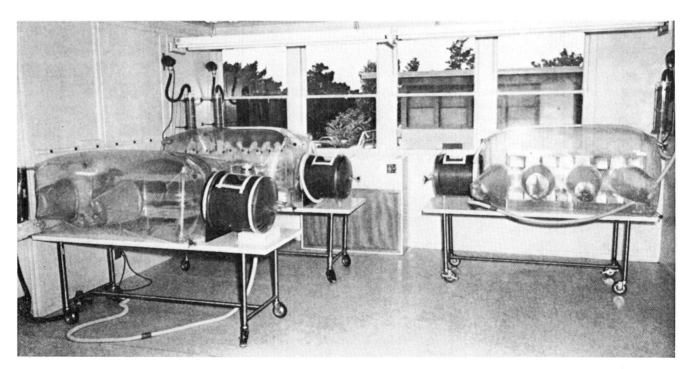

NUTRITIONAL NEEDS OF SMALL ANIMALS are studied in a trace-element isolator, a modification of the apparatus originally conceived to maintain animals in a germ-free environment. To prevent unwanted introduction of trace elements the isolator is built completely of plastics. It holds 32 animals in separate cages, individually supplied with food of precisely known composition. The system was designed by Klaus Schwarz and J. Cecil Smith of the Veterans Administration Hospital in Long Beach, Calif.

tified as being essential is fluorine. Even with tin and vanadium added to highly purified diets containing all other elements known to be essential, the animals in Schwarz's plastic cages still failed to grow at a normal rate. When up to half a part per million of potassium fluoride was added to the diet, the animals showed a 20 to 30 percent weight gain in four weeks. Although it had appeared that a trace amount of fluorine was essential for building sound teeth, Schwarz's study showed that fluorine's biochemical role was more fundamental than that. In any case fluoridated water provides more than enough fluorine to maintain a normal growth rate.

Although there were earlier clues that silicon might be an essential life element, firm proof of its essentiality, at least in young chicks, was reported only three months ago. Edith M. Carlisle of the School of Public Health at the University of California at Los Angeles finds that chicks kept on a silicon-free diet for only one or two weeks exhibit poor development of feathers and skeleton, including markedly thin leg bones. The addition of 30 parts per million of silicon to the diet increases the chicks' growth more than 35 percent and makes possible normal feathering and skeletal development. Considering that silicon is not only the second most abundant element in the earth's crust but is also similar to carbon in many of its chemical properties, it is hard to see how evolution could have totally excluded it from an essential biochemical role.

Nickel, nearly always associated with iron in natural substances, is another element receiving close attention. Also a transition element, it is particularly difficult to remove from the food used in special diets. Nickel seems to influence the growth of wing and tail feathers in chicks but more consistent data are needed to establish its essentiality. One incidental result of Schwarz's work has been the discovery of a previously unrecognized organic compound, which will undoubtedly prove to be a new vitamin.

Synergism and Antagonism

The interaction of the various essential metals can be extremely complicated. The absence of one metal in the diet can profoundly influence, either positively or negatively, the utilization of another metal that may be present. For example, it has been known for nearly 50 years that copper is essential for the proper metabolism of iron. An animal deprived of copper but not iron develops anemia because the biosynthetic machinery fails to incorporate iron in hemoglobin molecules. It has only recently been found in our laboratories at Florida State University that ceruloplasmin, the copper-containing protein of the blood, is a direct molecular link between the two metals. Ceruloplasmin promotes the release of iron from animal liver so that the iron-binding protein of the serum, transferrin, can complex with iron and transfer it to the developing red blood cells for direct utilization in the biosynthesis of hemoglobin. This represents a synergistic relation between copper and iron.

As an example of antagonism between elements one can cite the instance of copper and zinc. The ability of sheep or cattle to absorb copper is greatly reduced if too much zinc or molybdenum is present in their diet. Evidently either of the two metals can displace copper in an absorption process that probably involves competition for sites on a metal-binding protein in the intestines and liver.

The recent discoveries present many fresh challenges to biochemists. One can expect the discovery of previously unsuspected metalloenzymes containing vanadium, tin, chromium and selenium. New compounds or enzyme systems requiring fluorine and silicon may also be uncovered. The multiple and complex interdependencies of the elements suggest many hitherto unrecognized and important facts about the role and interrelations of metal ions in nutrition and in health and disease.

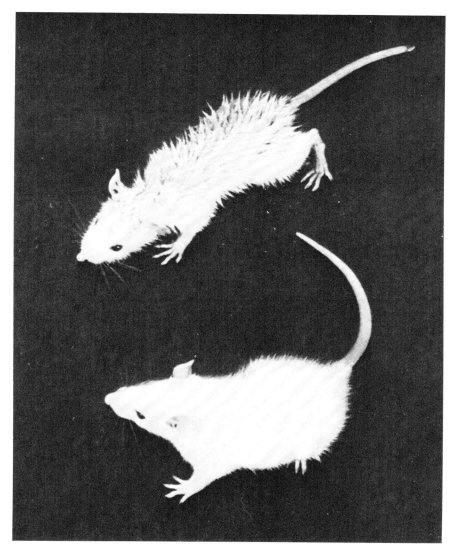

TRACE-ELEMENT DEFICIENCY developed when the rat at the top of this photograph was kept in the trace-element isolator for 20 days and fed a diet from which fluorine, tin and vanadium had been carefully excluded. The healthy animal at the bottom was fed the same diet but was kept under ordinary conditions. It was evidently able to obtain the necessary trace amounts of fluorine, tin and vanadium from dust and other contaminants.

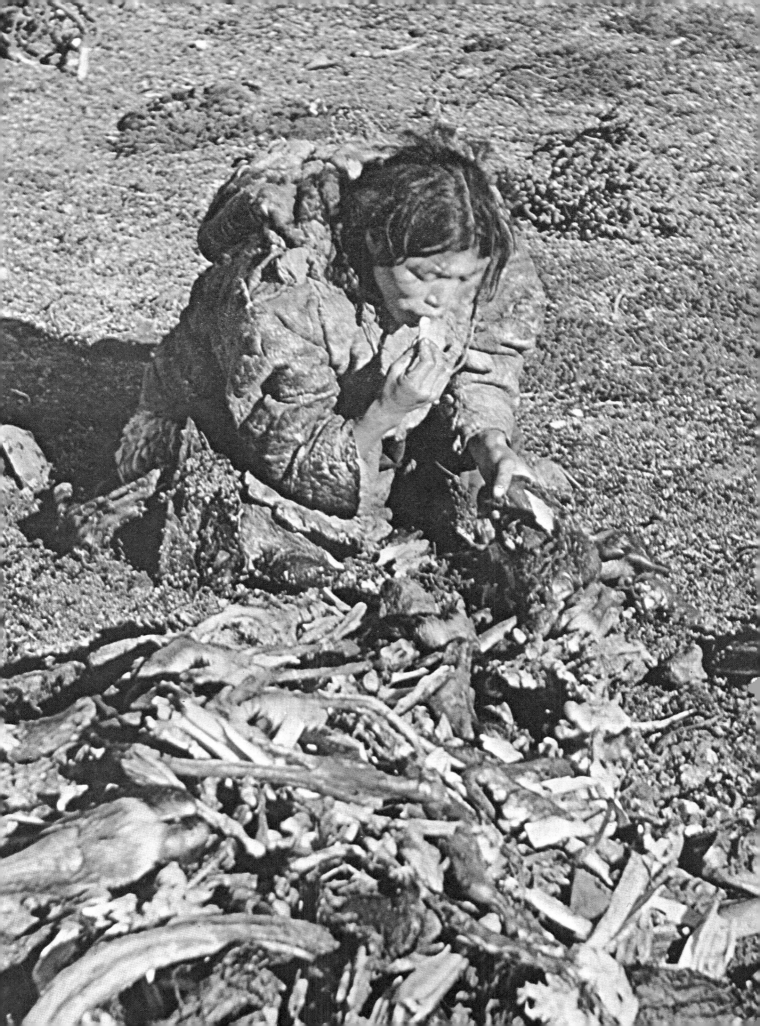

The Requirements of Human Nutrition

by Nevin S. Scrimshaw and Vernon R. Young
September 1976

*Environmental, dietary and physiological factors all
interact to set nutritional needs of individuals and
populations. Recommended energy and nutrient
allowances are thus statistical approximations*

Human beings lack the biochemical machinery to manufacture a variety of carbon compounds required for the formation and maintenance of tissues and for the metabolic reactions that sustain life. These compounds, which all animal cells and organisms must obtain preformed from the environment, together with a number of mineral elements, are termed the essential nutrients. Over the past few million years of evolutionary time the competitive struggle to obtain them in sufficient amounts has favored the emergence and dominance of the human species and has profoundly influenced man's social and cultural ascent. At the same time man's inability to manufacture the essential nutrient compounds has exposed him to deficiency diseases that continue to threaten hundreds of millions of people in today's world.

How did the diverse nutritional requirements of animals, including man, evolve? A significant clue was provided some 30 years ago when the pioneering studies of George W. Beadle and Edward L. Tatum of Stanford University with the red mold *Neurospora* demonstrated that gene mutation can bring about alterations in the needs of cells and organisms for an external supply of compounds. Like all other plants, *Neurospora* normally requires no vitamins or amino acids for its metabolism and growth; it makes them itself. When Beadle and Tatum exposed the mold cells to X rays, however, the resulting mutations caused a loss in the cells' ability to synthesize vitamins such as thiamine, pyridoxine and para-aminobenzoic acid and the amino acids histidine, lysine and tryptophan.

Evolutionary biologists now believe a similar series of mutations occurred in the remote past to give rise to the nutrient-synthesizing deficiencies of animals. The earliest forms of life appear to have been simple bacteriumlike organisms that were capable of manufacturing all the compounds they needed from mineral salts, nitrogen, simple compounds of carbon and of course water. This ability entailed the storage of an enormous amount of genetic information, and cells that could reduce the metabolic costs of replicating and maintaining genes gained a selective advantage. With natural selection favoring mutations that eliminated the "unnecessary" enzymatic synthesis of readily available nutrients, primitive forms of life evolved and ultimately developed into animal cells.

When the first single-cell animals appeared about a billion years ago, they lacked a number of the biosynthetic pathways found in plant cells, notably the photosynthetic pathway that enables a plant to convert the energy of sunlight into the energy-rich compounds that drive the metabolism of cells. All the animal species that subsequently emerged from these ancestral beginnings had similar deficiencies, but they survived by obtaining the energy and nutrients they needed from external sources. For example, plants have retained the ability to make all the 20 amino acids found in their proteins from simple carbon and nitrogen compounds, whereas animals depend on their diet to supply about half of these amino acids.

An interesting and quite recent evolutionary development of nutritional significance is the inability of certain animals to synthesize ascorbic acid (vitamin C). I. B. Chatterjee of the University College of Science in India has estimated that some 350 million years ago the capacity for synthesizing this vitamin arose in amphibians, but that a gene mutation about 25 million years ago in a common ancestor of man and other primates led to a loss of the enzyme L-gulono oxidase, which catalyzed the terminal step in the conversion of glucose to ascorbic acid. Linus Pauling has suggested that the loss of this pathway was selectively advantageous in that it freed glucose for energy use by the body. In any case the mutation was not lethal because the missing compound was present in the food of the mutant animals. Their evolution could thus continue.

Man's need to obtain an adequate supply of essential nutrients through his diet not only is a part of his biological evolution but also has shaped his social evolution. It has been suggested that the migration of human groups to the northern regions of the earth was slowed by the limited amounts of ascorbic acid in the foods available in those areas during the long winter months. Moreover, man's dependence on an adequate supply of nutrients meant that he initially had to be a hunter and gatherer, which circumscribed his cultural development. With the domestication of the cereal grains and other plants, along with a limited number of animal species, he was able to organize a stable way of life and secure the essential nutrients without foraging over substantial areas. This freed his energies for new kinds of so-

PREGNANT CARIBOU ESKIMO WOMAN chews caribou bones to extract the last scraps of nutrient-rich marrow in this photograph made in 1955 by Fritz Goro in the Canadian Northwest Territories. Scattered over barren taiga south of the Arctic Circle, small bands of these inland Eskimos subsisted entirely on the caribou, relying on the animal for food and clothing and even using the bones for projectile points and other tools. Although the caribou were once plentiful, in the late 1950's they changed their migration route, causing a disastrous famine among the Caribou Eskimos. In 1960 the Canadian government airlifted the survivors to the coast, where they mixed with other Eskimos and went to work in a nickel mine. Today the Caribou Eskimos do not exist as a distinct population, victims of their single-source diet.

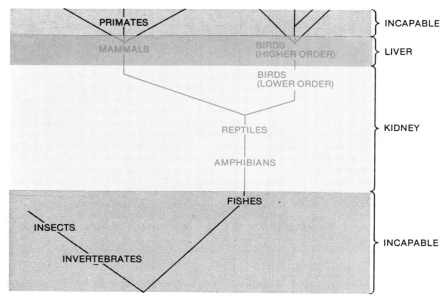

ABILITY OF ANIMALS TO SYNTHESIZE VITAMIN C and the type of cell performing the synthesis have varied over the span of evolution. Some 25 million years ago a mutation in an ancestor of primates (including man) and other mammals resulted in a loss of the terminal enzyme in the synthetic pathway. For this reason primates, guinea pigs, bats and some birds require a dietary source of the vitamin to prevent development of nutritional disease.

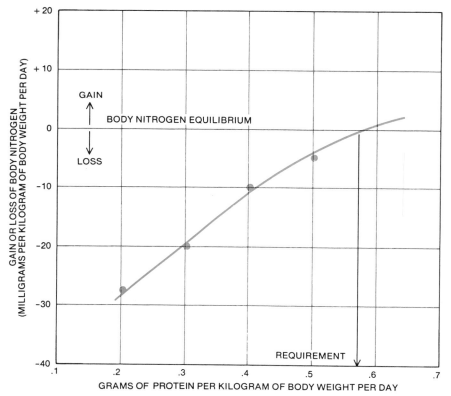

MINIMUM PROTEIN REQUIREMENT for a population of privileged young men was determined in the authors' laboratory with the metabolic-balance technique. Students at the Massachusetts Institute of Technology were studied at various protein (nitrogen) intakes for 15-day periods. They received a constant diet in which the entire protein source was whole dried-egg powder. Nitrogen-balance values (intake minus excretion equals balance) for the seven subjects were measured at each intake level; data points shown are statistical mean of individual numbers. Amount of protein sufficient to maintain nitrogen balance, where subjects were neither losing nor gaining body nitrogen, was judged to be minimum requirement.

cial, economic and artistic activities.

At least 45 and possibly as many as 50 dietary compounds and elements are now recognized as essential for a human being to live a full, healthy life. Plant and animal foods cannot, however, be directly utilized by the cells of human tissues. The nutrients contained in foods are released by digestion, absorbed in the intestine and transported to the cells by the blood. As long as the overall diet supplies all the essential nutrients, the cells and tissues of the body are capable of synthesizing the many thousands of additional compounds required for life.

Since the body is dependent on a regular supply of nutrients, intricate biochemical mechanisms have evolved to regulate the availability of the nutrients to the cells so that the organism can adjust to a wide range of intakes. Those nutrients that have been acquired in excess of cellular needs are handled by catabolic pathways that bring about their breakdown. The breakdown products are then eliminated in the urine, bile, sweat and other body secretions so that they do not accumulate and reach toxic levels.

The importance of regulating nutrient levels is dramatically illustrated in certain human diseases. In the genetic disorder known as maple-syrup-urine disease infants cannot adequately metabolize the branched-chain amino acids (leucine, isoleucine and valine). In another genetic disorder, phenylketonuria, the enzyme for breaking down the amino acid phenylalanine is lacking. Both conditions cause a buildup of amino acids in the blood and the tissues, particularly the brain, leading to cell death and mental retardation. The management of patients with these diseases consists of special diets containing a low level of the offending nutrient.

Another example of the accumulation of nutrients to toxic levels is hemochromatosis, a severe form of liver disease usually resulting from a combination of high iron and alcohol intakes that give rise to an excessive accumulation of iron in the liver. Vitamins A, D and K are also toxic in high concentrations. Hypervitaminosis from an excessive dietary intake of vitamin A, usually from the misguided use of high-potency vitamin pills, results in thickening of the skin, headaches and increased susceptibility to disease.

On the other hand, if the nutrient intake is so low that it is insufficient to meet the normal needs of cells, changes occur within the cells and tissues that act to conserve the limited supply. These changes may involve a more effective absorption of nutrients from the intestine and the activation of biochemical mechanisms that enhance the retention of the nutrient once it is inside the body.

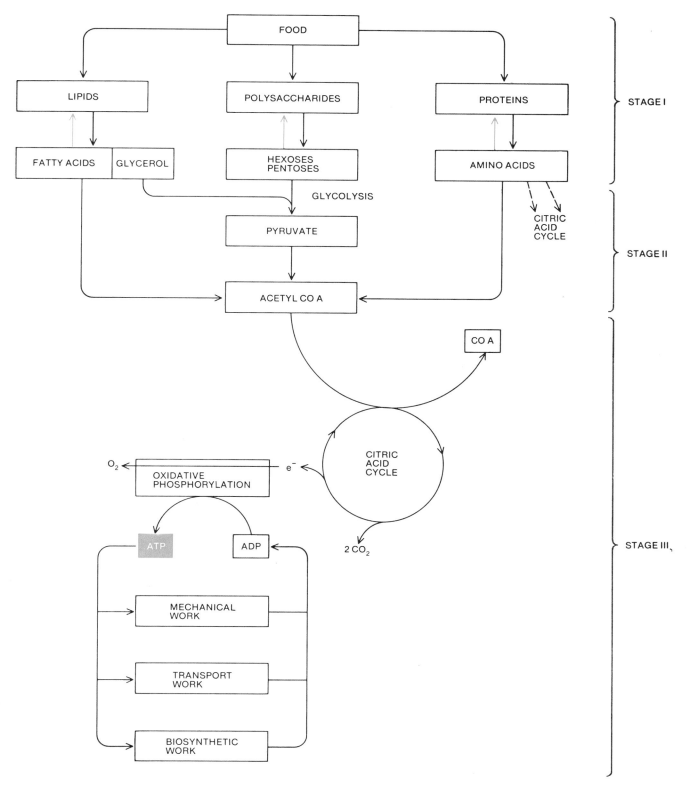

METABOLISM OF ENERGY-CONTAINING NUTRIENTS in the body proceeds in three major stages. In the first stage the large nutrient molecules of food are degraded into their main building blocks by digestive enzymes in the alimentary tract. In the second stage the many different products of the first stage are absorbed by the intestine and transported by the blood to the tissue cells. There they can either be incorporated into cellular molecules by anabolic pathways (*colored arrows*) or converted by catabolic pathways into a small number of intermediates that play a central role in metabolism. Glucose, glycerol, fatty acids and many amino acids are converted into a single two-carbon species: the acetyl group of the carrier molecule coenzyme A (CoA). In the third stage, which is localized in the mitochondria of cells, coenzyme A brings acetyl units into the citric acid cycle, where they are completely oxidized to carbon dioxide, concurrently releasing four pairs of electrons. The energy-rich compound adenosine triphosphate (ATP) is generated as the electrons flow down a transport chain to oxygen, the ultimate electron acceptor. Oxidation of a single glucose molecule can result in the formation of 36 molecules of ATP. Once generated, ATP provides the energy for the numerous physiological and synthetic activities of cells.

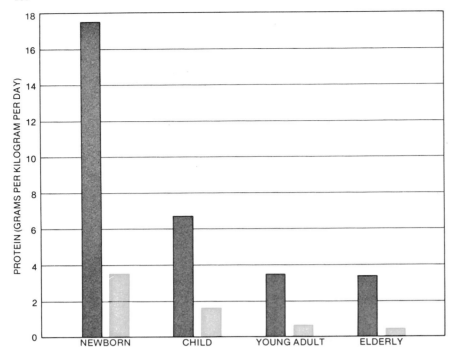

DECLINE IN DIETARY PROTEIN REQUIREMENT per unit of body weight (*color*) approximately parallels the change in rate of whole-body protein synthesis during the stages of life (*gray*). The early phase of rapid development in infants requires high levels of protein turnover and dietary intake, but both fall off as the rate of growth decreases. (Since 70 percent or more of the amino acids utilized in protein synthesis are provided by breakdown of other body proteins, dietary need is small in relation to turnover.) Data for infants, young adults and elderly subjects were obtained at the Clinical Research Center at M.I.T.; those for one-year-old children were provided by D. Picou of the Tropical Metabolism Research Unit in Jamaica.

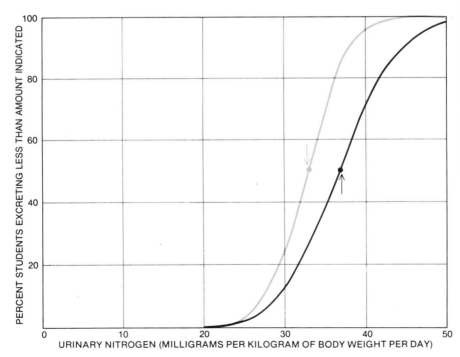

VARIATION IN PROTEIN METABOLISM of two genetically and geographically different population groups was revealed to a statistically significant degree by the distribution of obligatory urinary nitrogen losses in young men fed on a protein-free diet for 12 days. Daily urinary nitrogen excretion during the last four days of the experimental period was measured in 83 male college students studied at M.I.T. by the authors (*black curve*) and in 50 students subsequently studied by P.-C. Huang at the National Taiwan University College of Medicine (*colored curve*). The graph shows the mean excretion for each population (*vertical arrows*) and the cumulative distribution of urinary nitrogen losses within the two groups of students.

If the dietary intake continues to be inadequate, these metabolic adaptations break down and deficiency disease rises above the "clinical horizon," with characteristic symptoms that can lead to disability and death.

In addition to essential nutrients the body needs a supply of energy, that is, energy-rich compounds whose energy content is measured in calories. The assessment of the quantitative requirements for calories and the essential nutrients is clearly of great practical importance in human nutrition. The task is far more difficult than is generally realized. In animal husbandry the minimum needs of the animal for individual nutrients can be judged in relation to certain productive functions, such as rapid growth in meat-producing animals, high milk yield in dairy cows and maximum fleece production in sheep. The nutrient requirements of the human organism cannot be defined as readily because its well-being is more difficult to measure. What are the appropriate yardsticks? Maximum physical fitness and disease resistance would seem to be logical criteria for assessing the requirements for individual nutrients, but because we cannot quantify physical well-being as precisely as we can the growth of experimental animals, we must seek more objective measures.

Some nutrients or their breakdown products are excreted daily in the urine, feces and sweat and are lost through the shedding of small amounts of skin and hair. For the body to remain in metabolic equilibrium the total gain of a nutrient in food must equal the total loss. Therefore by measuring the intake required to balance the amount lost daily by the body it is possible to estimate the minimum metabolic need for a given nutrient. For example, nitrogen, a characteristic and relatively constant component of protein, is measured to determine protein needs. The metabolic-balance approach has also been followed in measuring the requirements for calcium, zinc and magnesium, but it is not suited to nutrients that are oxidized and whose carbon is eliminated in the respired air, such as fats and vitamins. For those nutrients the requirement can be estimated by determining the minimum amount of the nutrient that prevents the onset of subclinical deficiency disease, although the technique has its methodological and ethical restrictions.

Even when the metabolic-balance method is applicable, it does not provide information on where in the body the nutrient is being retained or utilized; overall nutrient balance might be achieved with a given intake of the nutrient being examined, but this does not prove that the tissues are functioning optimally and that health will be maintained. In addition it is difficult to carry out balance studies for prolonged dietary periods; such studies call for sophisticated facilities and a team of trained workers. The need to carefully control nutrient-intake levels requires that the daily menu be monotonous. Losses in the urine and feces (and ideally in sweat, skin and hair as well) must be assayed quantitatively, which means additional inconvenience for the subjects and technical problems for the investigators, particularly when the subjects are infants, young children or elderly people. For these reasons metabolic-balance studies are usually of short duration: a week or less in children and two or three weeks in adults. The long-term nutritional and health significance of these brief study periods has not been critically determined, so that the adequacy of our current estimates of nutrient requirements, which have been based on short-term studies, is uncertain. This is not a satisfactory state of affairs.

In the Department of Nutrition and Food Science at the Massachusetts Institute of Technology, working with Edwina E. Murray as research nutritionist and several physician graduate students, we have been able to complete a series of long-term metabolic-balance studies with highly motivated and cooperative students. These subjects have adhered to monotonous diets and have followed strict regimens for the complete daily collection of urine and feces for periods lasting up to 100 days, a significant increase over the usual 14- to 21-day balance period.

In one study six volunteer subjects lived on a diet providing protein at a level equal to the safe practical intake recommended by the 1973 Joint Food and Agriculture Organization–World Health Organization Expert Committee on Energy and Protein Requirements. By the end of three months metabolic measurements on these subjects indicated that there were decreases in lean body and muscle mass and/or changes in liver metabolism. These results

IRON IS RELEASED FROM FOODS during digestion. In the ferrous (Fe^{++}) oxidation state it passes from within the intestine into the cells of the intestinal mucosa, where it is oxidized to the ferric (Fe^{+++}) form. Ferric ion then combines with the protein apoferritin to form the complex known as ferritin. The amount of iron bound up in ferritin at any given time helps to stabilize the level of iron in the blood and protect the cells from iron toxicity. At the surface of the mucosal cell ferric ion is reduced to the ferrous form and enters the bloodstream, where it is reoxidized. It then combines with the protein transferrin, which transports it to the various tissues. Relatively little iron is excreted; the iron liberated by the breakdown of hemoglobin is recycled for the manufacture of hemoglobin.

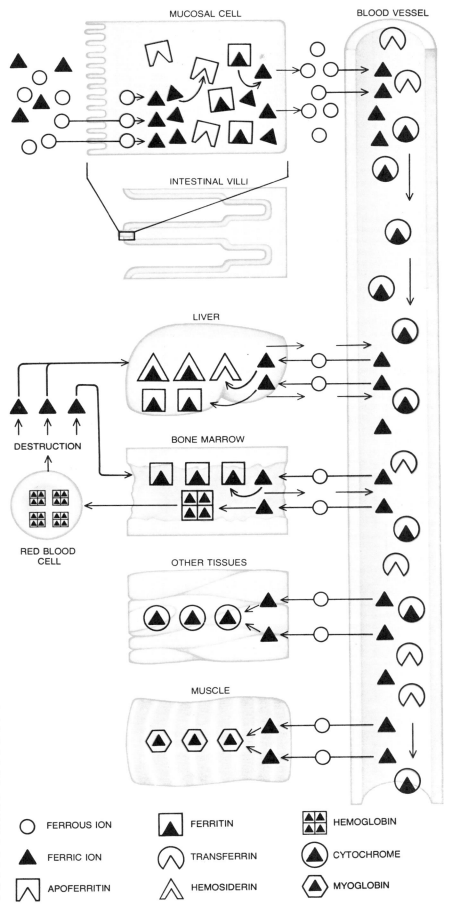

MUCOSAL CELL

BLOOD VESSEL

INTESTINAL VILLI

LIVER

DESTRUCTION

BONE MARROW

RED BLOOD CELL

OTHER TISSUES

MUSCLE

○ FERROUS ION

▲ FERRIC ION

⌈ APOFERRITIN

▣ FERRITIN

⋀ TRANSFERRIN

⋀ HEMOSIDERIN

HEMOGLOBIN

⬤ CYTOCHROME

⬡ MYOGLOBIN

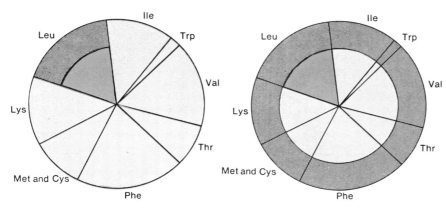

NINE ESSENTIAL AMINO ACIDS must be present simultaneously and in correct relative amounts for protein synthesis to occur. If one or more of the essential amino acids are partially missing (*dark color*), the utilization of all other amino acids in the cellular pool will be reduced in the same proportion. Leftover amino acids cannot be stored and are metabolized for energy. The amino acid abbreviations are Leu, leucine; Val, valine; Phe, phenylalanine; Thr, threonine; Ile, isoleucine; Lys, lysine; Met, methionine; Cys, cystine; Trp, tryptophan.

strongly suggest that short-term metabolic balance studies are not sufficient as the sole criterion for assessing human protein requirements and that the current recommendations for dietary protein intake for large population groups are inadequate. Although our own balance studies have involved experimental diet periods significantly longer than those employed for the FAO–WHO estimates, the fact remains that the experimental subjects are few in number and are confined to privileged American males, and that the duration of the study is still limited.

For some of the essential nutrients none of these approaches has been followed, and only vague epidemiological data are available. Here we must depend mainly on data obtained in animal experiments and extrapolate the results cautiously to humans, or attempt to assess how much well-nourished groups consume and consider that as an adequate intake level.

The many difficulties faced in determining the amounts of nutrients required by an individual are compounded by the problem of determining the variation in the requirements of that individual over a period of time, and with the variation encountered among individuals. It is easy to establish that physiological states such as growth, pregnancy and lactation call for greater amounts of most nutrients than those needed by healthy adults for maintenance alone. It is harder to measure the subtle changes in requirements that occur in the aging adult, a problem often complicated by the cumulative effects of both acute and chronic diseases that can affect requirements for nutrients by interfering with their absorption or utilization.

Knowledge of nutrient requirements in infants and in young children is also on uncertain ground. There is a tendency for investigators to regard such individuals as little adults and, with a small allowance for their growth, to extrapolate their requirements proportionately by weight from studies of older individuals. This approach does not take into account changes in the metabolic activities of cells and in the rates of nutrient turnover with age. For body protein, studies in our laboratory demonstrate high rates of turnover in newborn infants that diminish rapidly during the early weeks and months of infancy. Thereafter the decline is less rapid, but on a whole-body basis it probably continues with the passage of time during the adult years. Although protein requirements are not determined entirely by metabolic-turnover rate, the direction of change in the requirements for total dietary protein is the same as that for body protein turnover.

There is also variation in nutrient requirements among individuals of the same age, sex and physiological state because of the interaction of genetic and environmental factors. The important variation in nutritional requirements is the one that is due to the actual expression of genes in the individual, rather than the potential expression of genes under ideal circumstances. For example, in Japan there has been an increase in the height of adults over the past 30 years, when a progressively greater proportion of the full genetic potential was expressed as dietary and environmental conditions improved.

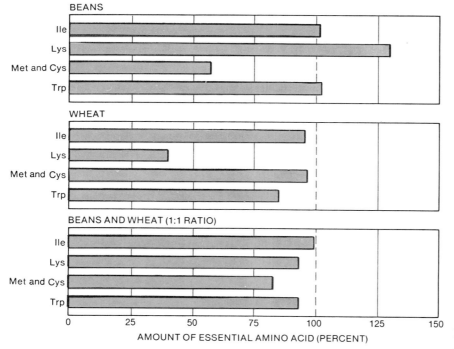

PROTEIN COMPLEMENTARITY can come about when a "poor quality" protein inadequate in certain essential amino acids but adequate in others is mixed with another protein having opposite strengths and weaknesses. If the two kinds of protein are ingested simultaneously or within a short time, the mixture can yield an overall amino acid balance comparable to that of a "high quality" protein ingested alone. The broken line represents 100 percent of the essential amino acid levels in a standard reference protein that is considered by a Food and Agriculture Organization–World Health Organization expert committee to best meet human requirements. Complementary protein combinations are found in almost all cultures.

One problem in knowing the appropriate variation to assign to nutrient requirements in normal individuals is the lack of data on the populations of different countries. In a study at M.I.T. we have given students a protein-free but otherwise adequate diet for 12 days in order to estimate the minimum level of nitrogen excretion, known as the obligatory loss. The statistical means of this urinary nitrogen value were significantly higher than those found subsequently for university students in Taiwan, who were studied under comparable conditions by P.-C. Huang of the National Taiwan University College of Medicine. Whether this disparity is due to genetic differences or to environmental and experimental factors is currently undetermined, but the fact of the difference appears to be indisputable. The nutritional significance of this observation is not fully known, but it emphasizes the great need for a larger number of comparative studies on nutrient metabolism and requirements in populations of differing geographic, cultural and genetic backgrounds.

Nutrient requirements also depend on a variety of environmental factors that may be physical (for example average ambient temperature), biological (the presence of infectious organisms and other parasites) or social (physical activity, the type of clothing worn, sanitary conditions and personal hygiene and other patterns of behavior). Environmental factors can influence nutritional status by directly modifying dietary requirements or by their effects on the production and availability of food and on its consumption.

The major dietary factors influencing nutrient requirements are threefold. The first is that the form of a nutrient in food may have a significant effect on its degree of absorption and utilization. For example, the relatively low efficiency of the absorption of iron from vegetable foods is a major factor in the total iron intake required by human beings. Ferrous iron (reduced iron, as in ferrous sulfate or finely divided elemental iron) is more effectively absorbed than ferric iron (as in ferric chloride or iron pyrophosphate). Even ferrous iron, however, is absorbed less efficiently when it is ingested in combination with phytates and oxalates, which are found in leafy green vegetables and the whole-grain, unleav-

NET PROTEIN UTILIZATION values are an index of the "quality," or nutritional value, of proteins from various food sources. They are the percent of the amino acids ingested as protein that are retained in the body and incorporated into cellular proteins. Egg protein, along with that of milk and most meats, has excellent proportions of all the essential amino acids, and its net utilization by the body is accordingly high. Legumes, on the other hand, are deficient in one or more of the nine essential amino acids, which greatly reduces the proportion of total amino acids that are available for protein synthesis and thus gives rise to their low NPU values.

FOOD	ESSENTIAL AMINO ACIDS		NET PROTEIN UTILIZATION (PERCENT)
	POOR	ADEQUATE	0 25 50 75 100
DAIRY			
EGGS	—	Trp, Lys, Met, Cys	
COW'S MILK	—	Trp, Lys	
COTTAGE CHEESE	—	Lys	
SWISS CHEESE	—	Lys	
MEATS			
FISH	—	Lys	
TURKEY	—	Lys	
PORK	—	Lys	
BEEF	—	Lys	
CHICKEN	—	Lys	
LAMB	—	Lys	
VEGETABLES			
CORN	Trp, Lys	—	
ASPARAGUS	Met, Cys	—	
BROCCOLI	Met, Cys	—	
CAULIFLOWER	Met, Cys	Trp, Lys	
POTATO	Met, Cys	Trp	
KALE	Lys, Met, Cys	—	
GREEN PEAS	Met, Cys	Lys	
GRAINS AND CEREALS			
BROWN RICE	Lys	—	
WHEAT GERM	Trp	Lys	
OATMEAL	Lys	—	
WHEAT GRAIN	Lys	—	
RYE	Trp, Lys	—	
POLISHED RICE	Lys, Thr	Trp	
MILLET	Lys	Trp, Met, Cys	
PASTA	Lys, Met, Cys	—	
LEGUMES			
SOYBEANS	Met, Cys, Val	Lys, Trp	
LIMA BEANS	Met, Cys	Trp, Lys	
KIDNEY BEANS	Trp, Met, Cys	Lys	
LENTILS	Trp, Met, Cys	Lys	
NUTS AND SEEDS			
SUNFLOWER SEEDS	Lys	Trp	
SESAME SEEDS	Lys	Trp, Met, Cys	
PEANUTS	Lys, Met, Cys, Thr	—	

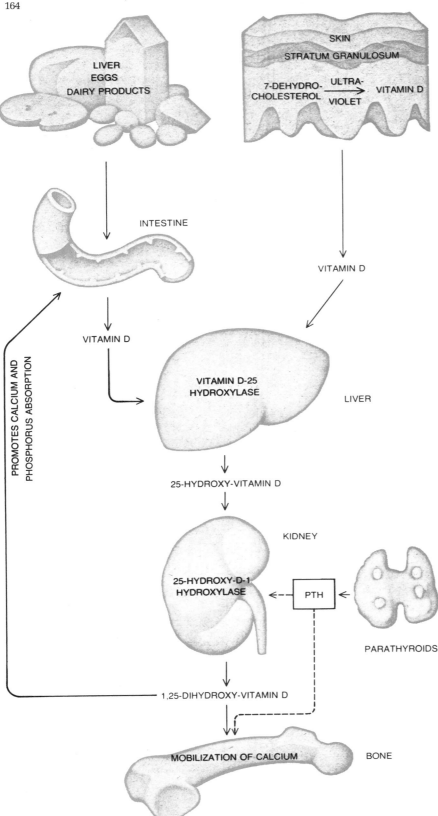

VITAMIN D is absorbed preformed from certain foods and is also synthesized in the stratum granulosum of the skin through the action of solar radiation on the closely related steroid 7-dehydrocholesterol. The physiological roles of the vitamin depend on its conversion to the active form 1,25-dihydroxy-vitamin D, which occurs in two enzyme-catalyzed steps, the first in the liver and the second in the kidney. Parathyroid hormone (PTH) serves to regulate the synthesis of the active form of the vitamin, and both act to mobilize calcium from bone. In addition the dihydroxylated vitamin alone stimulates calcium absorption from the small intestine.

ened bread of North Africa and the Middle East. The iron found in meat (heme iron) is much better absorbed than iron of vegetable origin, and small amounts of red meat markedly improve overall iron absorption.

The second major factor affecting nutrient requirements is that the presence or absence of one nutrient frequently affects the utilization of another. For example, when dietary protein intake is deficient, the two proteins that play a role in the transport of vitamin A (retinol-binding protein and prealbumin) are not made by the liver in adequate amounts. The esterified form of the vitamin remains stored in the liver, unavailable to the other body tissues. Signs of vitamin-A deficiency may then appear, in spite of the fact that the intake of the vitamin (or of its precursor, beta-carotene, which is present in plant foods) would be sufficient if protein nutrition were adequate.

The third factor is the presence in the human large intestine of bacteria that live on organic molecules not absorbed in the small intestine. In the course of their metabolic activities these bacteria manufacture vitamins that their human host absorbs; it is a symbiotic, or mutually beneficial, relationship. Vitamin K, a deficiency of which causes failure of blood clotting, is synthesized in this way, as are small quantities of some of the B vitamins.

The factors influencing the adequacy of dietary protein for an individual may be even more complex. In the first place, the normal requirement is not for protein per se but, depending on the individual's age, for some nine or 10 essential amino acids in adequate amounts and appropriate proportions. Whether an amino acid is utilized for the synthesis of new protein or is degraded for its energy content (a wasteful process) depends on a number of factors. First, each of the essential amino acids must be present simultaneously in the intracellular pool for protein synthesis to proceed. If a given amino acid is present only in a limited amount, the protein can be formed only as long as the supply of that amino acid (called the limiting amino acid) lasts. If one essential amino acid is missing from the pool, the remaining ones cannot be stored for later synthesis and will be catabolized for energy.

The level of nonprotein calories in the diet is also important. If it is high with respect to need, the ingested protein is spared from breakdown to meet energy requirements, but the individual tends to become obese. If it is low, some of the protein will be preempted to meet energy requirements and will not be available to fulfill the actual protein needs of the body. It is sometimes mistakenly believed that it is not worth improving the protein content of a diet if caloric intake is deficient. Our studies of young adults indicate that some improvement in protein retention is achieved even under circumstances of deficient energy intake. Adequate nonspecific sources of nitrogen are also needed so that the nonessential amino acids and other metabolically important nitrogenous compounds can be synthesized in the body.

Various proteins differ in their essential amino acid concentration and balance. A nutritionally "complete" protein source such as meat, eggs or milk supplies enough of all the essential amino acids needed to meet the body's requirements for maintenance and growth. A low-quality or nutritionally "incomplete" protein such as the zein of corn, which lacks the amino acids tryptophan and lysine, cannot support either maintenance or growth. A somewhat less inferior protein such as the gliadin of wheat provides enough lysine for maintenance but not enough for growth. Plant proteins usually contain inadequate amounts of one essential amino acid or more. Lysine and threonine levels in cereals are generally low, and corn is also deficient in tryptophan. Legumes are good sources of lysine but are low in the sulfur-containing amino acids methionine and cystine; leafy green vegetables are well balanced in all the essential amino acids except methionine.

In spite of these shortcomings of individual foods it is possible to devise meals containing acceptable proportions of essential amino acids by combining proteins from several sources. In general, cereals that are deficient in lysine are complemented by legumes that are deficient in methionine. Every culture has evolved its own mixtures of complementary proteins. In the Middle East wheat bread, which lacks adequate levels of lysine, is eaten with cheese, which has a high lysine content. Mexicans eat beans and rice, Jamaicans eat rice and peas, Indians eat wheat and pulses, and Americans eat breakfast cereals with milk. This kind of supplementation, particularly in infants and growing children, only works, however, when the deficient and complementary proteins are ingested together or are ingested separately within a few hours.

Acute or chronic infections or other disease processes that cause decreased gastrointestinal function increase the need for dietary protein, because less of it will be absorbed. Trauma, anxiety, fear and other causes of stress have an even more pronounced effect in altering protein requirements. Stress results in an increase in the catabolism of muscle protein with respect to synthesis, leading to the transport of amino acids away from muscle and peripheral tissues to the liver, where they are converted to glucose for energy pur-

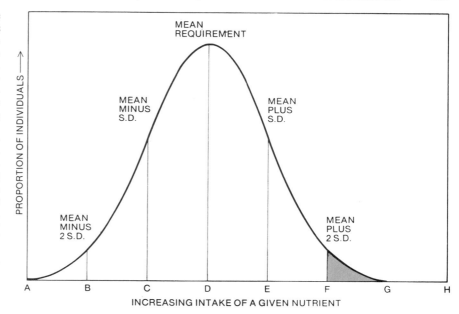

DISTRIBUTION OF NUTRIENT REQUIREMENTS in a hypothetical population of healthy individuals is bell-shaped. D is the mean requirement for the population. The statistical unit of variation from the mean is known as the standard deviation (S.D.), which is calculated from the sum of the squares of each individual's replacement values, minus the square of the average value, divided by the square root of the total number of observations. An intake of F, obtained by adding two standard deviations to the mean value, would cover the requirements for nearly all (97.5 percent) of the individuals in this population. Colored region shows the small minority of healthy individuals (2.5 percent) not covered by the allowance. This approach has been followed by international committees in estimating dietary allowances.

poses. This process creates a deficit in the protein content of the body, which must be compensated for by increased protein retention during the recovery period.

With any infection, even immunization with live-virus vaccines, there is a loss of appetite that leads to a decrease in food intake. The metabolic consequences of acute infections have been most extensively documented by William R. Beisel and his collaborators at the Army Medical Research Institute of Infectious Diseases. The first changes are increased synthesis of antibodies and other proteins characteristic of acute illness, followed by catabolic responses that result in increased losses of nitrogen (from body protein), vitamin A, vitamin C, iron and zinc, and probably other nutrients as well.

Disease may also directly upset the mechanisms controlling the metabolism of essential nutrients, thereby altering dietary nutrient requirements. The conversion of vitamin D into its metabolically active form, for example, depends on the activities of the liver and the kidneys. If the kidneys are diseased, the normal utilization of the vitamin is compromised. It is for this reason that many individuals suffering from kidney disease show skeletal abnormalities similar to those seen in rickets, a disease of vitamin D deficiency. When these patients are given a synthetic form of the active

derivative of the vitamin, they show a marked improvement in health.

The absorption of nutrients is reduced whenever the gastrointestinal tract is significantly affected by acute or chronic infections, by a high concentration of intestinal parasites or by malaria (which interferes with the mesenteric circulation). Chronic infections and parasitic infestations are also capable of increasing nutrient requirements in other ways. Even with a diet that would otherwise be adequate iron-deficiency anemia can develop as a result of the intestinal blood loss associated with hookworm, schistosomiasis and certain protozoal infections. In northern European countries where the eating of raw fish commonly leads to heavy infestations of fish tapeworm, vitamin B-12 deficiency disease (anemia and neurological damage) often develops in affected individuals because the parasite has a particularly large requirement for the vitamin.

For these reasons young children in developing countries who are subject to intestinal, respiratory and other infections that increase nutrient requirements, and who at the same time have a poor diet, are particularly likely to develop acute nutritional disease. The ideal public-health approach would be to eliminate the infections rather than to provide the extra amounts of nutrients these conditions require, but that is frequently not possible because of a lack of resources or for social reasons.

All these sources of variation in nutrient requirements make it impossible to generate precise values for nutrient requirements in either individuals or population groups. Instead nutrient allowances must be viewed statistically, on the assumption that individual variation in a nutrient requirement is distributed in a bell-shaped curve above and below the mean requirement for that population group.

It is not practical to attempt to arrive at nutritional recommendations suffi-cient to cover 100 percent of a population, because this would require far more nutrition than is necessary for most people. There will always be a few normal individuals in a population, two or three per 100, who need more of a nutrient than can be recommended in

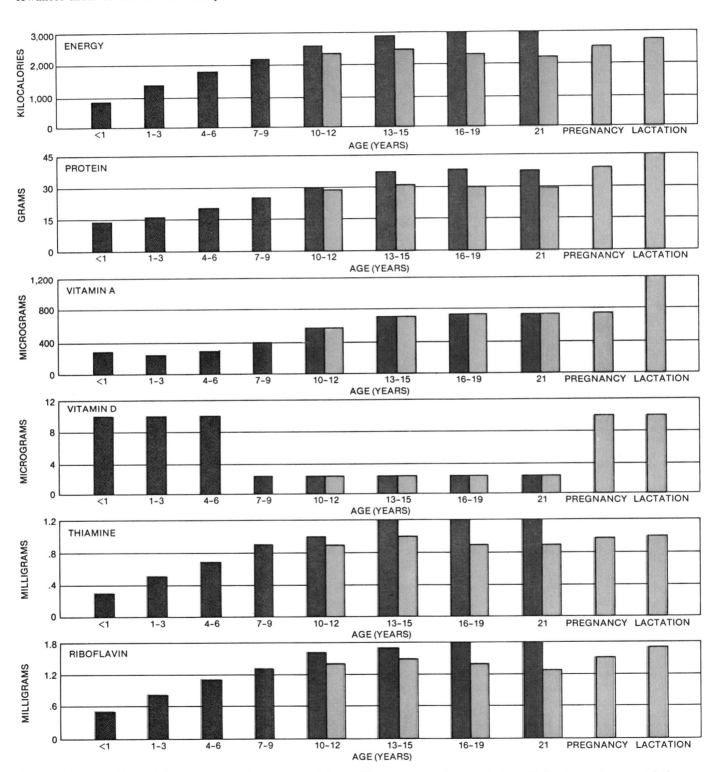

RECOMMENDED DAILY ALLOWANCES for energy, protein and selected vitamins and minerals shown here were agreed on by an FAO–WHO expert committee in 1974. Requirements vary marked-ly with age, and those of males (*gray*) are significantly different from

a practical dietary allowance, and a smaller number at the extreme tail of the bell curve, two or three per 1,000, whose metabolic abnormalities significantly increase their requirements. Finally, recommended daily allowances (RDA's) are intended only to cover healthy individuals and are often not adequate for people suffering from acute or chronic diseases.

The major limitation to the practical use of RDA's is that they are based on data from small and possibly unrepresentative samples that have been extrapolated to populations of all types. In developing countries, where a large fraction of the population is likely to be suffering from disease, children have a greatly reduced weight and height for their age because of the combined effects of repeated infections and malnu-

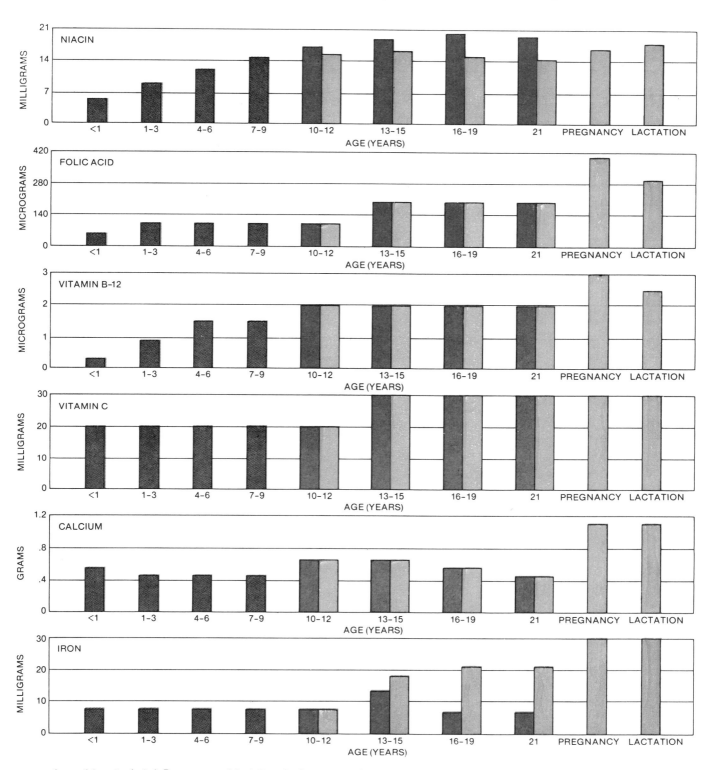

those of females (*color*). Pregnancy and lactation also increase nutritional needs. Recommended allowances are not absolute for individuals; they can be justifiably applied only to reasonably healthy populations and may well be subject to revision as knowledge advances.

trition. As a result the body size of adults is also small. For them the age-specific nutritional figures derived from well-nourished populations may be unnecessarily high and estimated caloric requirements may be excessive. It is therefore preferable to calculate allowances for adults in developing countries on the basis of kilograms of body weight.

Per-kilogram allowances are not sufficient, however, for children whose growth has been stunted by malnutrition and disease. Such allowances will be too low for maximum catch-up growth and will perpetuate the existing poor nutritional state of the children. A compromise in countries where nutritional dwarfism among children is common is to estimate the specific requirements of children on a per kilogram

ESSENTIAL AMINO ACIDS	RDA FOR HEALTHY ADULT MALE (MILLIGRAMS)	DIETARY SOURCES	MAJOR BODY FUNCTIONS	DEFICIENCY	EXCESS
AROMATIC					
PHENYLALANINE	1,100				
TYROSINE					
BASIC					
LYSINE	800				
HISTIDINE	Not known				

BRANCHED CHAIN		FROM PROTEINS
		
		GOOD SOURCES
		
		  Legume grains
		  Dairy products
		  Meat
		  Fish
			Precursors of structural protein, enzymes, antibodies, hormones, metabolically active compounds
			
			Certain amino acids have specific functions:		

ISOLEUCINE	700		(a) Tyrosine is a precursor of epinephrine and thyroxine	Deficient protein intake leads to development of kwashiorkor and, coupled with low energy intake, to marasmus.	Excess protein intake possibly aggravates or potentiates chronic disease states.

LEUCINE	1,000	ADEQUATE SOURCES
		
		  Rice
		  Corn
		  Wheat
			(b) Arginine is a precursor of polyamines		

VALINE	800	POOR SOURCES
		
		  Cassava
		  Sweet potato
			(c) Methionine is required for methyl group metabolism
			(d) Tryptophan is a precursor of serotonin		

SULFUR-CONTAINING					
METHIONINE	1,100				
CYSTINE					
OTHER					
TRYPTOPHAN	250				
THREONINE	500				
ESSENTIAL FATTY ACIDS					
ARACHIDONIC		Vegetable fats (corn, cottonseed, soy oils) Wheat germ Vegetable shortenings	Involved in cell membrane structure and function. Precursors of prostaglandins (regulation of gastric function, release of hormones, smooth-muscle activity)	Poor growth Skin lesions	Not known
LINOLEIC	6,000				
LINOLENIC					

ESSENTIAL AMINO ACIDS AND FATTY ACIDS cannot be synthesized in the body and must be present in food. Amino acids are the building blocks of body proteins; essential fatty acids are in- volved in the maintenance of cell membrane structure and function and serve as precursors of the prostaglandins, a family of hormone-like compounds that have diverse physiological actions in the body.

basis and add a modest extra allowance for catch-up growth.

When acute infections are prevalent in a population, extra allowance must be made for the individual during recovery, although because of reduced food intake during the acute phase of the illness and increased retention of some nutrients in depleted individuals, the overall food requirements of the group suffering from infections may be little affected. Increased dietary allowances may nonetheless be needed to compensate for continuing high nutrient losses or for the impaired absorption associated with intestinal-parasite load and chronic disease.

In sum, recommended allowances cannot serve as an absolute indicator of the adequacy of a given intake for a given individual. They can justifiably be

VITAMIN	RDA FOR HEALTHY ADULT MALE (MILLIGRAMS)	DIETARY SOURCES	MAJOR BODY FUNCTIONS	DEFICIENCY	EXCESS
WATER-SOLUBLE					
VITAMIN B-1 (THIAMINE)	1.5	Pork, organ meats, whole grains, legumes	Coenzyme (thiamine pyrophosphate) in reactions involving the removal of carbon dioxide.	Beriberi (peripheral nerve changes, edema, heart failure)	None reported
VITAMIN B-2 (RIBOFLAVIN)	1.8	Widely distributed in foods.	Constituent of two flavin nucleotide coenzymes involved in energy metabolism (FAD and FMN)	Reddened lips, cracks at corner of mouth (cheilosis), lesions of eye	None reported
NIACIN	20	Liver, lean meats, grains, legumes (can be formed from tryptophan)	Constituent of two coenzymes involved in oxidation-reduction reactions (NAD and NADP)	Pellagra (skin and gastrointestinal lesions, nervous, mental disorders)	Flushing, burning and tingling around neck, face and hands
VITAMIN B-6 (PYRIDOXINE)	2	Meats, vegetables, whole-grain cereals	Coenzyme (pyridoxal phosphate) involved in amino acid metabolism	Irritability, convulsions, muscular twitching, dermatitis near eyes, kidney stones	None reported
PANTOTHENIC ACID	5–10	Widely distributed in foods.	Constituent of coenzyme A, which plays a central role in energy metabolism	Fatigue, sleep disturbances, impaired coordination, nausea (rare in man)	None reported
FOLACIN	.4	Legumes, green vegetables, whole-wheat products	Coenzyme (reduced form) involved in transfer of single-carbon units in nucleic acid and amino acid metabolism	Anemia, gastrointestinal disturbances, diarrhea, red tongue	None reported
VITAMIN B-12	.003	Muscle meats, eggs, dairy products, (not present in plant foods)	Coenzyme involved in transfer of single-carbon units in nucleic acid metabolism	Pernicious anemia, neurological disorders	None reported
BIOTIN	Not established. Usual diet provides .15–.3	Legumes, vegetables, meats	Coenzyme required for fat synthesis, amino acid metabolism and glycogen (animal-starch) formation	Fatigue, depression, nausea, dermatitis, muscular pains	Not reported
CHOLINE	Not established. Usual diet provides 500–900	All foods containing phospholipids (egg yolk, liver, grains, legumes)	Constituent of phospholipids. Precursor of putative neurotransmitter acetylcholine	Not reported in man.	None reported
VITAMIN C (ASCORBIC ACID)	45	Citrus fruits, tomatoes, green peppers, salad greens	Maintains intercellular matrix of cartilage, bone and dentine. Important in collagen synthesis.	Scurvy (degeneration of skin, teeth, blood vessels, epithelial hemorrhages)	Relatively nontoxic. Possibility of kidney stones.
FAT-SOLUBLE					
VITAMIN A (RETINOL)	1	Provitamin A (beta-carotene) widely distributed in green vegetables. Retinol present in milk, butter, cheese, fortified margarine.	Constituent of rhodopsin (visual pigment). Maintenance of epithelial tissues. Role in mucopolysaccharide synthesis.	Xerophthalmia (keratinization of ocular tissue), night blindness, permanent blindness	Headache, vomiting, peeling of skin, anorexia, swelling of long bones
VITAMIN D	.01	Cod-liver oil, eggs, dairy products, fortified milk and margarine.	Promotes growth and mineralization of bones. Increases absorption of calcium.	Rickets (bone deformities) in children. Osteomalacia in adults.	Vomiting, diarrhea, loss of weight, kidney damage
VITAMIN E (TOCOPHEROL)	15	Seeds, green leafy vegetables, margarines, shortenings	Functions as an antioxidant to prevent cell-membrane damage.	Possibly anemia	Relatively nontoxic
VITAMIN K (PHYLLOQUINONE)	.03	Green leafy vegetables. Small amount in cereals, fruits and meats	Important in blood clotting (involved in formation of active prothrombin)	Conditioned deficiencies associated with severe bleeding, internal hemorrhages.	Relatively nontoxic. Synthetic forms at high doses may cause jaundice.

VITAMINS are organic molecules needed in very small amounts in the diet of higher animals. Most of the water-soluble (B complex) vitamins act as coenzymes, or organic catalysts; the four fat-soluble vitamins (A, D, E and K) have more diverse functions. Although low vitamin intake can result in deficiency disease, the misguided use of high-potency vitamin pills can also have undesirable effects.

applied only to a reasonably healthy population. In spite of their limitations, however, estimates of caloric requirements and recommended allowances for essential nutrients must be supplied. They guide the design of diets for individuals, the evaluation of the relative adequacy of diets for populations, the content of nutrition-education programs and the planning by government of nutrition-intervention programs.

There is no area of human health in which research is more urgently needed than the nutritional requirements of representative human populations over the full range of both health and disease. Clearly an adequate knowledge of the amount and kinds of food required by man is essential for food and nutrition policy planning and will be of major importance for the generations ahead.

MINERAL	AMOUNT IN ADULT BODY (GRAMS)	RDA FOR HEALTHY ADULT MALE (MILLIGRAMS)	DIETARY SOURCES	MAJOR BODY FUNCTIONS	DEFICIENCY	EXCESS
CALCIUM	1,500	800	Milk, cheese, dark-green vegetables, dried legumes	Bone and tooth formation Blood clotting Nerve transmission	Stunted growth Rickets, osteoporosis Convulsions	Not reported in man
PHOSPHORUS	860	800	Milk, cheese, meat, poultry, grains	Bone and tooth formation Acid-base balance	Weakness, demineralization of bone Loss of calcium	Erosion of jaw (fossy jaw)
SULFUR	300	(Provided by sulfur amino acids)	Sulfur amino acids (methionine and cystine) in dietary proteins	Constituent of active tissue compounds, cartilage and tendon	Related to intake and deficiency of sulfur amino acids	Excess sulfur amino acid intake leads to poor growth
POTASSIUM	180	2,500	Meats, milk, many fruits	Acid-base balance Body water balance Nerve function	Muscular weakness Paralysis	Muscular weakness Death
CHLORINE	74	2,000	Common salt	Formation of gastric juice Acid base balance	Muscle cramps Mental apathy Reduced appetite	Vomiting
SODIUM	64	2,500	Common salt	Acid base balance Body water balance Nerve function	Muscle cramps Mental apathy Reduced appetite	High blood pressure
MAGNESIUM	25	350	Whole grains, green leafy vegetables	Activates enzymes. Involved in protein synthesis	Growth failure Behavioral disturbances Weakness, spasms	Diarrhea
IRON	4.5	10	Eggs, lean meats, legumes, whole grains, green leafy vegetables	Constituent of hemoglobin and enzymes involved in energy metabolism	Iron-deficiency anemia (weakness, reduced resistance to infection)	Siderosis Cirrhosis of liver
FLUORINE	2.6	2	Drinking water, tea, seafood	May be important in maintenance of bone structure	Higher frequency of tooth decay	Mottling of teeth Increased bone density Neurological disturbances
ZINC	2	15	Widely distributed in foods	Constituent of enzymes involved in digestion	Growth failure Small sex glands	Fever, nausea, vomiting, diarrhea
COPPER	.1	2	Meats, drinking water	Constituent of enzymes associated with iron metabolism	Anemia, bone changes (rare in man)	Rare metabolic condition (Wilson's disease)
SILICON VANADIUM TIN NICKEL	.024 .018 .017 .010	Not established	Widely distributed in foods	Function unknown (essential for animals)	Not reported in man	Industrial exposures: Silicon – silicosis Vanadium – lung irritation Tin – vomiting Nickel – acute pneumonitis
SELENIUM	.013	Not established (Diet provides .05–.1 per day)	Seafood, meat, grains	Functions in close association with vitamin E	Anemia (rare)	Gastrointestinal disorders, lung irritation
MANGANESE	.012	Not established (Diet provides 6–8 per day)	Widely distributed in foods	Constituent of enzymes involved in fat synthesis	In animals: poor growth, disturbances of nervous system, reproductive abnormalities	Poisoning in manganese mines: generalized disease of nervous system
IODINE	.011	.14	Marine fish and shell-fish, dairy products, many vegetables	Constituent of thyroid hormones	Goiter (enlarged thyroid)	Very high intakes depress thyroid activity
MOLYBDENUM	.009	Not established (Diet provides .4 per day)	Legumes, cereals, organ meats	Constituent of some enzymes	Not reported in man	Inhibition of enzymes
CHROMIUM	.006	Not established (Diet provides .05–.12 per day)	Fats, vegetable oils, meats	Involved in glucose and energy metabolism	Impaired ability to metabolize glucose	Occupational exposures: skin and kidney damage
COBALT	.0015	(Required as vitamin B-12)	Organ and muscle meats, milk	Constituent of vitamin B-12	Not reported in man	Industrial exposure: dermatitis and diseases of red blood cells
WATER	40,000 (60 percent of body weight)	1.5 liters per day	Solid foods, liquids, drinking water	Transport of nutrients Temperature regulation Participates in metabolic reactions	Thirst, dehydration	Headaches, nausea Edema High blood pressure

ESSENTIAL MINERAL ELEMENTS are involved in the electrochemical functions of nerve and muscle, the formation of bones and teeth, the activation of enzymes and, in the case of iron, the transport of oxygen. The trace minerals nickel, tin, vanadium and silicon, previously considered to be health hazards, are now known to be essential for animals. Although they are so widely distributed in nature that primary dietary deficiencies are unlikely, changes in the balance among them may have important consequences for health.

Total Intravenous Feeding

by Stanley J. Dudrick and Jonathan E. Rhoads
May 1952

It is now possible to feed a person entirely by vein for prolonged periods. The technique provides sufficient calories, amino acids and other nutrients to promote growth, weight gain and wound healing

When the digestive system of a hospital patient cannot maintain his nutrition, it is a common practice to feed the patient through a peripheral vein in the neck, an arm or a leg. Although the technique of intravenous feeding has advanced in each decade of this century, there have been serious limitations in the daily amount of nutrient that can be administered. As a result many critically ill patients have been faced with slow starvation. In particular, individuals with diseases of the alimentary tract that usually can be alleviated or cured surgically often had a poor prognosis for recovery from the operation because of malnutrition. Such patients are highly susceptible to postoperative complications and failure of wound healing.

In the past few years a safe and effec-

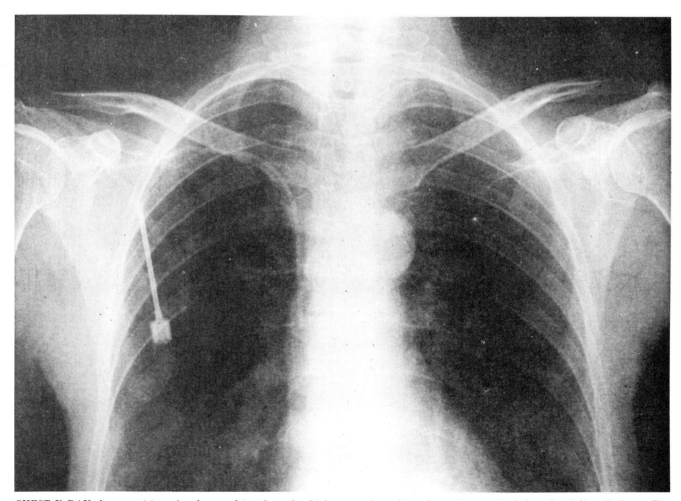

CHEST X RAY shows position of catheter tubing through which the nutrient solution is fed directly into a large vein near the heart. The thin catheter tubing still is attached to the needle used to introduce the catheter into a vein below the right collarbone. The tip of the inserted catheter can be seen near the spinal column. Infusion of nutrients through the catheter can begin immediately.

172

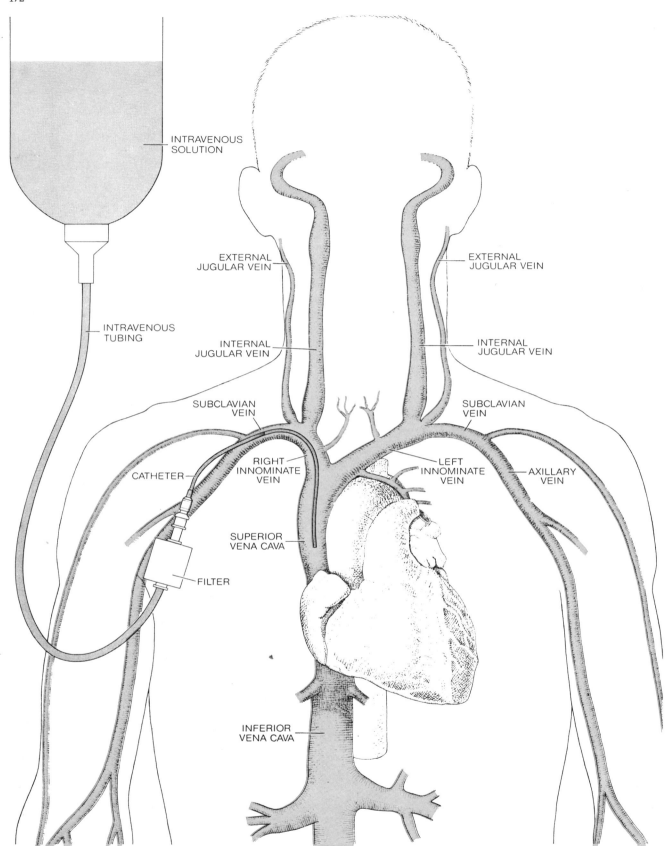

INTRAVENOUS
SOLUTION

INTRAVENOUS
TUBING

EXTERNAL
JUGULAR VEIN

EXTERNAL
JUGULAR VEIN

INTERNAL
JUGULAR VEIN

INTERNAL
JUGULAR VEIN

SUBCLAVIAN
VEIN

SUBCLAVIAN
VEIN

CATHETER

RIGHT
INNOMINATE
VEIN

LEFT
INNOMINATE
VEIN

AXILLARY
VEIN

SUPERIOR
VENA CAVA

FILTER

INFERIOR
VENA CAVA

CONCENTRATED NUTRIENT SOLUTION is infused through a catheter directly into the superior vena cava, the one-inch vein that returns blood to the heart from the upper part of the body. The high volume of blood flow in this large vein quickly dilutes the solution to a safe level. The catheter is inserted into the right sub-clavian vein and pushed along until the tip of the catheter is in the superior vena cava. The catheter can also be inserted through the left subclavian vein or one of the jugular veins. If the nutrient solution is continuously infused for 24 hours a day, the patient will receive enough nourishment for him to be able to gain weight.

tive technique for feeding a patient entirely by vein has been developed at the University of Pennsylvania School of Medicine. The technique of total intravenous feeding has proved to be a valuable adjunct in the treatment of virtually every disease of the alimentary tract where oral feeding is ill-advised. It also promises to become a tool of considerable usefulness in nutritional and biochemical research.

The idea of introducing substances directly into the bloodstream goes back to the discovery of the circulation of the blood by William Harvey in 1616. Physicians and scientists subsequently began to experiment with intravenous injection and blood transfusion in animals. In 1656 the architect Sir Christopher Wren, using a goose quill attached to a pig's bladder, injected ale, wine and opium into the veins of a dog. In 1667 a French physician, Jean Baptiste Denis, attempted a blood transfusion from a lamb to a man. Blood transfusions between men followed. The lack of proper sterilization techniques and the ignorance of blood chemistry led in many cases to complications and death.

Intravenous feeding had its beginning in 1843, when the French physiologist Claude Bernard infused sugar solutions into the veins of animals. By the end of the 19th century the intravenous infusion of saline or sugar solution into human patients was widely practiced. In the 1940's there were unsuccessful efforts to provide the total nutritional requirement with solutions of amino acids and glucose administered through one of the peripheral veins. In the 1950's the emphasis was on perfecting fat emulsions as a concentrated source of intravenous calories. Fat provides nine calories per gram, whereas sugars or proteins yield only about four calories per gram. Ethyl alcohol yields seven calories per gram but only limited amounts can be tolerated by intravenous infusion.

For a time it seemed that a mixture of fat emulsions, sugars, protein hydrolysates (proteins broken down into their constituent amino acids), vitamins and minerals could provide total intravenous feeding. Problems arose, however, with the fat emulsions. The fat had to be completely emulsified and the emulsion had to be stable under a variety of conditions. Fat particles that are too large will occlude capillaries in the lungs, brain and elsewhere, occasionally with fatal results. The U.S. Food and Drug Administration withdrew intravenous fat emulsions from the market in 1964.

One of the limitations of intravenous feeding is the total amount of water the

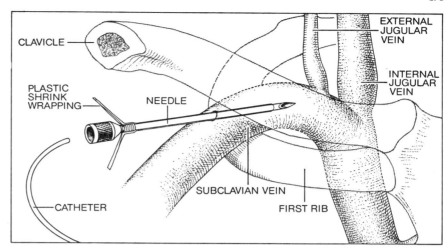

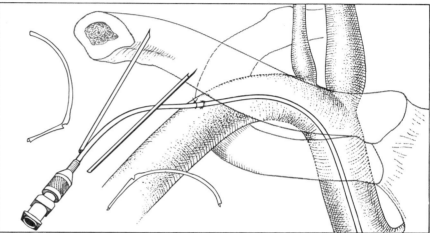

SPLIT NEEDLE specially developed for total intravenous feeding vein puncture is held together by a shrink-wrap plastic. After the hollow needle has been inserted into the vein (*top*) a catheter is pushed through the needle and into the superior vena cava. The needle is pulled out and its plastic wrapping is peeled off (*bottom*), thus allowing the needle to split apart. The tube from the nutrient solution is connected to the exposed end of the catheter.

average sick adult can handle in a day: about three liters. Larger amounts carry the threat of pulmonary edema, which is extremely dangerous. Moreover, when the solution is infused, as is customary, through one of the veins of the neck, arms or legs, the concentration of the nutrients is limited to about 10 percent. Higher concentrations frequently lead to inflammation and occlusion of the veins and blood clotting.

Thus the few safe nutrients—glucose and amino acids—that the body can assimilate from the blood yield only four calories per gram. These nutrients must be diluted to a tenth of their maximum concentration, so that each liter of 10 percent intravenous solution provides about 400 calories. Since the limit in standard intravenous feeding is three liters per day, the total caloric intake normally is limited to 1,200 calories per day. This falls short even of the basic energy requirements of the body. An in-

dividual at rest and not digesting food consumes about 1,400 calories per day.

When the patient has a fever, the metabolic energy expenditure increases about 8 percent per degree Fahrenheit. After major surgery, such as the removal of a stomach ulcer, the energy needs run at least 5 percent above the basal level. Daily requirements in the range of 7,000 to 10,000 calories have been recorded in patients who had suffered burns over half of the body's surface.

The principal energy stores of the body are in the form of fat. To convert fat into energy efficiently, however, the body requires some carbohydrate. The carbohydrate sources are glucose in the blood and glycogen in the liver and skeletal muscles. These carbohydrate stores are exhausted by a day or two of starvation. Thereafter the body produces the carbohydrate it needs by breaking down its protein, and a protein deficiency may quickly develop. In general, standard intrave..ous feeding through a peripheral vein is adequate for short-term supplementary nourishment. In the average patient it can supply adequate amounts of water, electrolytes, vitamins and minerals but only enough food energy to maintain the functioning of the central nervous system. For its additional energy needs the body must cannibalize its own tissues.

With the development of better drugs for increasing urine output it became possible to give larger volumes of the 10 percent nutrient solution and to remove the excess liquid by the use of diuretics. In this way the volume of intravenous feeding was increased to five or even seven liters per day in patients with good kidneys. The drawback is that constant attention must be paid to the patient's dynamic balance of water and electrolytes.

It occurred to us at the University of Pennsylvania School of Medicine that infusing the solution directly into a large vein would allow the use of a higher nutrient concentration. Theoretically the high blood flow in a large vein would promptly dilute the solution to a safe level. In 1965 we demonstrated the validity of this concept by feeding beagle puppies exclusively by vein for periods of up to 36 weeks and achieving normal growth and development. The puppies received a 30 percent nutrient solution through a plastic catheter that had been inserted into the superior vena cava, the large vein in the chest that returns blood from the upper half of the body to the heart.

The success of total intravenous feeding in animals led to the formulation of intravenous diets for human patients. The first person to respond to long-term total intravenous feeding was a female infant who had been born with a useless cordlike fibrous structure in place of a major portion of her small and large intestines. The infant underwent massive surgery shortly after birth. In spite of heroic efforts to feed her intravenously by conventional methods her weight declined continuously, and 19 days after birth she appeared to be at the point of death. Her weight had declined from five pounds two ounces at birth to four pounds. Then a catheter was inserted into her superior vena cava and infusion of a concentrated nutrient solution was begun. After 45 days her weight had nearly doubled to seven and a half pounds, and the infant had begun to grow. At six months of age she had received 97 percent of all her nutrition by vein and continued to grow and develop normally [see illustration on page 79]. At one year she had more than tripled her weight at birth. She eventually achieved a maximum weight of 18½ pounds during 22 months of intravenous feeding.

In another case a 17-year-old boy with a history of gastrointestinal problems developed abdominal pain and fever. In three months his weight had dropped from 205 to 145 pounds. X-ray studies revealed severe intestinal inflammation in the lower right abdomen and an associated mass that completely obstructed

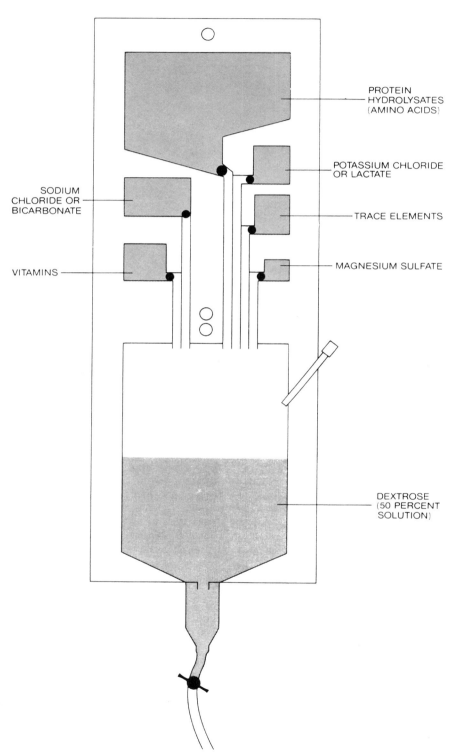

PROTEIN HYDROLYSATES (AMINO ACIDS)

POTASSIUM CHLORIDE OR LACTATE

SODIUM CHLORIDE OR BICARBONATE

TRACE ELEMENTS

VITAMINS

MAGNESIUM SULFATE

DEXTROSE (50 PERCENT SOLUTION)

CONTAINER for mixing components of a total intravenous diet solution is shown schematically. Development of prepackaged plastic containers with individual compartments for each component would lessen the risk of contamination from airborne microorganisms.

his right ureter: the tube from the kidney to the bladder. After three days of total intravenous feeding the abdominal mass was reduced sufficiently for the ureter to have opened, and the boy's pain and fever had disappeared. During seven weeks of intravenous feeding at 5,000 calories per day he gained 12 pounds, and the intestinal inflammation had also disappeared. He was discharged on no therapy other than a low-roughage diet and tranquilizers. He returned to his original weight and has had no further problems for more than a year.

The value of being able to feed a person entirely by intravenous transfusion, particularly when the digestive system is impaired, was demonstrated again in the case of a 46-year-old man who had had three feet of his bowel removed by surgery. He developed signs of a bowel obstruction and within two weeks underwent another operation in which another foot of bowel was removed. For a time after the operation he appeared to be doing well, but the sutures in his bowel did not hold and about three weeks later fecal material began to leak through the wound. Even though he had lost 30 pounds by this time, oral feeding had to be stopped. He was started on a regimen of total intravenous feeding and broad-spectrum antibiotics. Ten days later the fecal leakage had stopped, the wound began to heal and the patient began to gain weight. Within 40 days he was able to eat again. Total intravenous feeding had significantly reduced the ravages of the "short-gut syndrome" by providing a rest period for the alimentary tract. The patient had received a total of 176 liters of intravenous nutrient solution and had gained 11 pounds without eating or drinking at all. Following his discharge from the hospital he returned to his normal weight in three months and resumed his previous employment and activities.

The basic nutrient solution for total intravenous feeding is about six times more concentrated than blood and consists of 20 to 25 percent dextrose, 4 to 5 percent protein hydrolysate and 5 percent minerals, vitamins and other necessary nutrients. Pure crystalline amino acids can be used in place of the protein hydrolysate. The nutrient solution must be sterile and must not produce fever. The food in it must be in the forms that are normally found in the blood. The ingredients must not result in blood clotting or the occlusion of blood vessels. Finally, the solution must enable the body to maintain its normal concentrations of various essential ions such as

BASE SOLUTION	ADULT	INFANT
VOLUME (MILLILITERS)	1,100	720
CALORIES	1,000	660
COMPONENTS	GRAMS	
GLUCOSE	212	20
PROTEIN HYDROLYSATE (AMINO ACIDS)	37	20
	MILLIEQUIVALENTS	
SODIUM	40–50	20
POTASSIUM	30–40	25
CALCIUM	4.5–9	20
MAGNESIUM	4–8	10
PHOSPHATE	4–10*	25

VITAMINS (ADDED ONCE A DAY)	ADULT	INFANT
	USP UNITS	
VITAMIN A	5,000–10,000	3,000–4,000
VITAMIN D	500–1,000	300–400
	INTERNATIONAL UNITS	
VITAMIN E	2.5–5	1.5–2
	MILLIGRAMS	
VITAMIN C (ASCORBIC ACID)	250–500	150–200
NIACIN	50–100	30–40
VITAMIN B-1 (THIAMINE HYDROCHLORIDE)	25–50	15–20
VITAMIN B-2 (RIBOFLAVIN)	5–10	3–4
VITAMIN B-3 (PANTOTHENIC ACID)	12.5–25	7.5–10
VITAMIN B-6 (PYRIDOXINE HYDROCHLORIDE)	7.5–15	4.5–6
VITAMIN K (PHYTONADIONE)	5–10*	1–1.5
FOLIC ACID	5–1.5*	.5
	MICROGRAMS	
VITAMIN B-12 (CYANOCOBALAMIN)	10–30*	1

MINERALS (ADDED ONCE A DAY)	ADULT	INFANT
	MILLIGRAMS	
IRON	2–3*	.5–1
TRACE ELEMENTS	—	—

*OPTIONAL

TYPICAL NUTRIENT SOLUTIONS for the average adult and average infant are shown. The base adult solution can be prepared in single units by mixing 750 milliliters of 5 percent dextrose and 5 percent protein hydrolysate with 350 milliliters of 50 percent dextrose and then adding vitamins and minerals. Mixing must be aseptic and preferably should be done under a laminar-flow, filtered-air hood. Solutions for infants are prepared the same way.

sodium, calcium, magnesium, potassium, chloride, phosphate and bicarbonate.

Strict aseptic procedure during preparation of the nutrient solution must be followed to avoid contamination by bacteria, fungi and other harmful agents. The basic solution can be formulated in bulk lots or in individual units. At the Hospital of the University of Pennsylvania the basic solution is prepared in bulk and sterilized immediately after mixing by passing it into sterile bottles through a cellulose membrane filter with pores .22 micron in diameter. The solution cannot be sterilized by the usual steam-autoclaving method because heating tends to cook it. (It turns brown.) Samples from each lot of solution are tested for the presence of bacteria, fungi and fever-producing substances.

The minerals are added to the basic solution just before infusion. The vitamins are added daily to one bottle of the solution. The necessary trace elements (such as cobalt, copper, iodine, manganese, molybdenum and zinc) are present as contaminants in most intravenous solutions, particularly those containing protein hydrolysates.

For normal growth and development in newborn infants, who have no appreciable nutrient stores, more complete mixtures are required for daily infusion [*see illustration on preceding page*]. The standard adult formula must be modified for patients with heart disease, liver disease or kidney dysfunction. Morover, it is often necessary to modify the nutrient solution during the course of intravenous feeding, depending on the patient's metabolic response. No single intravenous nutrient solution can be ideal for all conditions in all patients at all times, or for the same patient during the various phases of treatment.

The solution is administered through a polyvinyl (or siliconized rubber) catheter inserted into the superior vena cava by way of a subclavian vein or an external or internal jugular vein [*see illustration on page 74*]. Insertion of the catheter can be accomplished safely and effectively in 99 percent of the patients if the proper procedures are followed. Strict aseptic techniques, including sterile surgical gloves and instruments, are crucial. The skin of the lower neck, shoulder and upper chest is shaved, cleaned with ether or acetone to remove skin oil and prepared with tincture of iodine, just as the skin is prepared for a major surgical operation. A local anesthetic is injected; then a split hollow needle specially developed for the purpose is inserted into the subclavian vein. An eight-inch catheter is introduced into the vein through the needle and pushed into the superior vena cava, which is about an inch in diameter. The needle is withdrawn and split away, leaving five and a half inches of catheter within the central venous system. The catheter is fixed in place firmly with a suture. After chest X ray has confirmed the accurate positioning of the catheter the infusion of the nutrient solution can begin.

In infants who weigh less than 10 pounds the relatively small subclavian vein can make percutaneous puncture of the vein difficult and hazardous. A safer procedure is to insert a smaller catheter into an external or internal jugular vein at the base of the neck. The exposed portion of the catheter can be tunneled under the skin behind the ear to prevent the tube's being kinked by the infant's movements.

Safe long-term intravenous feeding calls for meticulous care of the catheter. The intravenous tubing is changed at

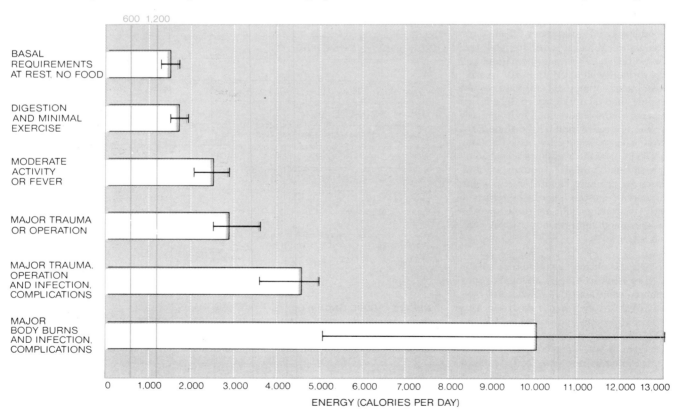

METABOLIC ENERGY REQUIREMENTS for the average adult under various conditions of stress are shown by the bars in this graph. The black lines indicate the range of variation for different individuals. The basal requirement of an adult at rest and not eating is about 1,400 calories per day. Standard intravenous feeding with 5 percent dextrose can supply about 600 calories per day. When the solution concentration is doubled to 10 percent, feeding through a peripheral vein can provide only about 1,200 calories per day. With total intravenous feeding the patient can normally obtain 3,000 calories per day and in some cases up to 4,000 calories per day. Intake of 10,000 calories per day has been possible only with a combination of oral food intake and total intravenous feeding.

least three times a week. With proper
maintenance each catheter can be left
in place safely for about 30 days. The
catheter should not be used for taking
blood samples, measuring blood pressure or administering medication. Indeed, it should be regarded as the patient's lifeline.

Although blood clotting is theoretically a possibility with the use of long-
term catheters and concentrated nutrient
solutions, we have not observed any clotting of the superior vena cava in the
more than 1,400 patients treated in this
way at the Hospital of the University of
Pennsylvania. The large blood flow in
the vein provides a dilution factor of
2,000 or 3,000. Well-maintained aseptic
conditions can practically eliminate the
hazard of blood clotting. Of course,
much care must be taken to avoid the
accidental puncture of a major blood
vessel or the lung.

The concentrated nutrient solution
must be continuously infused 24 hours a
day at a constant rate to maintain maximum assimilation of the nutrients without exceeding the patient's metabolic
capacities for water, dextrose, amino
acids or minerals. The sugar is either
broken down immediately to release energy and carbon dioxide and water or is
converted into glycogen, which is stored
in the muscles and liver. The amino acids
are utilized for the synthesis of proteins
and body tissue or are broken down to
release energy, carbon dioxide, water
and urea.

The carbon dioxide, water and urea
are easily excreted through the lungs,
kidneys and in sweat. There are virtually no solid wastes to be eliminated
through the bowel. The infrequent stools
of patients on total intravenous feeding
consist of mucus, bile, bacteria and cells
sloughed off from the intestines. The
activities of the digestive tract can be
reduced to about 10 to 25 percent of
normal with total intravenous feeding.
The stomach and bowel shrink in length
and in diameter, and a condition of true
"bowel rest" can be achieved. It may
take from several days to a few weeks
for the alimentary tract to be restored to
normal on resumption of oral feeding,
but no long-term adverse effects have
been observed.

If the solution is infused too rapidly,
the capacity of the kidney to retain dextrose can be exceeded and the sugar can
be lost in the urine, carrying with it some
of the minerals, vitamins and amino
acids. This not only is wasteful but also
can lead to dehydration with convul-
sions or coma. In patients with impaired

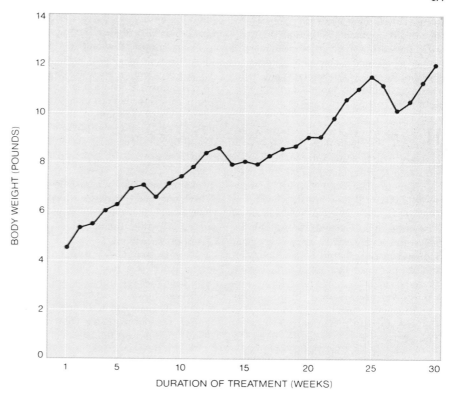

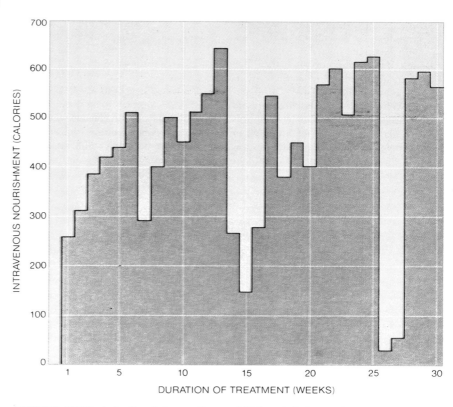

WEIGHT GAIN of the first infant to be nourished entirely by total intravenous feeding
paralleled the normal rate for infants. The infant girl underwent massive intestinal surgery
shortly after birth, and in spite of great efforts to feed her intravenously by conventional
methods her weight dropped from five pounds two ounces to four pounds. She began to gain
weight immediately with total intravenous feeding; within four weeks she surpassed her
birth weight. During the 22 months of intravenous feeding the infant reached a weight of
18.5 pounds. The lower graph shows the weekly average of calories given intravenously.

kidneys the amino acids may aggravate an already excessive retention of urea; such patients are given solutions with only the minimal amounts of the essential amino acids. The amino acid composition should be modified if the patient has a certain type of liver disorder.

Basic guidelines for safe intravenous feeding include daily measurement of body weight and water balance. Serum electrolytes, blood sugar and urea nitrogen in the blood should be measured daily until they are stabilized and then measured every two or three days. The urine sugar concentration should be measured every six hours. Liver and kidney function should be evaluated initially and then every two or three weeks. Periodic measurement of arterial and central venous pressure, blood acidity and dissolved gases may be indicated in the management of patients with heart, kidney, lung or metabolic disorders.

In newborn infants the nutrient solution can be best delivered at a constant rate by means of an external-action pump. Syringe pumps cannot be employed because the risk of contamination is high. A fine filter between the pump tubing and the catheter prevents the transmission of microorganisms and other contaminants. The filter also prevents air embolism, because air cannot pass through the filter pores after the filter has been moistened. Similar filters with larger pores can be used with adult patients. With patients who are capable of walking, the intravenous-feeding bottles (or plastic bags) can be attached to rolling poles so that the patient can engage in the exercise essential for optimal nutrition and recovery.

The prevention of infection is of paramount importance to the success of long-term total intravenous feeding. If the necessary aseptic and antiseptic procedures are followed conscientiously, the chances of infection are low. In addition, since the nutrient solution is a good culture medium for bacteria and fungi, the preparation of the solution, the changing of bottles and the replacement of tubing should be handled under conditions that ensure asepsis.

Fever or infection in a patient does not rule out total intravenous feeding. On the contrary, in a critically ill patient infection intensifies the need for nutritional support. Although seeding of the catheter by microorganisms circulating in the blood is a possibility, it has not been a significant problem. It is a cardinal rule, however, that whenever it is suspected that an infection may be caused by the catheter, the catheter should be removed immediately.

Total intravenous feeding has proved itself in the treatment of 1,300 adults, some for as long as a year, and in the treatment of more than 100 infants, some for as long as 22 months. Weight gain, wound healing and improved health have been observed in the large majority of cases. Before total intravenous feeding had been developed, patients with severe inflammation or ulceration of the digestive tract had a poor prognosis for survival. Often food taken by mouth is not properly absorbed by the diseased intestine, and the food can actually exacerbate the disease. With total intravenous feeding such individuals can now be given sufficient nourishment to achieve a state of tissue synthesis and weight gain. Patients with a deep ulcer or fistula (leak) of the alimentary tract that has perforated through the abdominal wall, so that food and fluid are actually lost through the opening, have in the past been extremely resistant to both surgical and nonsurgical treatment. With total intravenous feeding more than half of the patients have shown spontaneous healing of the fistula and the rest have improved sufficiently to be better risks for surgery. Patients with severe inflammatory disease of the intestinal tract may also show spontaneous remission of the disease on this regimen.

Patients with impaired liver function or with kidney failure have been supported adequately by the total intravenous feeding of specially formulated solutions. In patients with complicated major burns as much as 6,000 nutrient calories per day has been given by vein to supplement oral or tube feedings of 4,000 to 5,000 calories. In infants total intravenous feeding has proved capable of supporting normal growth and development until oral feeding can begin.

There are many other applications of total intravenous feeding in internal medicine, pediatrics and surgery. In addition the technique promises to be a powerful tool for basic investigations in biochemistry, pharmacology and nutrition. The role of hormones, amino acids, vitamins, minerals and fatty acids can be studied in animals and in man under conditions of control formerly unattainable. The degree to which immune mechanisms can be altered by intravenous diets of selected amino acids may be of significance in facilitating successful tissue transplants. Most potential applications of total intravenous feeding remain to be explored.

Prostaglandins

by John E. Pike
November 1971

These recently isolated hormone-like substances show much clinical promise. They affect a wide range of physiological processes, from the contraction of the uterus to secretion from the stomach wall

In the early 1930's several investigators studying human semen and animal seminal tissues discovered that these materials contained substances showing high physiological potency. Two gynecologists in New York, Raphael Kurzrok and Charles C. Lieb, examining the effects of fresh semen on strips of uterus from hysterectomized women patients, found that the seminal fluid caused the uterine tissue to relax or contract, depending on whether the woman was fertile (having borne children) or was sterile. At about the same time Maurice W. Goldblatt in England and Ulf S. von Euler in Sweden obtained other striking effects in experiments with human semen and with extracts from the seminal vesicular gland of sheep. They reported that the active substance could stimulate muscle tissue to contract or, on injection into an animal, could produce sharp lowering of the blood pressure. To this previously unknown, remarkably potent material von Euler gave the name prostaglandin.

Actually the term was a misnomer. The active substances had come not from the prostate gland but from the seminal vesicles, glands that also contribute to the semen. It was eventually learned that "prostaglandins" could be found in other body fluids and tissues, including the menstrual fluid of women. The prostaglandins are now known to be a family of substances showing a wide diversity of biological effects. They give promise of pharmacological uses in many medical areas. Although they resemble other known hormones in their dramatic effects, chemically they are a quite different class of compounds. Von Euler deduced from his investigations, and studies have since confirmed, that the prostaglandins are fatty acids. This was a considerable surprise, as fatty acids had not previously been suspected of playing the kind of role the prostaglandins are now observed to perform.

For some 20 years after the original discovery of the prostaglandins little was learned about their chemistry or their specific properties. One of the reasons is that the body produces these highly potent substances in very small quantities; for example, a man normally synthesizes only about a tenth of a milligram per day of two of the most important prostaglandins. Furthermore, prostaglandins are rapidly broken down in the body by catabolic enzymes. Consequently the amount in the tissues is so small that the prostaglandins could not be obtained in quantity or studied chemically until refined techniques were developed for isolating and analyzing them.

Interest in the prostaglandins grew, however, as extracts of crude acidic lipids (fatty substances) obtained from a variety of other sources proved to owe their biological activity to their prostaglandin content. By the late 1950's biochemists began to achieve success in purifying prostaglandins and examining their molecular structure. Sune Bergström and his associate Jan Sjövall in Sweden crystallized two of these substances, called PGE_1 and PGF_1-alpha. Working with minute amounts, they were able to decipher the structure of the two compounds, including some details of their three-dimensional configuration, with the help of gas chromatography, mass spectroscopy and X-ray analysis. With Bengt I. Samuelsson and other investigators they proceeded to work out the structure of several additional prostaglandins. They were all seen to be closely akin, and the distinctive biological effects of the various compounds in the family could be related systematically to their structural variations [see illustration on page 186].

It is now well established that the prostaglandins are 20-carbon carboxylic acids (that is, incorporating the COOH group) and that they are synthesized in the body from certain polyunsaturated fatty acids by the formation of a five-member ring and the incorporation of three oxygen atoms at certain positions [see top illustration on pages 180 and 181]. The enzymes involved in their synthesis have been found to be widely distributed in a variety of tissues, and the synthesis of prostaglandins has been demonstrated in many tissues, from the vesicular gland of sheep to the lung tissue of guinea pigs. It has also been established that after "primary" prostaglandins have been formed from fatty-acid precursors they can be converted into other members of the family by changing the primary structure.

The linking of the prostaglandins to polyunsaturated fatty acids provided clues to some of the prostaglandins' important functions. For example, one of the common fatty-acid precursors for prostaglandin is arachidonic acid. The main source of this substance is the phospholipids, which constitute a principal component of the cell membrane. Consequently it appears that the conversion of arachidonic acid to prostaglandin may play an important role in the regulation of the membrane's functions. It seems that the cell membrane is a prime site for the formation of the prostaglandins. Since there is no indication that any cells carry a store of prostaglandin, the likelihood is that the substance is produced by the membrane as needed. The tiny amount of prostaglandin we find in most tissues may therefore represent just the amount produced in the interval between the removal of the tissue and its preparation for extrac-

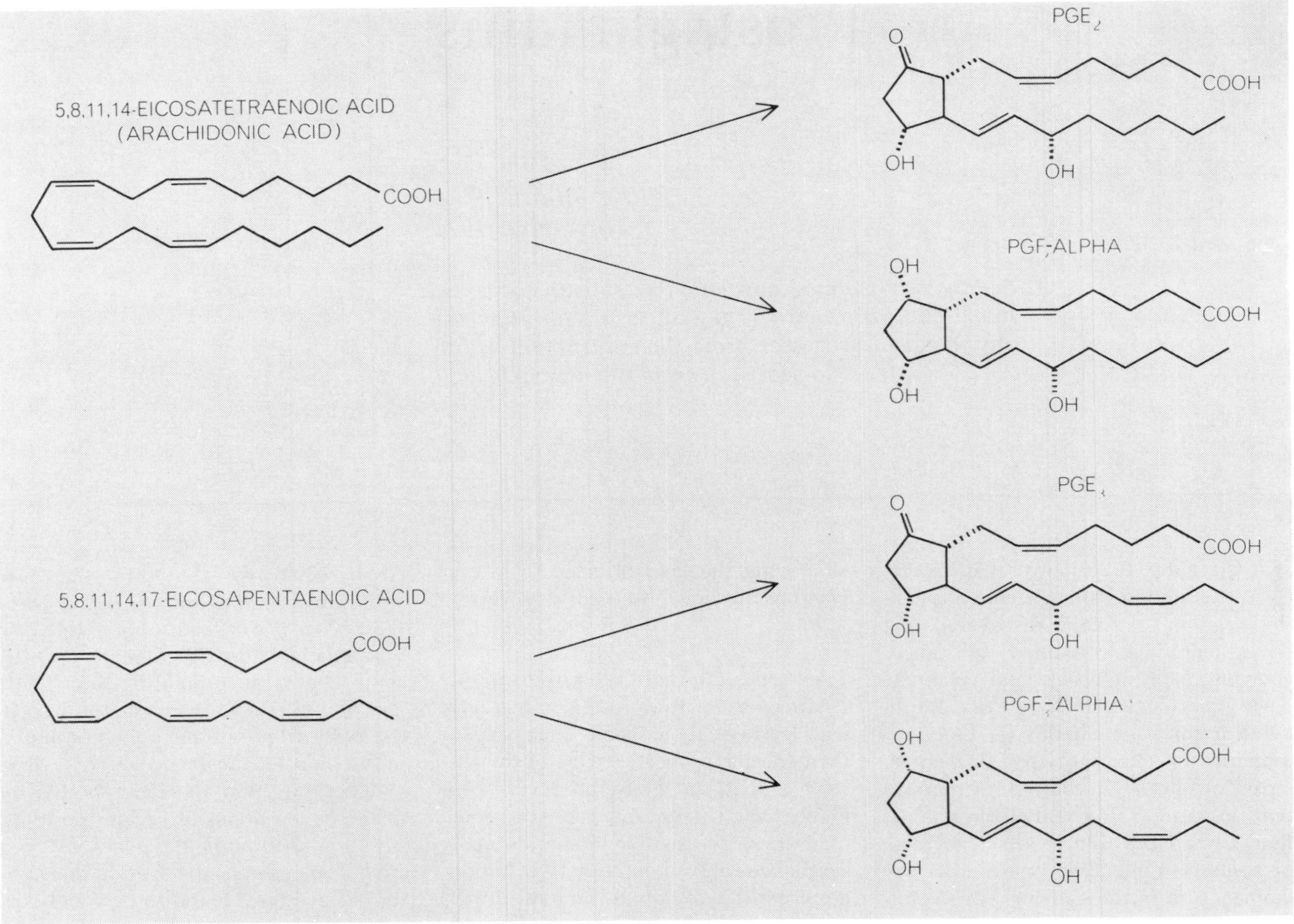

5,8,11,14-EICOSATETRAENOIC ACID
(ARACHIDONIC ACID)

COOH

PGE_2

COOH

OH   OH

PGF_2-ALPHA

OH

COOH

OH   OH

5,8,11,14,17-EICOSAPENTAENOIC ACID

COOH

PGE_3

COOH

OH   OH

PGF_3-ALPHA

OH

COOH

OH   OH

PROSTAGLANDINS ARE SYNTHESIZED in the body from certain polyunsaturated fatty acids by the formation of the five-member ring and the incorporation of three oxygen atoms at certain positions. For example, either PGE_2 or PGF_2-alpha can be formed directly from arachidonic acid (*top diagram at left*), whereas PGE_3 or PGF_3-alpha can be formed from a closely related fatty-acid pre-

tion of the substance. This amount typically is only about one microgram per gram of wet tissue. The seminal fluid of man or the extract from a seminal gland, on the other hand, usually contains 100 times this concentration of prostaglandins. Were it not for this rela-

tively rich source, the prostaglandins might still be awaiting discovery.

In addition to the involvement of the cell membrane, another fascinating question raised by the interrelation of fatty acids and prostaglandins has to do with diseases arising from dietary de-

ficiencies. It has long been known that certain polyunsaturated fatty acids are essential in a mammal's diet. Rats fed a fat-free diet suffer a stunting of growth, inability to reproduce and a characteristic skin lesion. The question arises: Could the administration of prostaglan-

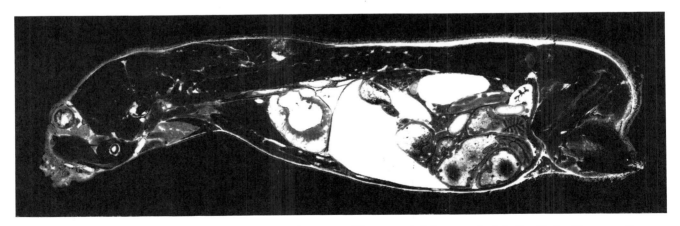

RAPID DISTRIBUTION of prostaglandin in the body is demonstrated by these two autoradiograms made by Bengt I. Samuelsson of the Royal Veterinary College and Eskil Hanson of the Astra Pharmaceutical Company, both in Stockholm. The autoradiograms show the distribution of radioactivity (*light areas*) in a female mouse (*left*) and a male mouse (*right*) 15 minutes after each had

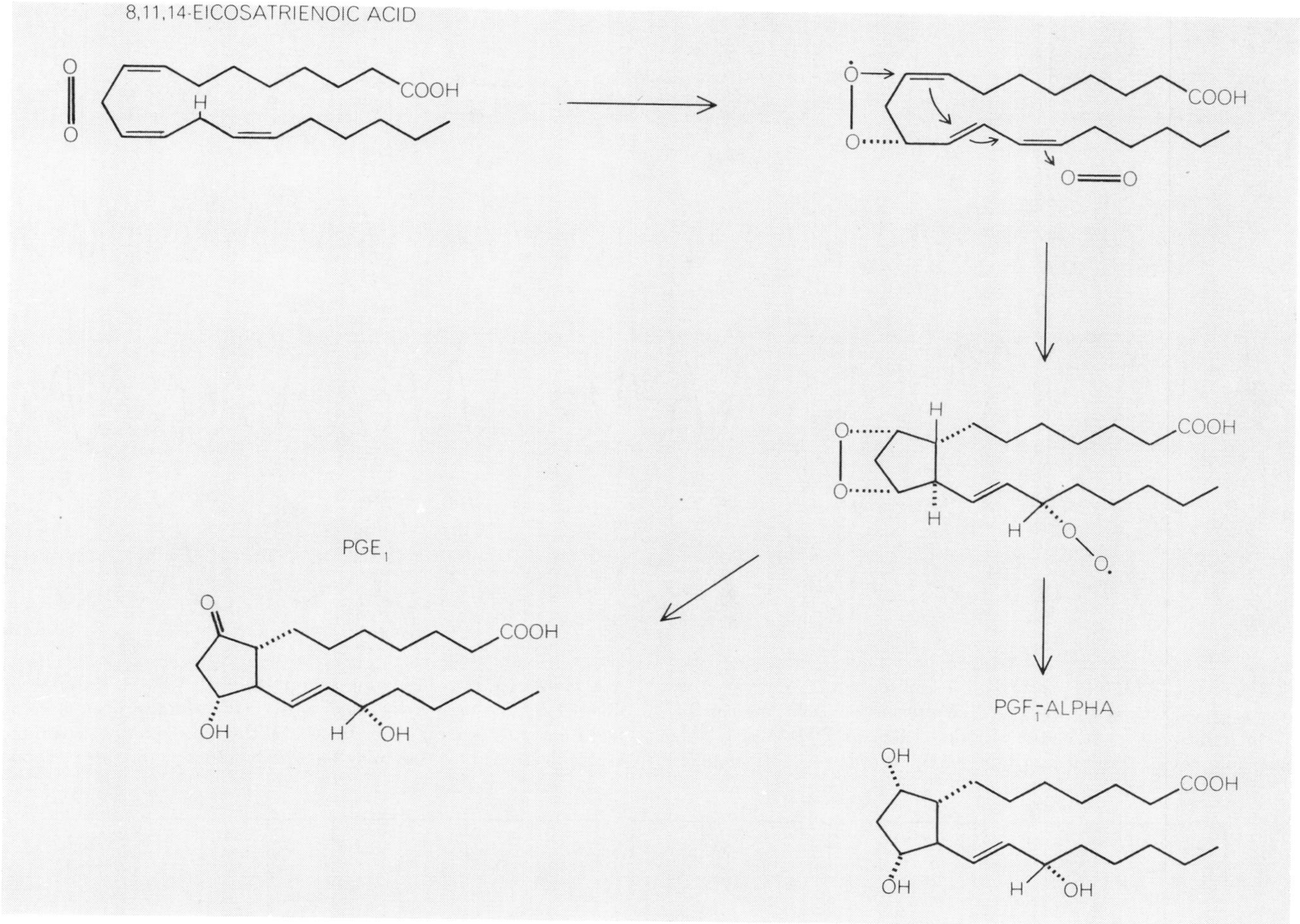

8,11,14-EICOSATRIENOIC ACID

PGE₁

PGF₁-ALPHA

cursor (*bottom diagram at left*). The probable mechanism of this type of biosynthesis is illustrated at the right. Two molecules of atmospheric oxygen provide three new oxygen atoms to a hypo-

thetical intermediate structure, which then leads to either the PGE or the PGF structure. These primary structures can thereafter be converted into other members of the prostaglandin family.

dins remedy the fatty-acid deficiency? James R. Weeks of the Upjohn Company found that treatment of deficient rats with prostaglandins had no effect on the external signs of deficiency. David A. van Dorp and his co-workers in the Netherlands have found a clear connec-

tion, however, between prostaglandins and the fatty acids that are essential in the diet. Only those fatty acids that serve as precursors for the synthesis of prostaglandins are effective in curing rats that have been subjected to a fatty-acid deficiency. This suggests that some

less obvious, perhaps metabolic, aspect, of the deficiency disease in rats deprived of the essential fatty acids may be due in part to failure to synthesize necessary prostaglandins.

Once it was recognized that the prostaglandins are formed from fatty acids

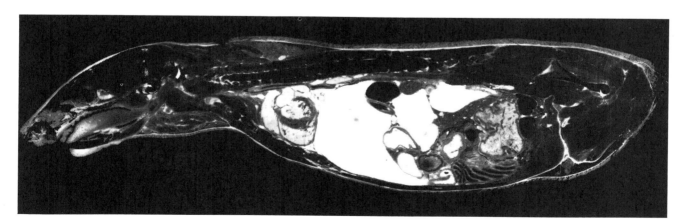

been injected intravenously with a small amount of radioactively labeled PGE₁. High concentrations of the prostaglandin are evident in the liver, the kidney and the subcutaneous connective tis-

sue of both animals and also in the uterus of the female and the thoracic duct of the male. The autoradiograms were made by placing a cross section of each animal on a radiation-sensitive plate.

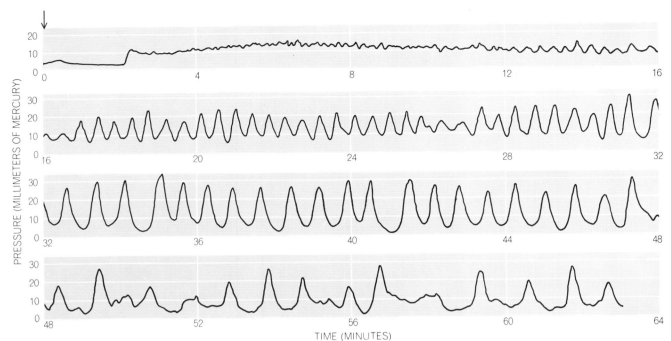

STRIKING EFFECT of prostaglandins on the female reproductive system is evidenced by the fact that uterine contractions can be stimulated by a very low dose of either PGE$_2$ or PGF$_2$-alpha. This particular trace, divided into four parts, records pressure changes in a monkey uterus following an injection of PGE$_2$ at the time indicated by the arrow. Prostaglandins have already been used to facilitate childbearing labor in several thousand women, and there are indications that they may be widely adopted for this purpose.

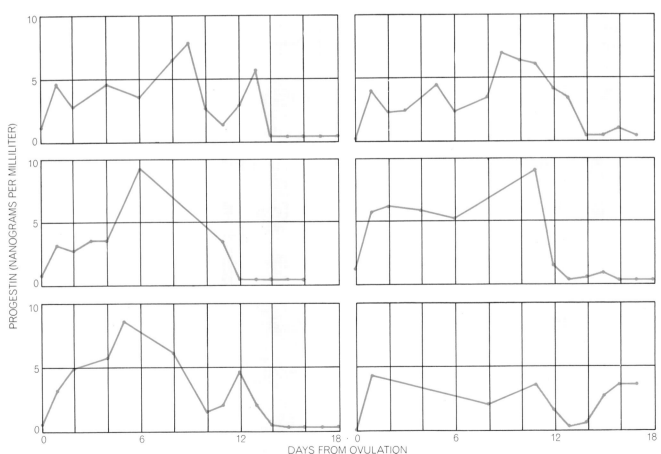

DRAMATIC REDUCTION in the secretion of progesterone by the ovaries of mated female monkeys followed the administration of PGF$_2$-alpha. In these graphs of the progestin levels in six such monkeys the prostaglandin was administered during the periods indicated by the colored bands. Since progesterone is needed to ensure implantation of a fertilized ovum in the wall of the uterus, there seems to be a strong possibility that prostaglandins may become important agents in helping to control population growth.

it became possible to turn to laboratory production of these scarce and expensive substances for experimental work. It was found that a fatty acid (gamma-linolenic acid) extracted from seeds of the borage plant (a European herb) could be converted into a polyunsaturated fatty acid that was a precursor for a prostaglandin biosynthesis. Enzymes for the biosynthesis were obtained from the seminal vesicular glands of sheep. This resort to artificial biosynthesis produced gram quantities of the prostaglandin and supported studies for several years. Recently chemists at the Upjohn Company and Elias J. Corey and his co-workers at Harvard University developed methods of total synthesis of prostaglandins from more common materials, so that the problem of supply of the substances for research is no longer so acute.

Incidentally, remarkably high concentrations of a prostaglandin isomer were found by Alfred J. Weinheimer and R. L. Spraggins of the University of Oklahoma in a type of coral, the sea whip or sea fan *Plexaura homomalla,* a primitive sessile animal found in coral reefs off the Florida coast. This isomer has been successfully converted to biologically important prostaglandins by Gordon Bundy, William P. Schneider and their co-workers at the Upjohn Company. Apparently prostaglandins once played more elementary roles than they do in mammals, and it is interesting to speculate on their origin and evolutionary development. Polyunsaturated fatty acids are absent in bacteria, but they do turn up in blue-green algae and some higher plants as well as in animals. The prostaglandins may represent an evolutionary step in which, thanks to the availability of molecular oxygen, these complex molecules were formed as agents for the regulatory functions of specialized cells.

The increase in the supply of prostaglandins for experiments has made possible a wide exploration of their effects and powers. These tests have demonstrated that the prostaglandins are among the most potent of all known biological materials, producing marked effects in extremely small doses, and that their existence in the body is remarkably ephemeral. For example, it is found that after a radioactively labeled prostaglandin is injected intravenously into a subject's arm, the injected material is metabolized very rapidly; in as short a time as a minute and a half 90 percent of the radioactivity is dispersed in

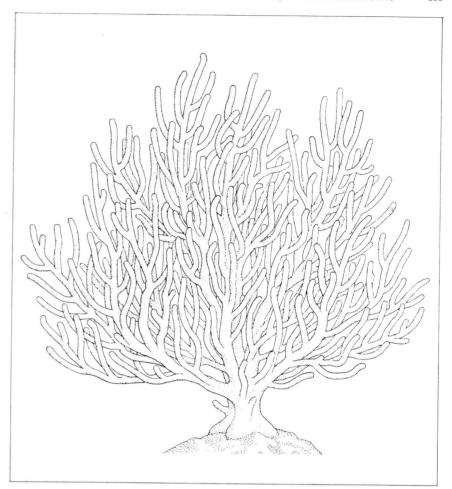

NONMAMMALIAN SOURCE of prostaglandins is represented by the sea whip or sea fan *Plexaura homomalla,* a type of coral found in reefs off the Florida coast. The coral contains high concentrations of a prostaglandin precursor, which has been converted to biologically important prostaglandins by workers at the Upjohn Company. There has been considerable interest in this primitive organism as a starting material for synthesizing prostaglandins.

metabolic products, as is shown in samples of venous blood taken from the other arm. Evidently the body's cells possess a copious supply of catabolic enzymes designed to confine the action of the prostaglandins to particular areas.

The principal interest in the prostaglandins has focused on their remarkable versatility and the wide range of their effects. The effects themselves may be quite specific; for example, one prostaglandin (PGE_2) lowers blood pressure, whereas a closely related member of the family (PGF_2-alpha) raises blood pressure. In general the effects of the prostaglandins are ·based on certain broad powers: regulation of the activity of smooth muscles, of secretion, including some endocrine-gland secretions, or of blood flow. Through these actions they are capable of affecting many aspects of human physiology, and this accounts

for the great current interest in their pharmacological possibilities.

Particularly striking are the effects on the female reproductive system. An intravenous injection of a very low dose of either PGE_2 or PGF_2-alpha was shown by Marc Bygdeman to stimulate contraction of the uterus. This finding, together with the finding by S. M. M. Karim, now at the Makerere University School of Medicine in Uganda, that prostaglandins are present in the amniotic fluid and in the venous blood of women during the contractions of labor, suggested that the prostaglandins may play an important role in parturition. The substances have been used to facilitate childbearing labor in several thousand women. Infusion of PGE_2 at the rate of .05 microgram per kilogram per minute has been found to induce delivery within a few hours. Oral administration of PGE_2 or PGF_2-alpha has also been reported to be effective. Further studies of the most effective dosage and route of administration of the drug, as well as evaluation in comparison with other methods of inducing labor, may lay a basis for wide adoption of the use of a prostaglandin for this purpose.

The possible use of prostaglandins as agents for abortion and for inducing menstruation (in cases of menstrual failure) is also being investigated. There is evidence that prostaglandins produce these effects by some process more complex than the mere stimulation of uterine contraction. Infusion of PGF$_2$-alpha in female monkeys after mating has been found by Kenneth T. Kirton to produce a dramatic reduction of the secretion of progesterone by the corpus luteum of the ovary, which is needed to ensure implantation of a fertilized ovum in the wall of the uterus. One suggested explanation is that the prostaglandin may induce regression of the corpus luteum, an event that generally does not occur after an ovum is fertilized. There seems to be a strong possibility that prostaglandins or perhaps synthetic analogues may become important agents in controlling population growth.

In an entirely different area of physiology, the prostaglandins, illustrating their versatility, seem to hold promise for the prevention of peptic ulcers. Andre Robert of the Upjohn Company has shown that the prostaglandin E$_1$ or E$_2$ can inhibit gastric secretions in dogs. The dogs were first given a stimulant for secretion (histamine, pentagastrin or food) and then were infused intravenously with one of the prostaglandins. The drug drastically reduced the digestive system's secretion of acid and pepsin throughout the infusion [*see illustration on opposite page*]. It is believed to have produced this effect by changing the chemical activity within the parietal cells of the stomach. Follow-up experiments have shown further that these two prostaglandins can prevent gastric and duodenal ulcers in rats. It seems well established that ulceration of the stomach and the duodenum is generally caused by prolonged exposure of their mucous membrane to gastric juice of high acidity and peptic potency. The stomach normally produces prostaglandins of the E series, and these may serve to regulate gastric secretion under normal circumstances and thus protect the stomach wall against ulceration. If the studies on dogs and rats are confirmed in man, the administration of E prostaglandins may be a helpful treatment for ulcer pa-

tients who lack this normal protection.

A number of other biological activities of prostaglandins suggesting possible pharmacological uses are under study. Among these potential applications are:

1. Opening the airways to the lungs. It has been shown experimentally in asthmatic subjects that breathing an aerosol preparation of the prostaglandin E$_1$ can improve the airflow by relaxing the smooth muscle of the bronchial tubes.

2. Regulating blood pressure. In experiments on dogs it has been found that infusion into the kidney artery of a very low dose of PGE$_1$ or another prostaglandin called PGA$_1$ produces an increase in the flow of urine and the excretion of sodium ions. This finding and others indicate that prostaglandins in the body normally help to regulate blood pressure. Tests have demonstrated that the infusion of PGA$_1$ can lower blood pressure in patients with essential hypertension.

3. Clearing the nasal passages. Applied topically to the nose, PGE$_1$ has been found effective in widening the passages by constricting the blood vessels.

4. Regulating metabolism. PGE$_1$ has been shown to counteract the effects of

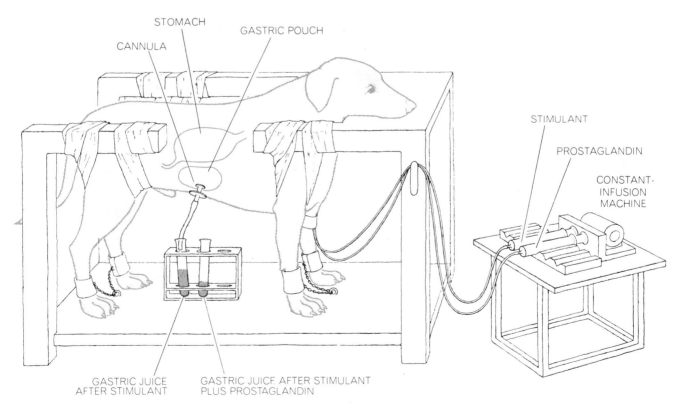

INFLUENCE OF PROSTAGLANDINS on the gastric secretions responsible for peptic ulcers was studied by Andre Robert of the Upjohn Company, who used dogs as experimental animals. The dogs were first given an intravenous infusion of a stimulant for secretion and then one containing the prostaglandin in addition. The output of gastric juice was reduced during the latter treatment.

many hormones in stimulation of metabolic processes, for example the breakdown of lipids in fatty tissues.

Many items of evidence now point strongly to the likelihood that the prostaglandins play a fundamental and critical role in the physiology of mammals. Production and release of these substances can be evoked by stimulation of nerves. Recent experiments by a group at the Royal Caroline Institute in Sweden (Per Hedqvist, Åke Wennmalm, Lennart Stjärne and Samuelsson) demonstrated a clear interrelation between the prostaglandins and the substances involved in the transmission of nerve impulses.

Testing preparations of isolated organs (the spleen of the cat and the heart of the rabbit), they found that infusion of the prostaglandin E_2 markedly inhibited the release of norepinephrine in response to nerve stimulation. In other words, the prostaglandin acted as a "brake" on the nerves' action in inciting release of the norepinephrine, a hormone that plays a key part in the transmission of nerve impulses in the sympathetic nervous system. When the preparation was infused, on the other hand, with an inhibitor of the formation of prostaglandins, the consequent removal of the brake from the tissues resulted in an abnormally large release of norepinephrine by nerve stimulation.

These and other results suggest that prostaglandins, playing a negative-feedback role, are part of the mechanism that normally controls transmission in the sympathetic nervous system. The inhibition of the production of prostaglandins in the body obviously invites further investigation. J. R. Vane and his coworkers at the Institute of Basic Medical Science of the Royal College of Surgeons recently conducted such a study and obtained results that suggest the anti-inflammatory action of aspirin and certain other agents may be explainable on the basis that they block the synthesis of prostaglandins.

Prostaglandin formation has been noted in many other apparently unrelated systems. For example, prostaglandins are formed by the lungs during anaphylaxis, by the kidney when its blood supply is restricted, by the surface of the brain when peripheral sensory nerves are stimulated, by the skin during human allergic contact eczema and during certain experimental inflammatory conditions. These diverse situations suggest that prostaglandins may play a fundamental role not only in normal physi-

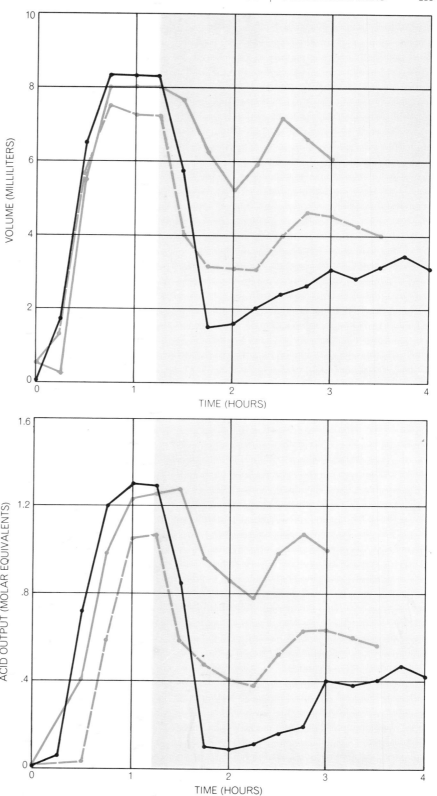

ABRUPT REDUCTIONS in gastric secretion were observed in dogs as a result of the administration of PGE_2. In this particular experiment the secretion of gastric juice was stimulated by the intravenous infusion of the histamine dihydrochloride at a dose rate of one milligram per hour. When PGE_2 was added to the infusion (*colored band*), both the volume (*top graph*) and the acidity (*bottom graph*) of the gastric secretion were reduced proportionately to the dose of PGE_2. In each graph solid colored curve represents a PGE_2 dose rate of 12.5 micrograms per minute, broken colored curve represents a dose rate of 18.75 micrograms per minute and black curve represents a dose rate of 25 micrograms per minute.

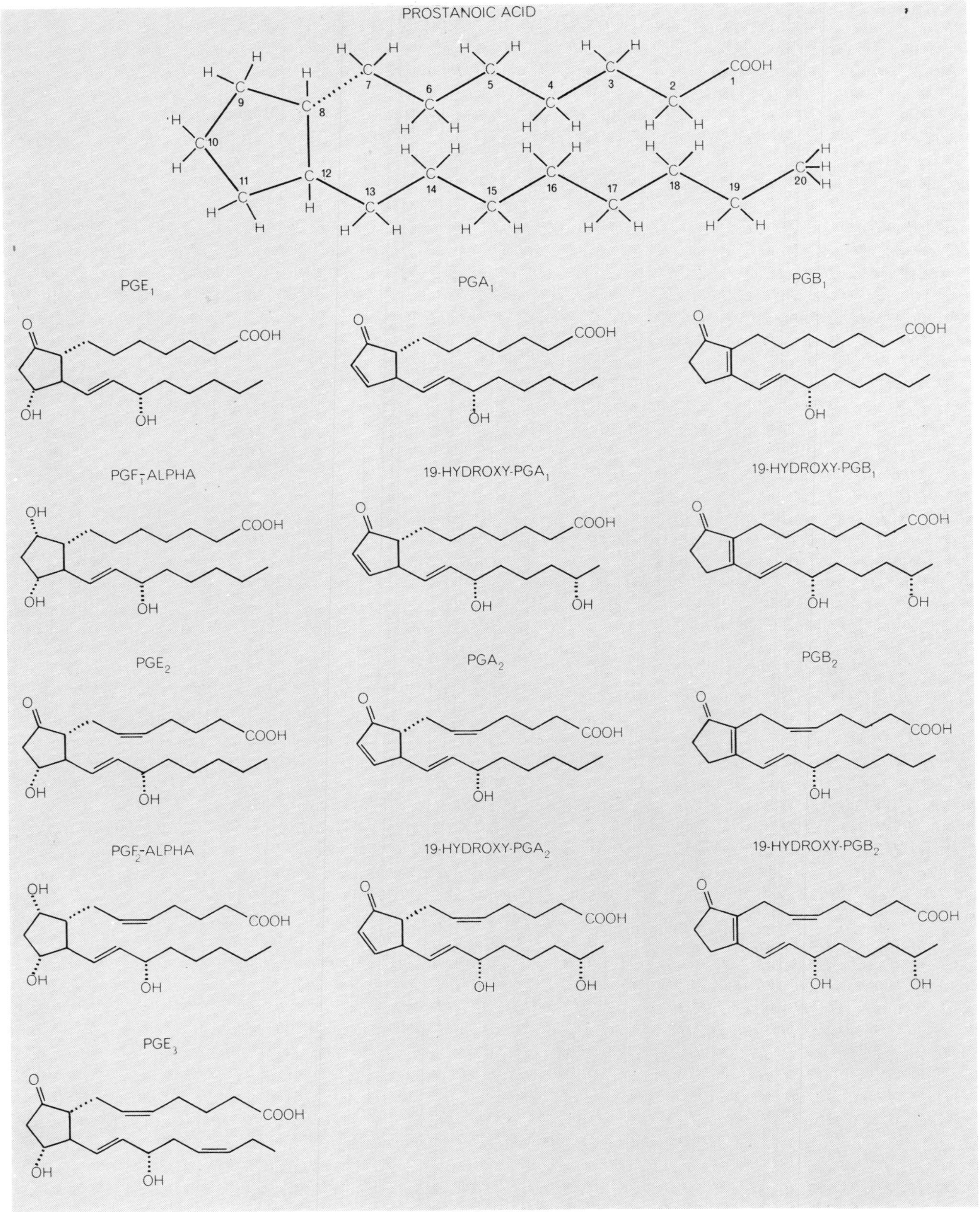

PROSTANOIC ACID

PGE₁

PGA₁

PGB₁

PGF₁-ALPHA

19-HYDROXY-PGA₁

19-HYDROXY-PGB₁

PGE₂

PGA₂

PGB₂

PGF₂-ALPHA

19-HYDROXY-PGA₂

19-HYDROXY-PGB₂

PGE₃

SOME IMPORTANT PROSTAGLANDINS are represented on this page by diagrams of their molecular structure. In general all the prostaglandins are variants of a basic 20-carbon carboxylic (COOH-bearing) fatty acid incorporating a five-member cyclopentane ring (top). Slight structural changes are responsible for quite distinct biological effects. Prostaglandins of the 1, 2 and 3 series respectively incorporate one, two and three double bonds. The molecules designated PGE and PGF are called primary prostaglandins; the PGE structures have an oxygen atom (O) attached to the cyclopentane ring at carbon site 9, whereas the PGF structures have a hydroxyl (OH) group at the same site. Dehydration of a PGE molecule leads to either a PGA or a PGB compound. Broken bonds are those that extend below the plane of the cyclopentane ring. Hydrogen atoms are shown only in top diagram.

ological functions but also in certain pathological conditions.

It appears that the prostaglandins are leading us to the meeting ground of the two main systems of communication in the body: the hormones and the nerves. They meet most directly, it seems, in the membrane of the cell. The cell membrane is indeed coming to be recognized as a most important crossroads for a great number of vital activities. Its complex biochemical apparatus controls the selective transport of all kinds of materials into and out of the cell, governs many aspects of the formation of products within the cell and is responsible for cell-to-cell communication, particularly the transmission of signals across the synapses in the nervous system, which is accomplished by chemical means. The discovery of the prostaglandins now lends new significance to the fact that the cell membrane is made up largely of phospholipids, along with proteins as the other main component. Since phospholipids supply the building materials—fatty acids—for the formation of prostaglandins, it can be supposed that the prostaglandins have a great deal to do with regulation of the functioning of the cell membrane itself. The membrane contains a common medium of communication—the chemical medium—for the chemical agents of the endocrine system and the nervous system. It will be fascinating, therefore, to explore the roles of the prostaglandins in mediating this communication, particularly with regard to their possible connection with the formation of cyclic AMP, the "second messenger," which is increasingly being recognized as a key actor in important functions such as translating the messages of specific hormones and regulating the growth and differentiation of cells.

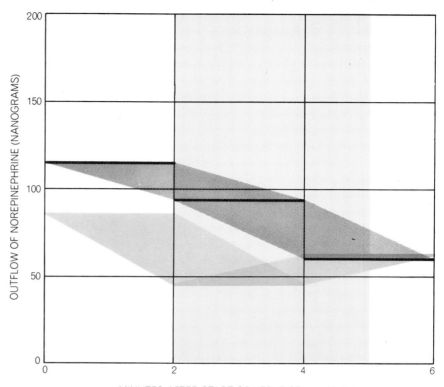

MINUTES AFTER START OF NERVE STIMULATION

INTERRELATION of the prostaglandins with the substances involved in the transmission of nerve impulses was demonstrated by a group of investigators at the Royal Caroline Institute in Sweden. In general they found that PGE$_2$ acted as a "brake" on the nerve's action in inciting the release of norepinephrine, a hormone that plays a key part in the transmission of nerve impulses in the sympathetic nervous system. In this experiment nerve stimulation of an isolated rabbit heart over a period of six minutes caused an outflow of norepinephrine, the amount of which was measured over three two-minute intervals and declined somewhat over this time span (*black lines*). In separate tests a known inhibitor of the formation of prostaglandin was infused during a three-minute period from the beginning of the second interval, and caused an increased outflow of norepinephrine during the second and third intervals (*colored lines*). Presumably the inhibitor removed the normal prostaglandin brake, resulting in an abnormally large release of norepinephrine.

V

IMPACT OF HUMAN NUTRITION ON HEALTH AND DISEASE

IMPACT OF HUMAN NUTRITION V
ON HEALTH AND DISEASE

INTRODUCTION

Health is dependent on a complex interplay of genetic and environmental factors. Among the latter, which also include shelter, sanitation, and psychological interaction, nutrition is one of the most important. The nutritional needs of an individual at any one time are dependent upon heredity, the stage of life, whether there is active growth, pregnancy, nursing, or aging, the amount of physical activity, the presence of certain diseases, and a host of unspecified factors. Requirements for calories, proteins, vitamins, and minerals may vary under all of these conditions. For example, as a result of the undeveloped state of its metabolic systems, the very young infant has special nutritional needs for optimal growth and development. Superimposed on these ontogenetic nutritional conditions are hereditary factors determining an individual's needs. Examples are the inability to tolerate milk or higher requirements for vitamins B_6 or D. Although these examples are variations from the average and are not unexpected in biology, when the variation is extreme it must be regarded as a disease.

Diet in the treatment or prevention of disease is a necessary adjunct of clinical care. The therapeutic or preventive approach may vary from the one extreme of, for example, administration of a single amino acid or vitamin to the other extreme of changing an entire life-style. The articles in this section discuss these extremes.

"Rickets" by W. F. Loomis indicates the close relationships between vitamin D, sunlight, calcium metabolism, and the general diet, and describes how the parathyroid gland, kidney, and intestine function in the normal physiology of vitamin D. "Night Blindness" by John E. Dowling explains the special relationship of vitamin A with visual function and physiology and also with inherited forms of night blindness. Studies of specific vitamin deficiencies such as those reported here have permitted scientists to explain and understand major disease entities and specific metabolic pathways.

The complexity of nutritional problems is illustrated in the article "Endemic Goiter" by R. Bruce Gillie. Knowledge of the importance of iodine in the diet goes back 5000 years, but detailed information concerning the intricate metabolism of iodine in the thyroid gland was obtained only recently. The use of iodine by the body is but one example of how trace elements participate in normal physiology.

There is little truth in the simple statement "we are what we eat." Diet is just one of the many factors in the progress and development of degenerative diseases, such as diabetes, atherosclerosis, and arthritis. This fact is well-documented in D. Spain's article, "Athersosclerosis." Recent studies in Finland and California have shown that diet works synergistically with economic class, work habits, and attitudes in the development of this disease. Recently it has beeen shown that 60 percent of premature deaths from coronary artery disease are suffered by people who have a genetic defect in fat metabolism; yet such people constitute less than one percent of the population.

by W. F. Loomis
December 1970

Although it is still widely regarded as a dietary-deficiency disease resulting from a lack of "vitamin D," it results in fact from a lack of sunlight. In smoky cities it was the first air-pollution disease

The discovery of the cause and cure of rickets is one of the great triumphs of biochemical medicine, and yet its history is little known. Indeed, it is so little known that even today most textbooks list rickets as a dietary-deficiency disease resulting from a lack of "vitamin D." In actual fact rickets was the earliest air-pollution disease. It was first described in England in about 1650, at the time of the introduction of soft coal, and it spread through Europe with the Industrial Revolution's pall of coal smoke and the increasing concentration of poor people in the narrow, sunless alleys of factory towns and big-city slums. This, we know now, was because rickets is caused not by a poor diet but by a deficiency of solar ultraviolet radiation, which is necessary for the synthesis of calciferol, the calcifying hormone released into the bloodstream by the skin. Without calciferol not enough calcium is laid down in growing bones, and the crippling deformities of rickets are the consequence. Either adequate sunlight or the ingestion of minute amounts of calciferol or one of its analogues therefore prevents and cures rickets, and so the disease has been eradicated.

That seems a clear enough story, and yet the textbooks speak of diet and vitamin D. How can that be? What happened is that the investigation of rickets proceeded along two quite independent lines. Intuitive folk medicine and then medical studies pointed in the direction of sunlight and calciferol. At the same time, however, common assumptions about poverty and poor nutrition and then studies by nutritionists pointed in the direction of diet and vitamin D. Now, with the inestimable advantage of hindsight, it is possible to trace these two chains of thought, to disentangle them and set the historical record straight.

Now that one knows what to look for, the evidence of a climatic influence on rickets can be discerned quite early. In the early 19th century G. Wendelstadt published *The Endemic Diseases of Wezlar,* a German town of 8,000 population with exceptionally narrow streets and dark alleys. The town was infamous for rickets, he wrote, with entire streets where in house after house individuals crippled by rickets could be found. "The children must sit indoors... which ends in death or if they continue to live, they develop thick joints, cease to be able to walk or have deformed legs. The head becomes large and even the vertebral column bends. It comes to pass that such children sit often for many years without being able to move; at times they cease to grow and are merely a burden to those about them." This terrible picture of an entire town afflicted with severe rickets leads one to guess that many of William Hogarth's sketches of frightfully deformed men and women may have depicted the crippling effects of rickets in London in the 18th century.

As early as 1888 the English physician Sir John Bland-Sutton found unmistakable evidence of rickets in animals in the London zoo—chimpanzees, lions, tigers, bears, deer, rabbits, lizards, ostriches, pigeons and many other species. He noted that "in spite of every care and keeping them in comfortable dens" lions in London developed rickets, whereas "in Dublin, Manchester, and some other British towns, lions can be reared successfully in captivity." It is clear in retrospect that the pall of coal smoke over London was the causative factor.

The geographical relation between rickets and cities was clearly noted in 1889 by the British Medical Association. After a survey of the incidence of the disease in the British Isles the associa-

tion published maps [*see illustration on page 195*] that supported its major conclusion: There was widespread and severe rickets "in large towns and thickly peopled districts, especially where industrial pursuits are carried on," whereas rickets was almost totally absent in rural districts. Specifically, the report added, "almost the whole of London and the greater number of its outlying suburbs" reported severe rickets among rich and poor alike.

Solar ultraviolet may be blocked by many means, among them being the industrial smog in London and the sunless alleys of Wezlar, but beneath such specific industrial and urban conditions there is a major underlying factor: the far northern location of the entire European land mass. The area is made habitable by the benign influence of the Gulf Stream, yet its winter sun, hanging low in the sky, is almost without potency in effecting the crucial conversion of 7-dehydrocholesterol into calciferol. Elsewhere in the world, lands as northerly as Europe are largely uninhabited—the Aleutian Islands, for example, or Labrador or northern Siberia. The long, dark winters of Europe therefore powerfully predisposed European infants toward rickets during the winter months.

The seasonal variation was noted as early as 1884 by M. Kassowitz in Germany, who attributed it to the prolonged confinement of infants indoors during the winter. Then in 1906 D. Hansemann noted that nearly all German children who were born in the fall and died in the spring had rickets; those who were born in the spring and died in the fall were free of the disease. Noting the progressive rise of rickets during the winter months, he concluded that rickets was primarily a disease of "domestication,"

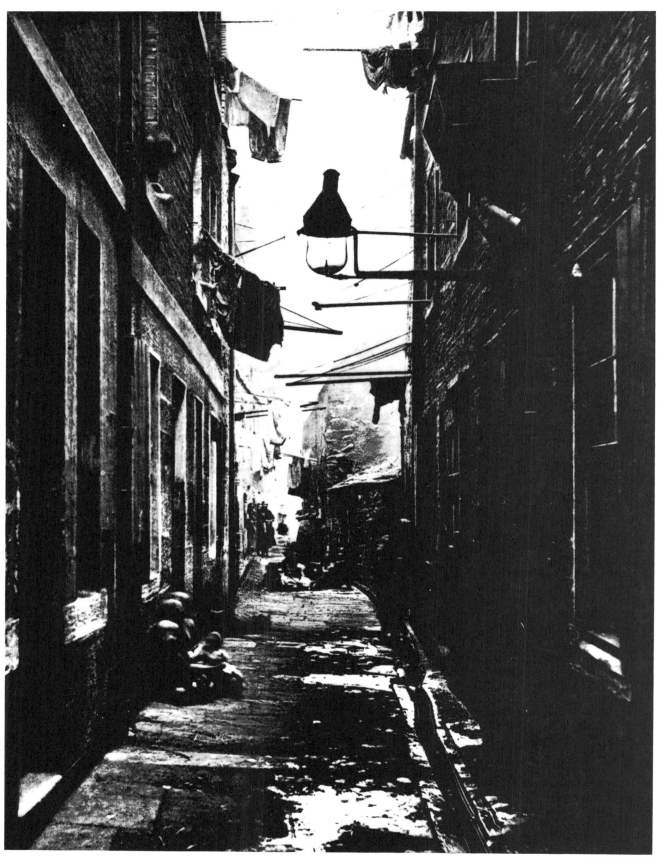

DARK ALLEY in Glasgow, photographed in about 1870, is typical of the environment in which rickets was once endemic. In such a setting children received little ultraviolet radiation, which is necessary for the synthesis of the hormone that prevents rickets. Along the left side of the alley are two groups of children. Images are blurred because the children moved during the time exposure.

for "I have learned that rickets never exists in wild tribes or in animals [that] live in complete freedom. Once caught, however, most of these formerly wild animals—and especially monkeys—show great disposition towards rickets. Hardly one young captured animal can avoid this danger. By observing rickets in people, who do not get this disease to such a degree as monkeys, one can also see that it is a sickness of *domestication*. We can say that in living locked indoors, with thick, heavy walls and windows facing brick walls in other houses, the natural habitat of a child is being disturbed—namely the outdoors." In 1909 G. Schmorl strongly documented this marked seasonal variation in the frequency of rickets with a series of 386 postmortem examinations carried out on children under four years old.

Perhaps the most brilliant investigation into the nature of rickets was made in 1890 by Theobald Palm, an English medical missionary who went to Japan and "was struck with the absence of rickets among the Japanese as compared with its lamentable frequency among the poor children of the large centres of population in England and Scotland." He wrote to other medical missionaries around the world, collated the results and was amazed to find that rickets was essentially confined to northern Europe and was almost totally absent from the rest of the world.

Dugald Christie wrote him from Mukden, for example, as follows: "I have met with not a single case of rickets during a residency of six years in Manchuria," and this in spite of the fact that there were "no sanitary conditions whatever" and the only articles of diet were millet, rice, pork and vegetables. C. P. Smith reported from Mongolia that he had not seen any rickets. "We have 10 months in the year of almost constant sunshine. In summer the children go practically naked, and even in winter, with the rivers frozen into a solid mass of ice, I have seen children running about almost naked, that is during the day while the sun is shining." From Java a Dr. Waitz reported what was a known fact there: European children suffering from rickets recovered from the malady within a few months of moving to Java and without any medical treatment.

From data such as this Palm deduced that rickets was caused by the absence of sunlight. "It is in the narrow alleys, the haunts and playgrounds of the children of the poor, that this exclusion of sunlight is at its worst, and it is there that

the victims of rickets are to be found in abundance." He proceeded to recommend "the systematic use of sun-baths as a preventive and therapeutic measure in rickets."

The first successful attempt to induce rickets experimentally in animals was

made at the University of Glasgow in 1908 by Leonard Findlay. He published conclusive pictures of puppies that had been confined in cages and developed rickets; unconfined animals did not become rachitic. His results convinced him that the cause of rickets was not any

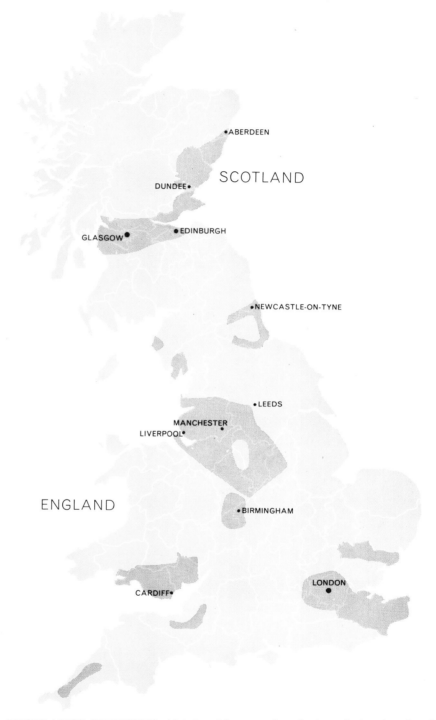

CORRELATION OF RICKETS with industrial areas and smoke from the burning of coal appeared in data assembled in 1889 by the British Medical Association. The map, which shows in gray the principal concentrations of rickets, is based on maps of England and Scotland prepared by the association. Since diets in these areas were in general better than those in poorer surrounding areas, the distribution of rickets is not what one would expect if the disease were of dietary origin. In actuality the cause was smoke that obscured sunlight.

defect in the diet, but he did not come to quite the right conclusion; he suggested that rickets was caused by "confinement, with consequent lack of exercise." More accurate was a brilliant experiment by Jan Raczynski of Paris in 1912. Raczynski pointed to lack of sunlight as the principal etiological factor in rickets. Two puppies, "newborn in the month of May from the same mother, were reared for six weeks, the first in sunlight from morning to evening, the second in deep shade in a large, well-ventilated cage. Both were fed in the same manner, that is exclusively on the milk of their mother." After six weeks the puppy kept out of the sunlight was markedly rachitic, a diagnosis confirmed by chemical analysis of its bones, which were found to contain 36 percent less calcium phosphate than the bones of the puppy that had been raised in the sun. Raczynski concluded that sunlight played a principal role in the etiology of the disease.

In 1918 Findlay returned to the problem with the assistance of Noel Paton. They did experiments with 17 collie puppies from two litters and reported that "all those kept in the laboratory showed signs of rickets to a greater or less degree. One which had been confined and had had butter was most markedly affected. It was unable to walk. Another of the confined animals which had had no butter was least affected." They concluded: "Pups kept in the country and freely exercised in the open air, although they had actually a smaller amount of milk fat than those kept in the laboratory, remained free of rickets, while the animals kept in the laboratory all became rickety." Findlay and Paton fed butter to some of their animals to check on the effect of diet, since the idea that rickets was a dietary-deficiency disease was already taking hold and milk fat was known as an important source of vitamin A. Their results argued against such a theory, of course. Moreover, it is known today that the adverse effect of butter they observed was due to the fact that "florid," or severe, rickets develops best in well-fed puppies; a poorly fed animal develops only mild rickets since the defect in calcification does not have as much effect in an animal whose bones are not growing. Rather than being a dietary-deficiency disease, therefore, florid rickets required a good diet, complete with vitamins A, B and C; only then could the puppy grow rapidly and hence develop incapacitating rickets.

Findlay's group had by now become known as the "Glasgow school," as op-posed to the "London school" of nutritionists. Their competing theories led to two important studies of human rickets, one in Scotland and one in India.

Margaret Ferguson studied 200 families living in Glasgow among whom marked rickets existed and decided that inadequate air and exercise appeared to be the most potent factors. "Over 40 percent of the rachitic children had not been taken out, while only 4 percent of the nonrachitic children had been confined indoors." It is clear now that being out of doors was the chief variable, for both sets of children were free to exercise at will.

The most clear-cut investigation was conducted by Harry S. Hutchinson in Bombay. He found no rickets at all among poor Hindus who subsisted on a pitifully inadequate diet but who worked outdoors all day "and while at work left their young infants at some nearby point in the open air." In contrast, he found that rickets was exceedingly common among the well-fed Moslems and upper-caste Hindus, whose women usually married at the age of 12 and entered purdah, where the ensuing infants usually remained with their mother for the first six months of life in a semidark room in the interior of the house. Hutchinson found that infants of both sexes kept in purdah suffered severely from rickets; the girls, who entered purdah when they were married, recontracted the disease then. He concluded that "the most important etiological factor in the production of rickets is lack of fresh air, sunlight, and exercise." He then proceeded to cure 10 such cases of purdah-induced rickets by taking the patients out into the open air, "showing that removal of the cause removes the effect. All other factors remained constant and no medicine was given."

Although it was becoming increasingly clear by 1919 to many physicians that sunlight had the power both to prevent and to cure rickets, no method of providing summer sunlight during European winters was available. Not only were such winters generally cloudy, with an ineffective sun less than 30 degrees from the horizon, but also the cold usually required exposure of children to the sun in glassed-in solariums whose windowpanes, it is now known, effectively filtered out the required ultraviolet rays. Folk custom had taught northern European mothers to put their infants out of doors even during January for "some fresh air and sunshine." The trouble was that in large cities with narrow streets even this became ineffective because of the intervening buildings and the pall of smoke.

With natural sunlight ineffective, doctors such as E. Buchholz in Germany turned to artificial illumination such as that provided by the carbon-filament electric bulb. Since the ultraviolet component of such light is very small, the treatments did little good. Then in 1919 a Berlin pediatrician, Kurt Huldschinsky, tried the light from a mercury-vapor quartz lamp, which includes the ultraviolet wavelengths, on four cases of advanced rickets in children. He obtained complete cures within two months.

Huldschinsky's discovery of the subtle fact that it is the invisible portion of the sun's rays that prevents rickets solved the problem of this disease for all time. In addition to providing a truly effective method of curing the disease, he proceeded to show that an endocrine hormone must be involved. He irradiated one arm of a rachitic child with ultraviolet. Then he showed, with X-ray pictures, that calcium salts were deposited not only in the irradiated arm but in the other arm as well. This proved that on irradiation the skin released into the bloodstream a chemical that had the needed power to induce healing at a distance—in other words, a hormone.

After World War I, Huldschinsky's findings were extended by Alfred F. Hess in New York. He showed that sunlight alone had the power to cure rickets in children. He then showed that this was true also of rats that had been made artificially rachitic by means of a low-phosphate diet. In June, 1924, Hess found that ultraviolet irradiation rendered linseed or cottonseed capable of curing rickets. Similar results were obtained on whole rat rations later that year by Harry Steenbock. Hess proceeded to show that a crude cholesterol and plant sterols, as well as the skin, acquired the property of curing rickets when irradiated by ultraviolet light. In 1927 Otto Rosenheim and Thomas A. Webster showed that the plant sterol ergosterol (derived from ergot, a fungus) became enormously antirachitic when irradiated with ultraviolet light. This is the process that has now become routine: Some .01 milligram per quart of ergocalciferol—or what is called "vitamin D_2"—is added to almost all the milk sold in the U.S. and most European countries.

A description of the nature of the skin hormone naturally released by irradiated skin was finally provided in 1936 by Adolf Windaus of the University of Göt-

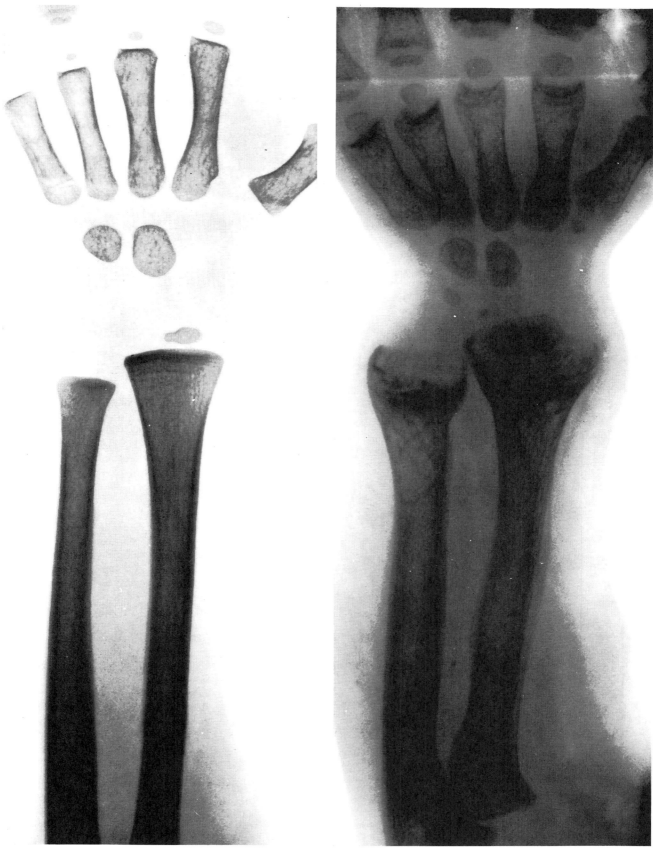

EFFECT OF RICKETS is deformation of bone for want of the calcifying hormone calciferol, which is synthesized on ultraviolet radiation. An X ray of normal arm and hand bones in an 18-month-old child (*left*) is compared with an X ray of the bones of a child of the same age with rickets (*right*). The disease can be prevented or cured by sunlight or the ingestion of small amounts of calciferol.

FOOD	WINTER	SUMMER
MILK	0	.025
BUTTER	0	4
CREAM	0	1
EGG YOKE	4	1.2
OLIVE OIL	0	0
CALF LIVER	0	0

CALCIFEROL IN FOOD is charted. The substance, which is often called vitamin D, is essentially absent from foodstuffs other than fish, particularly in winter. The numerals give the percentage of the minimum daily protective dose of calciferol in a gram of each food.

tingen. He demonstrated that 7-dehydrocholesterol is the natural prehormone that is found in the skin and showed how it becomes calciferol on ultraviolet irradiation.

The hormonal nature of calciferol had been recognized to some degree as early as 1923 by such an authority as the American pediatrician Edwards A. Park, who wrote a careful summary of the history of rickets in *Physiological Reviews*. He summarized his view of the complex situation by saying that rickets is best compared to the endocrine-deficiency disease diabetes rather than to the genuine vitamin-deficiency diseases such as scurvy, pellagra, xerophthalmia and beriberi. Hess shared this view. In the first sentence of a 1929 monograph he stated that rickets "must be regarded as essentially a climatic disorder."

How, then, has the London school's view that rickets is due to a deficiency of "vitamin D" prevailed even up to the present day? Why is the error almost universally found in modern textbooks of endocrinology, physiology, biochemistry and medicine and further propagated by the words printed on every carton of milk sold in the U.S. and many other countries: "400 U.S.P. units vitamin D added per qt."? The remainder of this article will attempt to explain briefly the origin of the mistake.

Modern studies such as those of G. A. Blondin of Clark University support the long-suspected fact that fish, unlike birds and mammals, are able to synthesize calciferol enzymatically without ultraviolet light. Shielded by water, fish receive essentially no ultraviolet (290-to-320-millimicron) radiation, and yet the bluefin tuna has up to a milligram of calciferol per gram of liver oil—enough to provide a daily protective dose of calciferol for 100 children. Cod-liver oil contains less than 1 percent as much, enough to protect against rickets if it is consumed in amounts equal to four grams per day. It is an effective antirachitic medicine because of calciferol's unusual stability: an oil or fat containing the hormone preserves its efficacy for a long time.

In the north of Europe fish has always been a staple of diet, and so the normal diet tended to protect children against rickets. Slowly, over the years, the people of Scandinavia and the Baltic regions became aware of the specific therapeutic value of cod-liver oil as a preventive and even as a cure for rickets. By the end of the 19th century this therapy had come to the attention of physicians, but it was not generally accepted because a number of variables made the evaluation difficult: the advent of spring, chance exposure to sunlight or some unrelated retardation of growth that reduced the severity of the rickets could mask the effect of the cod-liver oil. It remained for Hess to make the unequivocal demonstration. In 1917 he conducted a controlled test with Negro children in New York City, among whom rickets was severe and almost universal, and proved the prophylactic value of routine administration of cod-liver oil.

It was a significant finding but it helped to turn investigators away from sunlight and toward diet. In 1919, the very year in which Huldschinsky pointed directly to ultraviolet radiation as the crucial factor in preventing rickets, the British nutritionist Edward Mellanby re-

A	UNDER 20
B	20 TO 24
C	25 TO 29
D	30 TO 34
E	35 AND OVER

INDOOR LIVING had a marked effect on rickets in India, according to a survey conducted by Harry S. Hutchinson in Bombay. He found a high incidence (*left*) among rich, well-fed Moslems, whose married women entered purdah and whose infants remained indoors; less among well-to-do Hindus (*middle*), whose children got outdoors more; none among poor Hindus (*right*), who had bad diets but who worked (and whose babies played) outdoors.

ported on what he called a "rachitogenic" diet. Working in London, under its pall of industrial smoke, Mellanby found that puppies would rapidly develop florid rickets on a diet reinforced with yeast, milk and orange juice—a natural finding, considering that Bland-Sutton had shown that almost all the animals in the zoo in industrial London suffered from rickets. Mellanby's announcement of the "production" of rickets in dogs by means of a particular diet was in line with the new "vitamine" theories of Frederick Gowland Hopkins and Casimir Funk; Mellanby suggested that the efficacy of cod-liver oil was "most probably" due to vitamin A, which was presumably missing in his "rachitogenic" diet. The diet finding was greeted with enthusiasm—even though Findlay had produced rickets in dogs 11 years earlier by simply keeping them indoors.

Park has pointed out that the report of Mellanby's "first experiments was meagre and would probably have awakened little interest, had not the British Medical Research Committee endorsed the work and publicly committed itself to the view that rickets was a deficiency disease due to a lack in the diet of 'antirachitic factor.'" It is clear enough today that Mellanby's idea that the cod-liver oil factor was probably vitamin A was wrong, but it is not generally recognized that *no* specific medicine such as cod-liver oil can be called a dietary vitamin unless it is present in normal foods in significant amounts. (Orally administered thyroid, for example, cannot be regarded as a "vitamin T" even though patients with insufficient thyroid of their own are cured by thyroid extract. Both endocrine secretions require external factors, incidentally: ultraviolet radiation in the case of calciferol and iodine in the case of thyroxine.)

In 1921 the American nutritionist Elmer V. McCollum, who had just accomplished the separation of fat-soluble vitamin A from water-soluble vitamin B, turned his attention to the rickets problem, putting his laboratory rats on Mellanby's "rachitogenic" diet. At first he could not produce rickets; being nocturnal animals, rats have become adapted to survival without direct sunlight and are resistant to rickets. Eventually Henry C. Sherman and Alwin M. Pappenheimer came on the trick of artificially giving rats a diet low in phosphate. Under this artificial stress the bones of young rats failed to calcify—unless they were placed in direct sunlight or were given cod-liver oil.

McCollum went on to establish the difference between the active factor in cod-liver oil and vitamin A in 1922 by showing that, after having been aerated and heated, cod-liver oil could still cure rickets but had lost its ability to cure xerophthalmia, which is due to lack of vitamin A. On this basis he called the cod-liver oil factor "vitamin D." Final recognition of the uniqueness of fish-liver oils came from the finding that animal fats such as butter and lard have essentially no calciferol, particularly in winter; the conclusion was clear that no nonfish diet of any kind could protect against rickets in a sunless environment. It was quite clear then that cod-liver oil was a medicine and not a food.

Nevertheless, McCollum had called it "vitamin D," and in the flush of enthusiasm for these new-found dietary factors the name acquired general acceptance. Semantic confusion now entered the picture in overwhelming force. Circular verbal proof made it evident that if "vitamin D" cured rickets, then rickets was a vitamin-deficiency disease! All the careful work demonstrating that rickets

was primarily a climatic disorder was forgotten in the enthusiasm for the latest "vitamin." Chemists such as Windaus set about the task of deciphering its chemical structure. When Windaus received the Nobel prize in chemistry in 1928, it was "for his researches into the constitution of the sterols and their connection with the vitamins"—a curious citation in view of the fact that all biologically active sterols are manufactured by the body and are hormonal in character, whereas none of the known vitamins have a steroid structure. Even the discovery that calciferol was produced naturally in the skin in the presence of ultraviolet did not wipe out its classification as a vitamin or the definition of rickets as a dietary problem. Meanwhile the addition of ergocalciferol to milk had essentially eradicated the disease in Europe and America. Ironically, its effectiveness tended to buttress the dietary concept of the disease.

It took time for the correct view to emerge. In 1927 the chairman of the American Medical Association's section on the diseases of children remarked that "cod-liver oil is our civilization's excellent, economical and practical substitute—at least during the colder and darker half of the year—for exposure to sunlight. Is it not strange that the established vitamin deficiencies such as xerophthalmia, beriberi and scurvy are so rare in infants fed human milk from mothers and that rickets is so common? The great primary importance of the actinic [chemically active] rays to normal growth is evidenced by the fact that rickets occurs most severely and most frequently at the end of winter, and especially in those infants whose skins are pigmented. These observations strongly suggest that in human infants vitamins do not play a primary role in the development of rickets...."

CHEMICAL STRUCTURES of calciferol (*right*) and its precursor, 7-dehydrocholesterol (*left*), are closely related. The precursor is in the skin, and ultraviolet radiation from the sun is crucial in effecting its conversion to calciferol, which then enters the blood.

The fact that cod-liver oil, which contains the so-called 'vitamin D,' cures rickets does *not* prove that rickets observed in human infants primarily is a vitamin-deficiency disease."

It is interesting to consider the essential difference between the methods of the Glasgow school and those of the London school. Whereas the Glasgow school studied rickets in humans as well as in animals, and from a medical point of view, the London nutritionists studied it only in animals, believing only the results of their experiments and essentially ignoring such brilliant medical studies as those of Palm and Hutchinson. The methodological differences between clinical medical research and beginning biochemistry are therefore behind the whole tangled story, and it is only today, 50 years later, that hindsight can explain the errors of those days.

A word should be said in answer to those who may ask what difference it makes whether calciferol is called a hormone or a vitamin. The answer lies in the point of view from which one approaches this vital calcifying factor needed for the healthy development of

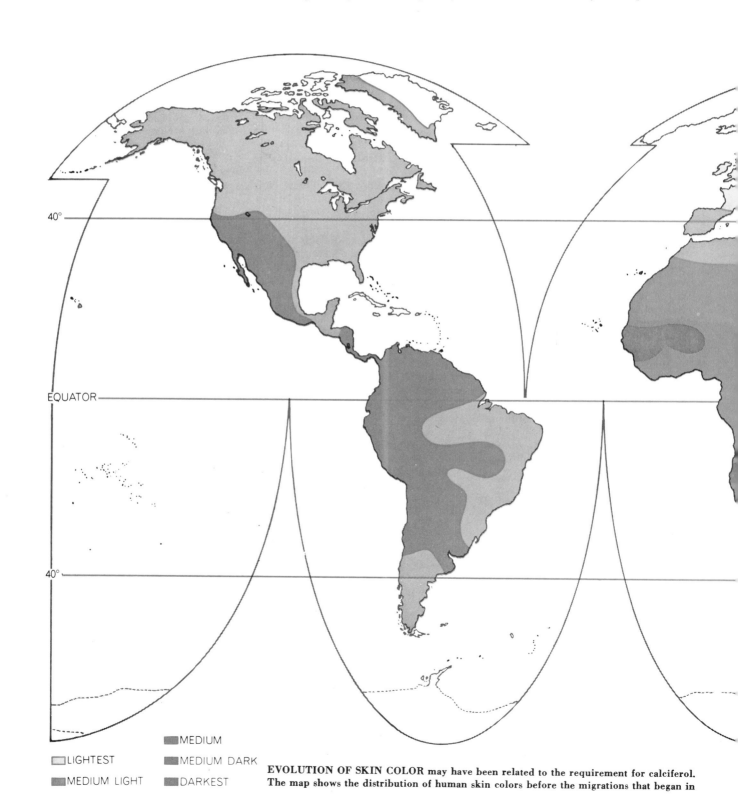

LIGHTEST

MEDIUM LIGHT

MEDIUM

MEDIUM DARK

DARKEST

EVOLUTION OF SKIN COLOR may have been related to the requirement for calciferol. **The map shows the distribution of human skin colors before the migrations that began in**

the skeleton. Calling calciferol "vitamin D" at least suggests that it forms the nucleus of some cellular coenzyme, as is the case with many vitamins. Calling calciferol a hormone, on the other hand, explains why three hormones, calciferol, thyrocalcitonin and the parathyroid hormone are linked together in the delicate control of the level of calcium in the blood [see "Calcitonin," by Howard Rasmussen and Maurice M. Pechet; SCIENTIFIC AMERICAN, October]. Since no other cases of hormones and vitamins working together are known to medicine, it should not be surprising that calciferol turns out to be a steroid hormone whose production rate is under physiological control rather than being left to the vagaries of diet.

Other leads opened up by the hormonal view include the evolutionary development of the hormone. Fish synthesize it without ultraviolet light. Amphibians, reptiles, birds and mammals each apparently have some ultraviolet-receptive area of the body where the hormone is made, such as the ears of rabbits and the feet of birds. By and large, northern animals avoid rickets by living out of doors and by bearing their offspring in

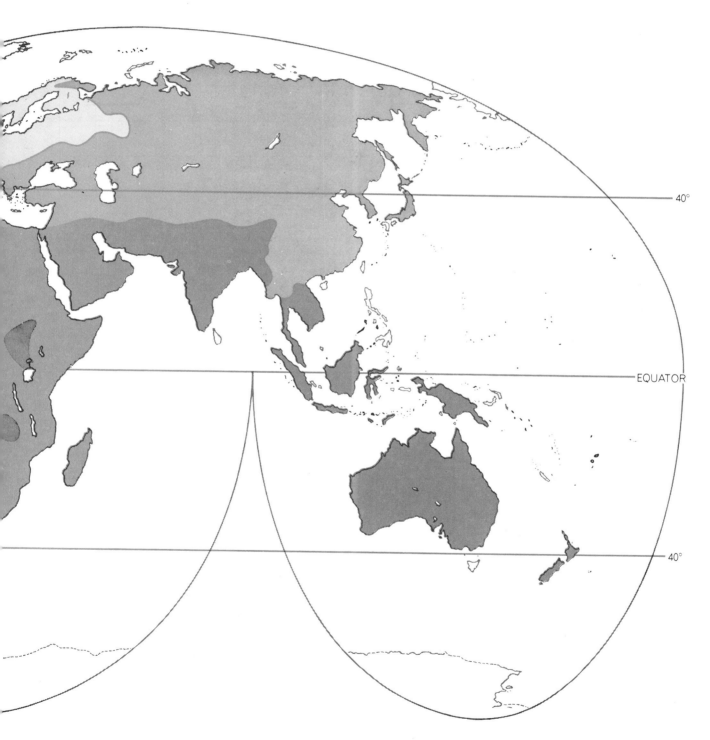

the 16th century. Dark skin presumably protected against overproduction of calciferol. In Europe, much of which is at very high latitudes, man needed all the ultraviolet he could get, particularly in winter, and was presumably selected for unpigmented skin.

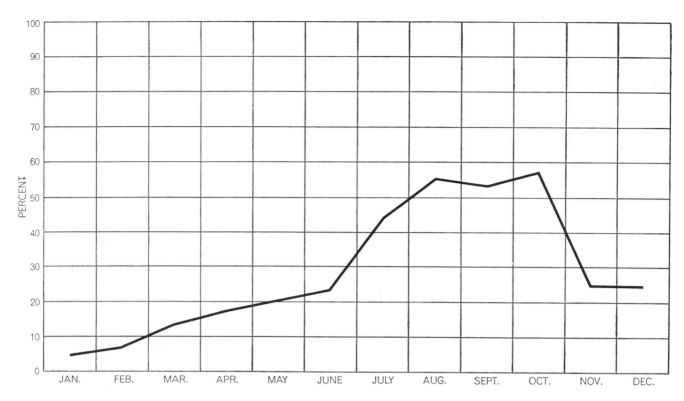

SEASONAL VARIATION in the frequency of rickets appeared in a series of 386 postmortem examinations of children with rickets conducted by G. Schmorl in 1909. Children were classified accord-ing to whether they had an active case of rickets at the time of death (*color*) or a "healing" case (*black*). It was clear that the se-verity of the disease increased in the fall and decreased with spring.

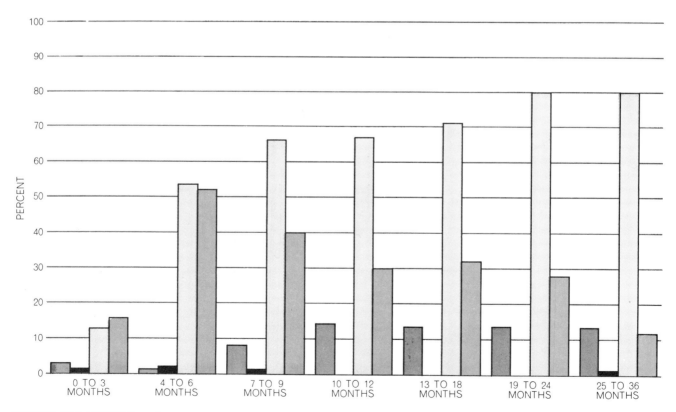

EFFECT OF LATITUDE on the incidence of rickets among chil-dren of various ages in Puerto Rico (*gray*) and New Haven (*color*) was demonstrated in a survey that was reported in 1933. The in-cidence is apparently related to the amount and strength of sun-light at 18 degrees of latitude and at 42 degrees. The light bars indicate clinical diagnosis of rickets, dark bars X-ray diagnosis.

the spring, so that they are exposed to the summer sun during their growing period. Truly arctic animals, such as the polar bear and the seal, that live the year round in an area of deficient ultraviolet obtain their calciferol orally from their staple diet of fish. (The same was true of the Eskimos, who were entirely free of rickets until they were placed on a European diet by missionaries—when they too rapidly developed the disease.)

The recognition of calciferol as an ultraviolet-dependent hormone gives fresh meaning to a number of seemingly unrelated physiological and cultural adaptations. Tropical man probably avoids the dangers of too much calciferol production by virtue of his dark skin; the melanin granules in the outer layers protect the lower layers of the skin. European man, on the other hand, needed to use all the scanty ultraviolet light available, and consequently was gradually selected for an unpigmented skin such as is present in extreme degree in the blond-haired, blue-eyed, fair-skinned and rosy-cheeked infants of the English, north German and Scandinavian peoples. Indeed, the northern European idea of female beauty fits this picture: a girl with trim ankles, straight legs, fair skin and rosy cheeks must never have suffered from rickets and hence would probably bear strong sons and daughters if chosen as a mate. The very phrase "a fair young damsel" implies that a girl who is beautiful in the eyes of northern beholders is the possessor of an unpigmented skin! Delicate wrists are further proof of the absence of a history of rickets, as is a free-swinging walk, which is only possible in the absence of the pelvic deformities of rickets that would later endanger the process of childbirth.

June weddings tend to bring the first baby in the spring; an infant born in the fall was almost certain to have rickets by the time he was six months old. The fish-on-Friday tradition was as adaptive as the scurvy-preventing eating of an apple a day. Taking the baby out of doors even in the middle of winter for "some fresh air and sunshine" became a northern folk custom. Pink cheeks are visible evidence of the thinness of the unpigmented skin in the one area left uncovered in babies wrapped up warmly and placed out of doors in winter. The ability of outdoor-living Europeans to become deeply bronzed by the sun prevents the synthesis of too much calciferol in summer; it is significant that this seasonal pigmentation is induced by the identical 290-to-320-millimicron radiation that produces calciferol. Clearly northern European man, bronzed in summer but crocus white in winter, has an epidermis well adapted to the seasonal variation in ultraviolet radiation. Only with the advent of industrial smog did rickets appear in England and northern Europe.

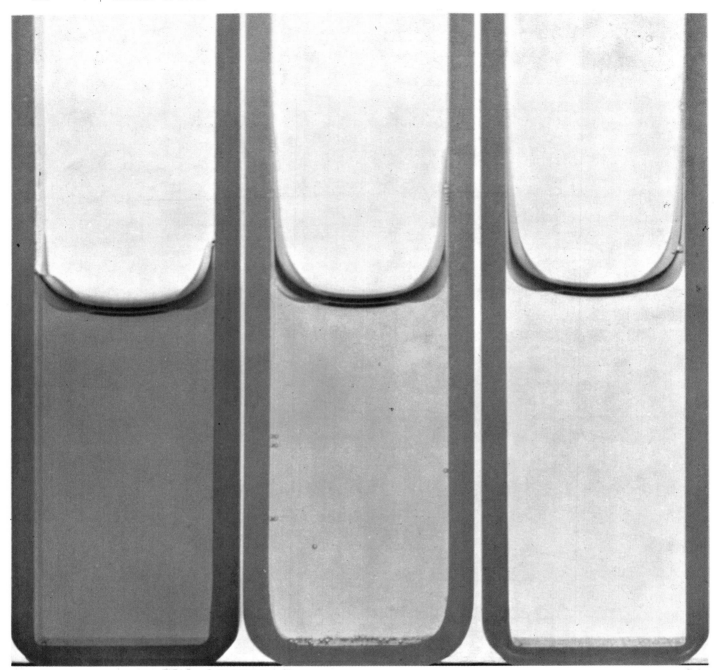

The three vessels contain extracts of the visual pigment rhodopsin in three states. Rhodopsin is the pigment found in the rod cells of the retina, which are responsible for vision in dim light. It is a complex of the protein opsin and the aldehyde form of vitamin A. When it absorbs light, it initiates excitation of the rod cell and is "bleached" from a purplish red to yellow. In the photograph the vessel at left contains unbleached rhodopsin that has been extracted from the retina of a bullfrog. The vessel in center contains the bleached pigment, which has been dissociated into opsin and vitamin A aldehyde. In the vessel at right the vitamin A aldehyde has been converted into colorless vitamin A. The extracts were prepared by John E. Dowling and Paul K. Brown at the Biological Laboratories of Harvard University.

Night Blindness

by John E. Dowling
October 1966

*It has long been known that poor vision in dim light
can be improved with vitamin A. Experiments
with rats have now clarified exactly what it is the
vitamin does*

Night blindness—insensitivity of the eye to dim light—is one of the oldest diseases known to man, and a cure for the disease has also been known since early times. Medical papyruses of ancient Egypt prescribed the eating of raw liver as a specific for restoring night vision. Early in this century investigators identified the curative factor in liver as vitamin A. Beginning in the 1930's, George Wald of Harvard University and other workers went on to elucidate in detail the critical role played by vitamin A in vision [see "Eye and Camera," by George Wald; Scientific American Offprint 46].

In his classic study Wald showed that the visual pigment in the rods, the retinal cells responsible for vision in dim light, is a complex called rhodopsin that consists of the aldehyde form of vitamin A (also called retinene and retinaldehyde) joined to a large protein molecule named opsin. This pigment, on absorbing light, initiates excitation of the rod cell. The absorption of light also splits the rhodopsin molecule into vitamin A aldehyde and opsin, and the pigment is thereby "bleached" from purplish red to yellow. The chemical conversion of the vitamin A aldehyde into vitamin A can also be detected by a change in the color of the retina from yellow to white [*see illustration on the cover of this issue*].

It then became evident that a deficiency of vitamin A would prevent rod cells from synthesizing sufficient rhodopsin and thus would produce night blindness. It has since been shown that a deficiency of the vitamin also reduces the sensitivity of the retinal cone cells, which serve for vision in ordinary light (such as daylight), because vitamin A is necessary for the synthesis of their visual pigments. The loss of cone sensitivity, however, is not usually great

enough to be noticed in daylight; it is only in the faint light of nighttime that a person deficient in vitamin A becomes blind.

Soon after Wald's discovery investigators proceeded to test the visual effects of vitamin A deficiency, and of

treatments with the vitamin, on human volunteers. Two puzzling findings emerged. Although some of the subjects who were fed an A-deficient diet showed signs of night blindness within a few days, others retained their normal visual sensitivity for months or even

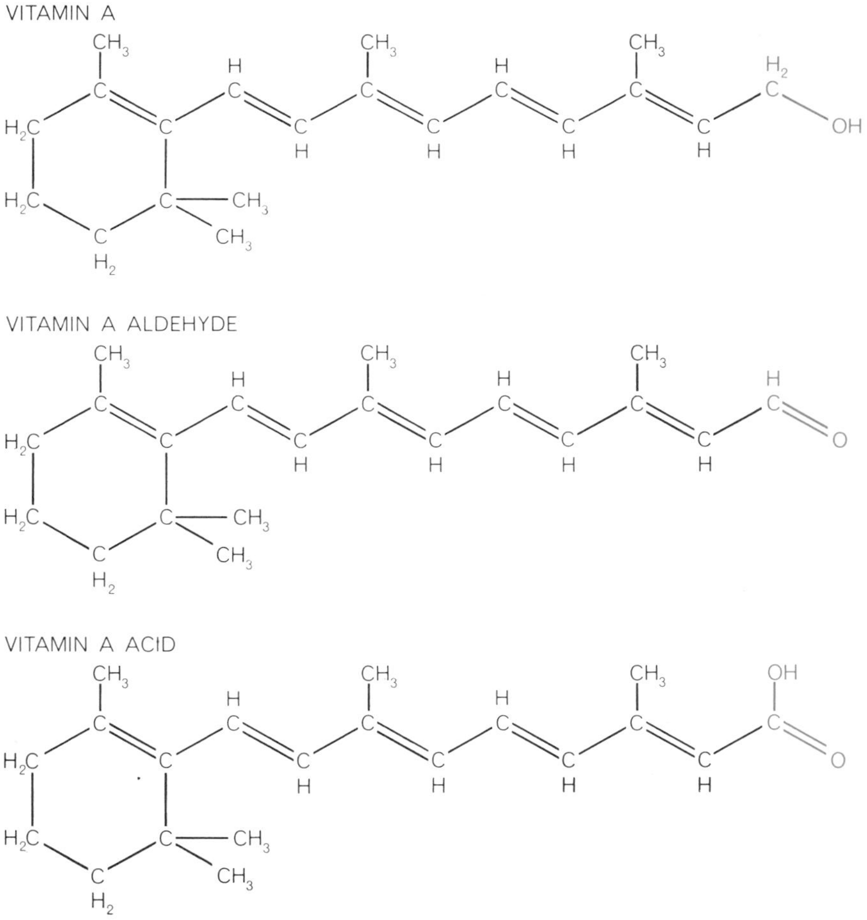

CHEMICAL STRUCTURES of three different molecular forms of vitamin A are depicted here; the parts of the molecules that differ are in color. The aldehyde form of vitamin A combines with a large protein molecule (opsin) to form a complex (rhodopsin) that is the visual pigment in the rods, the retinal cells responsible for vision in dim light. Vitamin A acid keeps rats healthy but is not converted into vitamin A or vitamin A aldehyde in rat tissues.

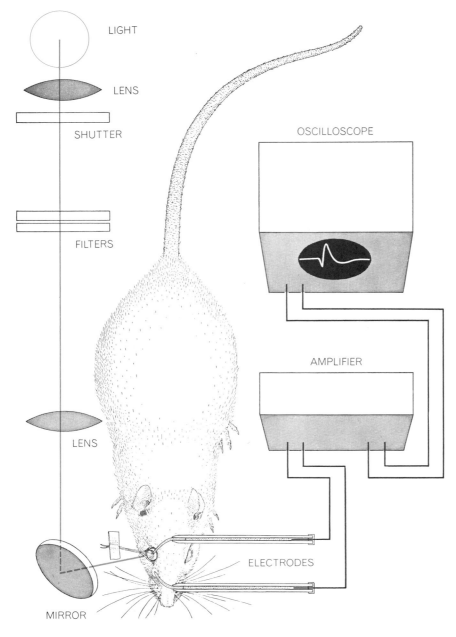

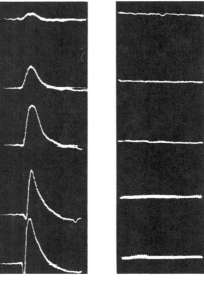

ELECTRORETINOGRAM (ERG) is used by the author to measure the visual sensitivity of rats' eyes to flashes of light of varying intensity. The optical system delivers a flash of light lasting a fiftieth of a second to the eye of an anesthetized rat. Cotton-wick electrodes inserted in the ends of glass pipettes filled with salt solution are placed on the edge of the cornea and on a shaved area of the cheek (the same as if the electrode were placed on the back of the eye). The eye's electrical response to a flash of light is amplified and recorded on an oscilloscope. Visual sensitivity is determined by the threshold of light intensity to which the eye will respond with a minimum ERG. The two sets of oscilloscope traces at right show the ERG responses of a normal rat (*left*) and a rat that has been on a vitamin-A-deficient diet for 10 months (*right*). The second rat is blind. Its loss of visual sensitivity increased exponentially, or at a logarithmic rate.

LIGHT

LENS

SHUTTER

FILTERS

LENS

MIRROR

OSCILLOSCOPE

AMPLIFIER

ELECTRODES

years. Secondly, of those who developed night blindness, some quickly recovered normal vision after vitamin A was restored to their diet, but in others the recovery was slow and occasionally was not complete even many months later. Not surprisingly, in view of the latter finding, the experiments with human subjects were discontinued.

A search began for possible explanations of these curious results. Thomas Moore of the Dunn Nutritional Laboratory in Cambridge, England, discovered one significant clue: adult human beings vary considerably in the amount of reserve vitamin A stored in their liver. Consequently a person with a large reserve might show no signs of deficiency for months after going on an A-deficient diet, whereas one with little storage of the vitamin would show effects almost immediately.

The second question—why some affected persons responded promptly to treatment with vitamin A while others did not—was less easy to answer. There were one or two suggestive findings. In the 1930's Katherine Tansley of University College London and others had found in experiments with animals that the visual cells in the retina degenerated when the animals were kept on an A-deficient diet for a prolonged period. More recently Ruth Hubbard of Harvard learned that opsin is rather unstable compared with rhodopsin. It seemed, therefore, that in the absence of a supply of vitamin A aldehyde for re-forming rhodopsin, opsin might break down with a consequent degeneration of the visual cell.

It was in the light of these findings that, as a student in Wald's laboratory at Harvard, I undertook a study of nutritional night blindness. As our experimental animal we used the rat, the retina of which contains mostly rod cells. We began by measuring the depletion of vitamin A, rhodopsin and opsin from the animal's body when it was fed a diet deficient in the vitamin. The results ran true to our expectations. First the animal drew on the store of vitamin A in its liver; in young rats this supply lasted about three to four weeks, and during that time the vitamin level in the animal's blood and the levels of rhodopsin and opsin in the retina remained normal. After the vitamin A reserve in the liver was used up the level of the vitamin in the blood fell precipitously. Within a few days the level of rhodopsin in the eye also began to decline; two to three weeks later the opsin level began to fall.

How did this depletion correlate with the animal's vision? As a measure of its visual sensitivity we resorted to the electroretinogram (ERG), a gross electrical response of the retina to a flash of light. Cotton-wick electrodes are placed on the eye of the anesthetized animal, and the eye's electrical response to a flash of light is amplified and recorded on an oscilloscope. The eye's sensitivity is determined by the threshold of light intensity to which it will respond with a minimum ERG.

During the first three to four weeks of a rat's subsistence on the vitamin-A-deficient diet, while the rhodopsin level in the eye remained normal, there was no detectable loss of visual sensitivity. By the fifth week, with a decline in the rhodopsin level, the ERG response also began to decline: it took more light to evoke the minimal electrical reaction. By the eighth week, when the rhodopsin level had dropped to 15 to 20 percent of normal, the ERG threshold had risen by a factor of almost 1,000, that is, the light intensity had to be 1,000 times stronger to produce a response. In general, as the rhodopsin level fell, the loss of visual sensitivity increased exponentially, or at a logarithmic rate.

Up to this point there was apparently no permanent damage to the eye. The retina could be restored to yield a normal ERG response within a few days simply by giving the rat a large dose of vitamin A. Thus the eye's loss and recovery of sensitivity was uncomplicated, in the sense that it paralleled the usual behavior of the organ in adapting to the dark after adapting to bright light. We found, by using the ERG test, that during the process of dark adaptation the sensitivity of the rat's eye bears a loga-

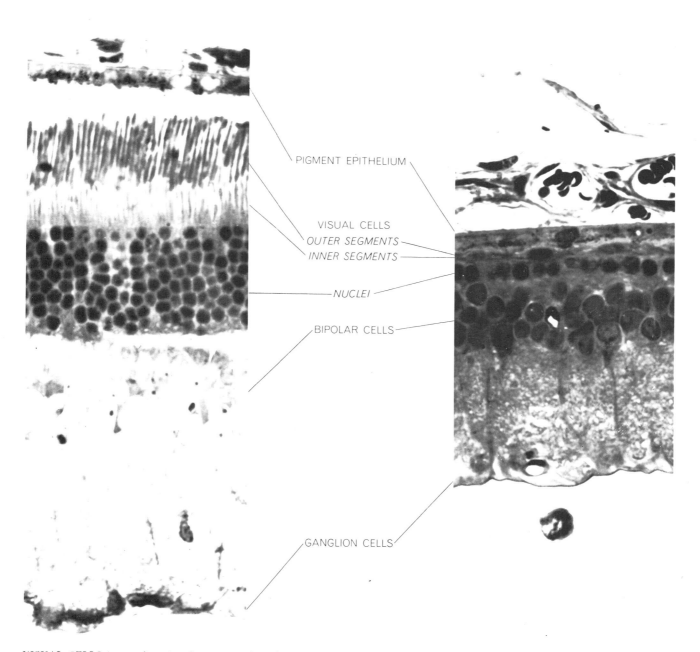

PIGMENT EPITHELIUM

VISUAL CELLS
OUTER SEGMENTS
INNER SEGMENTS

NUCLEI

BIPOLAR CELLS

GANGLION CELLS

VISUAL CELLS in a rat's retina degenerate when the animal is kept on a vitamin-A-deficient diet for a prolonged period of time. The retina shown in cross section at left is from a normal rat. The retina at right is from a totally blind rat that had been on a vitamin-A-deficient diet for 10 months. Its visual cells had been almost completely destroyed and could not have been regenerated later.

rithmic relation to the rhodopsin level, just as it does when the rhodopsin level is depleted by vitamin A deficiency. W. A. H. Rushton of the University of Cambridge has found that a similar relation between the logarithm of visual sensitivity and pigment concentration holds during the dark adaptation of the rods and cones in the human eye [see "Visual Pigments in Man," by W. A. H. Rushton; SCIENTIFIC AMERICAN Offprint 139].

What happens when the rat is kept on a vitamin-A-deficient diet beyond eight weeks? Investigation of the visual effects here runs into a serious difficulty: the problem of keeping the animal alive. Vitamin A is essential for maintaining epithelial tissues throughout the body, and a severe, prolonged deficiency will destroy the animal's health and eventually kill it. After eight to nine weeks on an A-deficient diet rats lose weight drastically, have difficulty breathing and become highly susceptible to infection; usually they do not survive beyond 10 to 12 weeks on such a diet. Fortunately we found a way to circumvent this difficulty. It was suggested by certain experiments reported by Moore in his superb book *Vitamin A*, published in 1957. Moore noted that two Dutch organic chemists, J. F. Arens and D. A. Van Dorp, had made the finding that a compound called vitamin A acid, which apparently was not converted into vitamin A in the tissues of rats, was highly effective in keeping the animals healthy. This looked like a possible answer to our problem. Perhaps we could maintain rats on the vitamin A acid and observe a decline in their vision because they lacked the vitamin itself.

This was, indeed, the way the experiment turned out. On a diet deficient in vitamin A but with a supplement of the acid, rats grew normally and remained generally healthy but became severely night-blind. After about two months on the deficient diet the visual cells in their retinas began to degenerate, and this breakdown was correlated with a loss of opsin from the retina. By about the tenth month the visual cells were almost completely destroyed. At that point the animals were totally blind; their eyes gave no ERG response to light at any intensity. Treatment with doses of vitamin A failed to restore sight to the animals. Visual cells, like other cells in the nervous system, cannot be regenerated once they are lost.

Before full destruction of the cells

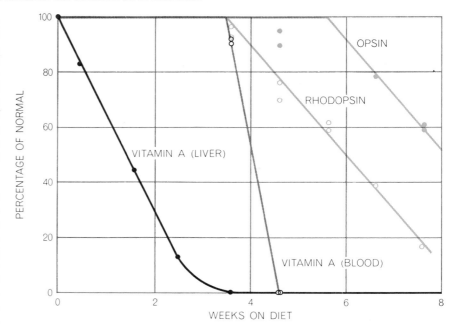

PROGRESSIVE DEPLETION of vitamin A, rhodopsin and opsin in the body of a rat fed a diet deficient in vitamin A is represented in this graph. The rat first drew on the store of vitamin A in its liver; in young rats this supply lasted about three to four weeks, and during that time the vitamin level in the animal's blood and the levels of rhodopsin and opsin in the retina remained normal. After the vitamin A reserve in the liver was used up the level of vitamin in the blood fell precipitously. Within a few days the level of rhodopsin in the eye also began to decline; two or three weeks later the opsin level began to fall.

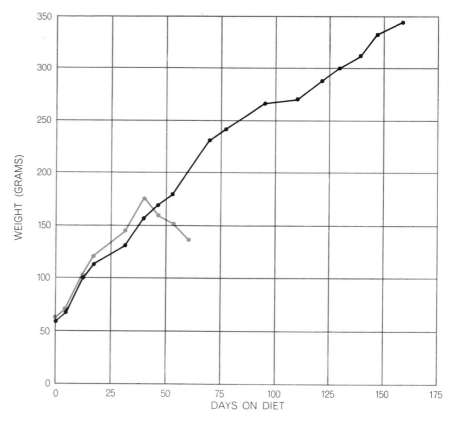

SUPPLEMENT OF VITAMIN A ACID given to a rat on a vitamin-A-deficient diet enabled the rat to grow normally and remain healthy while becoming severely night-blind (*black curve*). A rat on an identical diet without the vitamin A acid died (*colored curve*).

occurs, some recovery is possible. If a rat is given vitamin A at the six-month stage, for example, when the visual cells are only partly damaged, it can regenerate missing cell structures and regain a certain degree of night vision [*see illustration below*]. The ERG response of such an animal, however, is only about half the size of the normal ERG, which suggests that probably about half of the visual cells in the retina were lost beyond repair.

The breakdown of the A-deprived visual cell begins in the outer part of the cell, which contains the visual pigment. A study with the electron microscope that I carried out with Ian Gibbons at Harvard showed that the disks in the outer region, which give the cell its rod shape, swell and break apart into vesicles and tubules [*see upper illustration on page 209*]. The outer structure of the cell consequently loses its rod shape and becomes a spherical blob. Eventually it disappears altogether. If the animal is treated with vitamin A therapy while the inner part of the cell is still intact, it will regenerate the outer structure in a manner that is strikingly sim-

ilar to the growth of an embryonic visual cell during its normal development [*see lower illustration on page 209*]. Cilia-like structures grow out from the cell interior, slowly enlarge and become filled with membrane-covered disks that are characteristic of the outer part of the visual cell. The process of regeneration takes about two weeks, the same length of time the normal embryonic visual cell takes to differentiate its outer structure.

After the studies of nutritional night blindness, Richard L. Sidman of the Harvard Medical School and I decided to look into the hereditary forms of night blindness. In man the most common of these inherited disorders is the disease known as retinitis pigmentosa. The genetic disorder cannot be attributed to any shortcoming in the diet, yet it shows striking similarities to nutritional night blindness. The eye gradually loses visual sensitivity, the visual cells degenerate and eventually complete blindness results. The parallel to the progressive blinding that results from vitamin A deficiency is so close

that it seemed the inherited disorder might be due to a genetic defect in the metabolism of vitamin A or the synthesis of the visual pigments. Sidman and I undertook to investigate this hypothesis.

Our experimental subject, as before, was the rat. In this animal the inherited disease is carried by a recessive gene, and the disorder (called inherited retinal dystrophy) shows itself only in individuals that have received the defective gene from both parents. The disease begins to show its effects at about the 18th day of the young animal's life; tests by means of the ERG disclosed that its visual sensitivity gradually declines until by the age of 60 days the ERG response has disappeared. We reasoned that if the defect was related to vitamin A metabolism or rhodopsin synthesis, the decline in visual sensitivity should be paralleled by a decline in the rhodopsin content of the visual cells. To our great surprise we found that there was actually an *increase* of the rhodopsin level in the animals' eyes during the early stages of the disease. Rats with the inherited night blindness had much

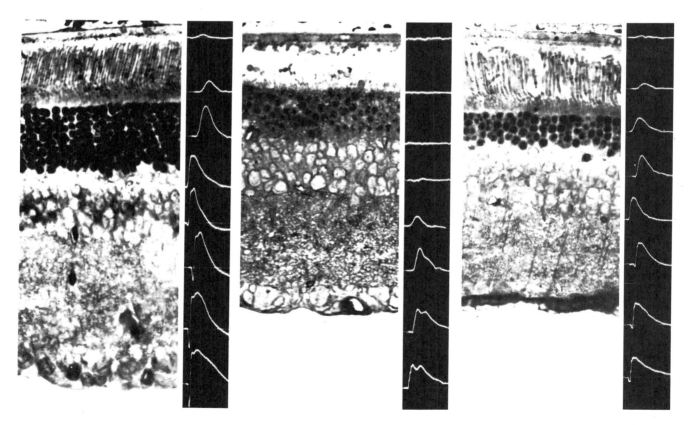

RECOVERY FROM NIGHT BLINDNESS is represented here in two different ways. The micrographs show cross sections of the retinas of a normal rat (*left*), a severely night-blind rat fed a vitamin-A-deficient diet with a vitamin-A-acid supplement for approximately six and a half months (*center*) and a partially recov-ered rat fed the identical vitamin-deficient, acid-supplemented diet for six and a half months and then given vitamin A for another 16 days (*right*). The accompanying ERG responses show that only about half of the normal ERG potential is recovered, which suggests that about half of the visual cells at right were lost.

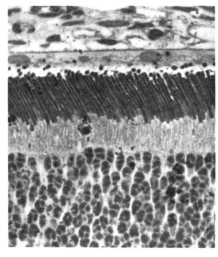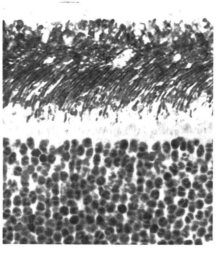

OVERDEVELOPED OUTER SEGMENTS of the visual cells in a 22-day-old rat with an inherited form of night blindness known as a retinal dystrophy (*right*) are almost twice as large as the outer segments in the eye of a normal 22-day-old rat (*left*). The inherited disease, which apparently arises from some failure of metabolic control, is also characterized by a decrease in ERG response and an increase in the rhodopsin content of the visual cells.

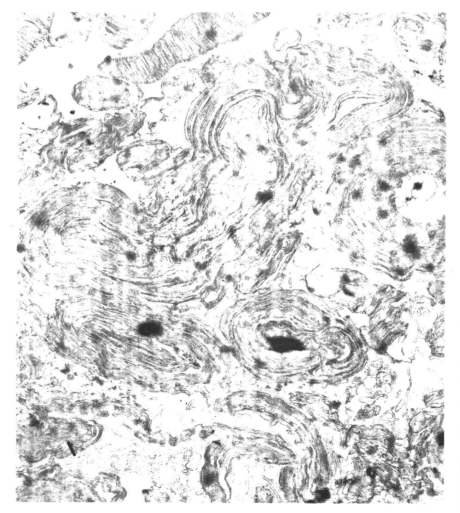

ENLARGEMENT of a small area near the surface of the outer segments of the visual cells in a rat with inherited night blindness reveals the spiral-shaped bodies that characterize this layer. The distorted structures appear to be formed by an overabundance of material produced by the diseased retina. An inner layer containing disks in the normal rodlike form (*not shown in this electron micrograph*) underlies the layer of distorted retinal structures.

more rhodopsin than is ever found in normal animals!

Along with the excess of rhodopsin there was a considerable overdevelopment of the outer structure of the visual cells. In a rat with the inherited disease this zone at 22 days of age, for example, was almost twice as large as it is in the normal eye [*see top illustration at left*]. It was divided into two layers: an inner layer containing structures in the normal rodlike form and an outer layer filled with spiral-shaped bodies instead of disks. It appeared that the diseased retinas produced an overabundance of material that formed distorted structures.

Evidently the inherited disease arises from some failure of metabolic control. In any event, the cause of the blindness is so unrelated to the simple case of vitamin A deficiency that we could see there was little hope of finding a simple cure in the form of therapeutic feeding. One of our observations, however, opened up an interesting new line of investigation. We found that when animals with the inherited disease were kept in darkness or dim light, the accumulation of rhodopsin in their visual cells was enhanced. This suggested that the progress of the disease might be influenced by the amount of light to which the eye was exposed.

To test this idea we reared groups of rats bearing the genetic defect under different conditions: one group was kept in darkness or in dim light 24 hours a day, the other was kept in the ordinary daily cycle of alternating daylight and darkness. The rats kept in darkness showed a much slower deterioration of visual sensitivity than those that were exposed to normal light. At the age of 60 days, when the latter animals had lost all sensitivity to light, the animals that had been kept in the dark still showed a considerable ERG response to light. In fact, they continued to give an ERG response up to the age of 120 days. Microscopic examination of the retinas also showed that the degeneration of the visual cells proceeded more slowly in the animals kept in darkness.

This finding led us to ask the question of what effect prolonged exposure to bright light might have on the normal eye. During World War II, Selig Hecht of Columbia University and his co-workers demonstrated that daily exposure to several hours of bright sunlight on the beach slightly impaired the dark-adapting abilities of human subjects. The effects were cumulative, and after several such sessions of exposure it took the subjects several days to recover their normal capacities for dark adaptation. In the laboratory where I am now working, at the Wilmer Ophthalmological Institute of the Johns Hopkins University School of Medicine, Robert Mittenthal and I recently conducted a similar experiment on rats. We found that albino rats with normal vision that were kept around the clock in light of ordinary brightness (two 75-watt fluorescent lamps) developed severe night blindness after only three to five days of exposure to this light. These animals, given long periods (up to three months) of dark adaptation afterward, recovered very little of their normal sensitivity to light, according to ERG measurements. The visual cells in their retinas were almost completely destroyed by several days of constant exposure to light. Werner K. Noell of the State University of New York at Buffalo School of Medicine has reported similar results in experiments he conducted with both pigmented and albino rats: short periods of exposure to bright light destroyed the visual cells in his animals also.

Probably the lighting to which human beings are customarily exposed rarely produces any permanent damage to normal eyes. It seems possible, however, that people with inherited night blindness (such as retinitis pigmentosa) or other retinal diseases may be more sensitive to excessive light. Thus the possibility exists—and it is well worth testing—that wearing dark glasses, particularly in bright light, may be helpful to such persons, much as dim light prolongs visual responses in rats with inherited blindness.

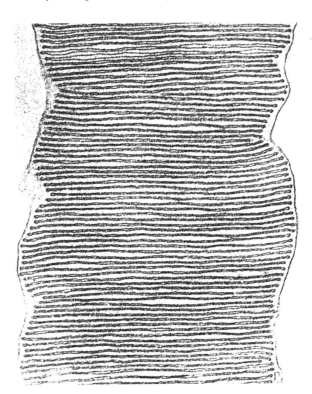
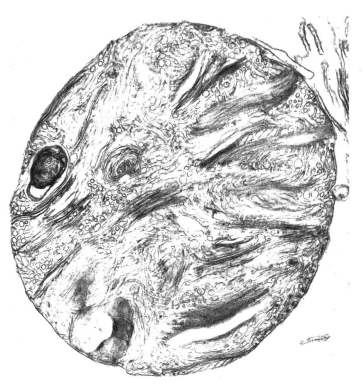

DEGENERATION of the outer segments of the rods in a rat's retina is the first stage in the breakdown of a vitamin-A-deprived visual cell. The electron micrograph at left shows the disks, enlarged about 45,000 diameters, in the outer region that give the normal cell its rod shape. In the electron micrograph of an A-deficient cell at right the disks, enlarged about 30,000 diameters, are swollen and broken apart into vesicles and tubules. The outer structure has consequently lost its rod shape and become a spherical blob.

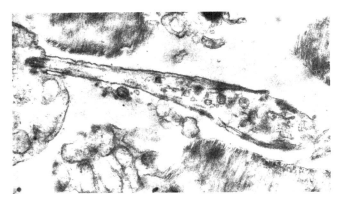
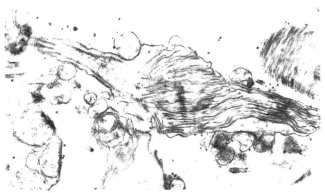

REGENERATION of the outer segments of a rod is possible if the animal is treated with vitamin A therapy while the internal part of the cell is still intact. The regeneration of the outer structure, which takes about two weeks, is strikingly similar to the growth of an embryonic visual cell during its normal development. Cilia-like structures grow out from the cell interior and form disks enclosed in membranes (electron micrograph at right). In both electron micrographs the outer segments of the rod are to the right.

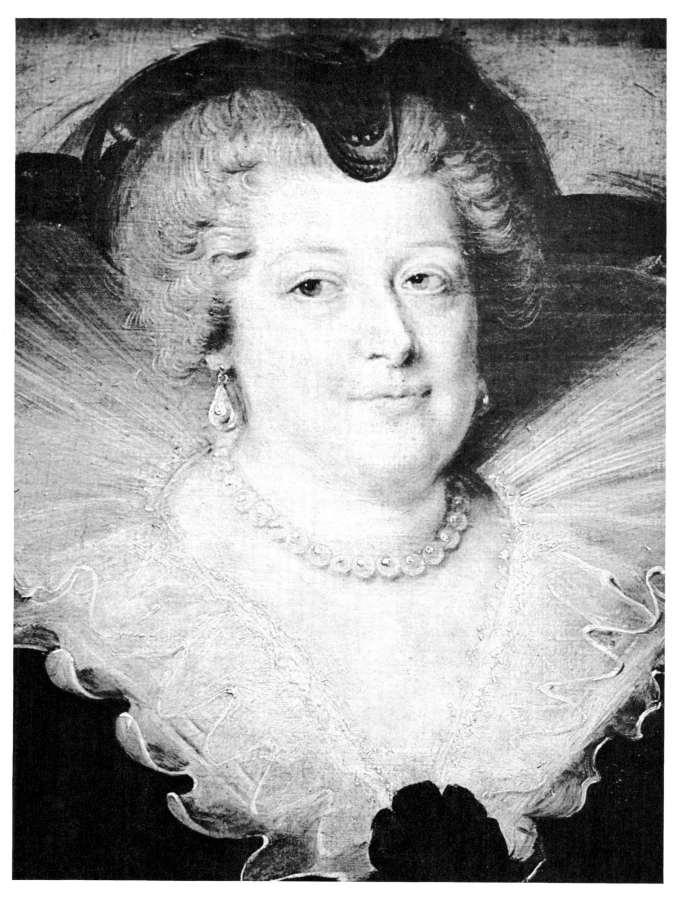

MODERATE GOITER is evident in this detail from a portrait of Maria de' Medici, wife of Henry IV of France. It was painted in 1625 by Rubens and now hangs in the Prado in Madrid. Moderate goiter was considered an adornment in the late Renaissance.

Endemic Goiter

by R. Bruce Gillie
June 1971

*The disorder has a long record because its principal
sign is so apparent. It is now a disease of the poor,
because an unbalanced diet often cannot correct for a
deficiency of iodine in the soil*

The "regular and rounded neck" with which Maria de' Medici was endowed by Rubens [*see illustration on page 212*] is a goiter, or compensatory hypertrophy of the thyroid gland. The thyroid is a pinkish pad of tissue wrapped partly around the trachea and esophagus; it is a ductless gland of vertebrates that secretes into the blood the hormones that regulate the rate of development and metabolism. Goiter is an unusually obvious manifestation of an endocrine disorder, and as such it has drawn attention, sometimes admiring and sometimes fearful, since man's earliest days.

There are many different causes of goiter: disease, developmental defects and environmental conditions. Endemic goiter, so designated because it affects a significant proportion of a given population, is almost always the result of a dietary deficiency of iodine, an essential substrate for the synthesis of the thyroid hormones thyroxine and tri-iodothyronine. Iodine-deficiency goiter is now easily prevented or cured by the ingestion of minute quantities of iodine, but over the centuries it has been one of the most persistent and ubiquitous diseases of mankind. As recently as 1960, 200 million people were still afflicted with it.

The secretion of thyroid hormones is a link in one of the exquisitely balanced feedback systems that regulate the internal environment of vertebrate organisms [see "The Thyroid Gland," by Lawson Wilkins; SCIENTIFIC AMERICAN, March, 1960]. Impulses from the nervous system cause the hypothalamus at the base of the brain to release a neurosecretion, the thyrotropin-releasing factor (TRF), into portal veins leading directly to the pituitary, the pea-sized master gland that regulates the activity of the thyroid and other endocrine glands. The thyrotropin-releasing factor stimulates the pituitary to secrete into the blood thyrotropin, or thyroid-stimulating hormone (TSH), which in turn causes the thyroid to synthesize and secrete its hormones. The system is self-regulating: an excess of thyroid hormones in the blood suppresses hypothalamus and pituitary activity and reduces the secretion of the thyroid-stimulating hormone; when the thyroid hormone concentration is too low, the pituitary responds by secreting more thyroid-stimulating hormone to restore the normal thyroid-hormone level [*see illustration on page 216*].

If the thyroid is healthy and there is enough iodide (ionic iodine) in the blood, the thyroid-stimulating hormone steps up the trapping of iodide by the thyroid and in other ways abets the synthesis of thyroxine and tri-iodothyronine within the follicles of the thyroid gland [*see illustration on page 218*]. In the absence of sufficient iodide thyroxine synthesis is inhibited; the flow of thyroid-stimulating hormone is unchecked and its effect is to increase the number and change the shape of the cells that form the follicles; in time the follicles become distended. This compensatory proliferation of cells and distention of the follicles, which constitute goiter, may restore thyroid-hormone production to a satisfactory level for normal life.

A Chinese document from about 3000 B.C. is the earliest known record of goiter. Remarkably, it not only described the symptoms but recommended an effective cure: the ingestion of seaweed and burned sponge, which contain large amounts of iodine. Speculating on the causes of what was apparently a common affliction, Chinese scholars listed poor quality of drinking water, mountainous terrain and emotional vicissitudes, all of which are indeed associated with a higher incidence of goiter. The Chinese even administered desiccated thyroid glands of deer as a treatment for goiter. (Nowadays extracts of beef, sheep or hog thyroid are given for hypothyroidism.)

The Ebers Papyrus of Egypt, dating from about 1500 B.C., described two possible treatments for goiter: surgical removal of the gland (which must have been a high-risk procedure if it was ever attempted) and the ingestion of salt (presumably containing iodine) from a particular site in lower Egypt.

Hippocrates blamed goiter on the drinking water in certain places. Juvenal, Vitruvius and Julius Caesar were impressed by the enlarged neck of residents of some alpine regions; Caesar, in fact, believed that the large neck was a national characteristic of the Gauls. The word "goiter," incidentally, is from the Latin *guttur*, or "throat."

Roman physicians noticed that even in a normal person the size of the thyroid may fluctuate somewhat during times of physiological stress such as puberty, menstruation and pregnancy. They noticed in particular that the physical and emotional circumstances surrounding the initial sexual activity of a bride brought about a slight swelling of her thyroid. The Romans thereupon originated the ritual of measuring the circumference of a bride's neck with a ceremonial ribbon before and after her first week of marriage. If the circumference increased, the marriage was considered consummated.

Because moderate goiter is quite compatible with normal life, causing no pain and often no impairment, it was not necessarily perceived as an affliction; if in some cultures it was considered a divine stigma, in others it was a mark of beauty. In Europe it was often attributed to some serious religious or social transgression—robbing the graves of saints, for example. In Germany during the Middle

Ages it was thought that the condition could be caused by strenuous work, including childbirth. That was the rationale for a now forgotten custom of tying a cord around the neck of a woman in labor. In India inhaling the odor of people dying of· malaria was said to cause goiter. At one time or another the condition has been blamed on indolence, drunkenness and debauchery. In 1867 a French student of the matter named J. Saint Leger listed more than 40 different possible causes then being cited—among them a lack of electricity in the atmosphere, incest, alcoholism and coitus interruptus.

Cures were not so easy to find. A procedure that appears to have persisted for many centuries was piercing the thy-roid gland with a red-hot needle. That presumably created an inflammation, and the resulting fibrosis may well have reduced the size of the gland. Actual surgery could not have been effective until the end of the 19th century. One reason is that the thyroid is so richly supplied with blood vessels that in the early days of surgery an incision would have resulted in excessive and uncontrollable bleeding. Even after the advent of satisfactory techniques surgical removal was dangerous at best before the discovery of the parathyroid glands. These tiny glands, nesting on the surface of the thyroid lobes, regulate the concentration of calcium in the blood, and their inadvertent removal along with the goitrous thyroid would threaten life.

The first attempt at an epidemiological survey was made at the request of Napoleon I, who was impressed (as Caesar had been) by the many cases he saw in the course of his alpine campaigns. Napoleon was also disturbed by the loss of potential recruits who had to be rejected because the military uniform would not fit their goitrous necks.

The basic mystery surrounding goiter, of course, was the function of the thyroid gland in health. The early anatomists were impressed by the gland's large blood supply and puzzled by the fact that (like the other endocrine glands) it had no duct and therefore, it seemed to them, could have no secretory function. In the Middle Ages some anat-

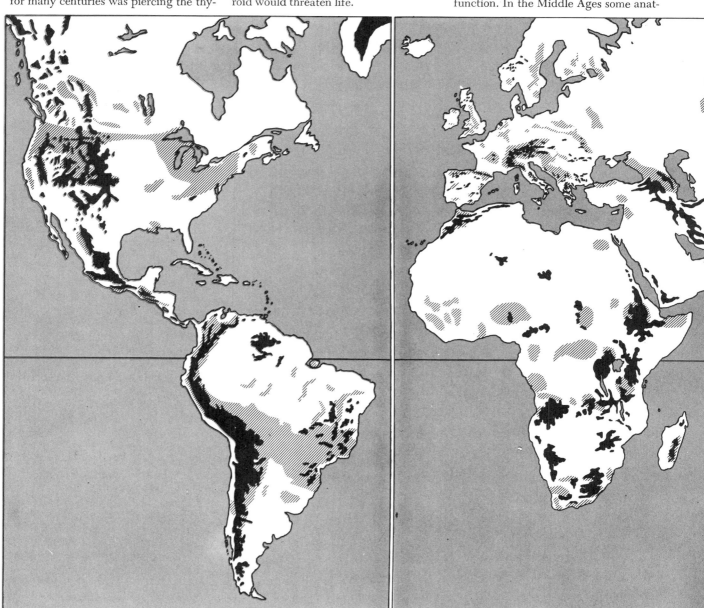

REGIONS OF ENDEMIC GOITER and the mountainous terrain with which it is often associated were mapped by the World Health Organization. Areas where iodine-deficiency goiter is endemic are indicated by the black hatching. Populations near seacoasts are sel-

omists thought of the thyroid as the seat of the soul. Others were more practical. The Italian anatomist Giulio Casserio wrote in 1600: "Kind nature has especially beautified the gentle female sex with many sorts of ornaments. And not the least among them is this one, that the empty spaces which exist around the larynx being filled up, they show to our eyes, to the great joy of our sight, a regular and rounded neck." Paintings by artists of the time, including Dürer and Rembrandt, suggest that Casserio's view was the general one, since madonnas and other female subjects are often depicted with moderately goitrous necks.

In 1656 the British anatomist Thomas Wharton wrote a complete description of the thyroid and also named it after the Greek word for a large oblong shield: *thyreos*. Wharton agreed with Casserio that it served to beautify the neck ("particularly in females to whom for this reason a larger gland has been assigned"), but he suggested that it might also keep the tracheal cartilages warm, since they were "rather of a chilly nature," and lubricate the larynx, rendering the voice more melodious. Other students believed the thyroid shunted blood away from the brain to protect it from sudden changes in blood pressure, or that it was a cushion to support and protect the structures of the larynx.

It was not until 1895, after surgeons had seen the effects of removal of the thyroid gland and after treatment with thyroid extract had been attempted, that Adolf Magnus-Levy of Germany demonstrated that the thyroid regulated the basal metabolic rate: the rate at which the cells of the body consume oxygen, which is to say the rate at which they convert nutrients into the energy of life. In the same year the German biochemist Eugen Baumann learned that the thyroid is particularly rich in iodine. It was a serendipitous discovery. Baumann was trying to analyze the protein content of thyroid tissue, and his usual procedure was to precipitate the protein from an extract with sulfuric acid. One day, reaching for the sulfuric acid on a shelf above his workbench, he picked up a bottle of nitric acid instead, and before he had realized his mistake he had added some of its contents to the extract. To his astonishment the characteristic brownish-purple fumes of iodine gas swirled up from the preparation. Baumann went on to describe the role of iodine in thyroid physiology. In 1914 Edward C. Kendall of the Mayo Foundation first crystallized some thyroid hormone. It was a large and difficult task: the 37 grams of crystallized hormone that Kendall subsequently obtained were derived from three and a quarter tons of pig thyroid! Finally in 1927 Charles Robert Harington of the University College Hospital Medical School in London and George Barger of the University of Edinburgh established the definitive structure of thyroxine, confirming Baumann's observations. Well before that time Baumann's work had led on the one hand to the understanding that endemic goiter was the result of environmental iodine deficiency and on the other to simple and effective iodine therapy.

As investigators looked into the ecology of goitrous populations they first found a correlation between goiter and the accessibility of a population to the sea and thus to a seafood diet rich in iodine. A map compiled by the World Health Organization makes it clear that it is in inland areas, particularly mountainous ones, that goiter may be endemic [*see illustration on these two pages*]. The Alps, the Pyrenees, the Himalayas and the Andes are strikingly goitrous. So are inland plains regions in Italy, in the Congo and in the Great Lakes basin of North America.

The geography of goiter is not simple, however. Many inland and mountainous regions do not support goitrous populations, and there are coastal areas that unpredictably have goitrous populations. A factor that is more closely correlated with the incidence of endemic goiter than mere distance from the ocean is the

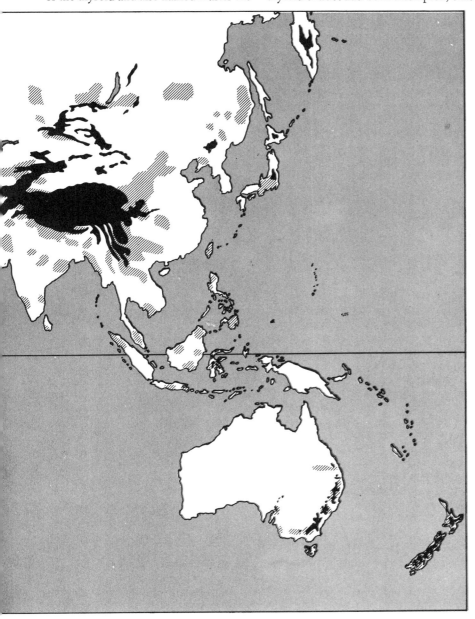

dom affected because of the iodine content of seafood. Not all inland areas are equally affected; the geology and remoteness of mountainous regions (*color*) make them most susceptible.

iodine content of the soil. As long as the soil content of iodine is adequate, enough iodine (about 100 to 200 micrograms per person per day) will be ingested in locally grown produce to prevent the onset of goiter. Although the iodine content of soils is generally higher in coastal regions than it is inland, soil content is determined by more complex factors than distance from the ocean alone. The most seriously depleted soils are in areas that were subjected to the most intense glaciation. Such glaciation did two things. By crushing virgin igneous rocks that had never been exposed to atmospheric iodine, it left behind vast amounts of new, iodine-poor topsoil, and

it leached the soluble iodine salts out of the original soil.

Leaching may also make soils along the shores of rivers that periodically overflow their banks deficient in iodine. An interesting example of this process was noted in a study of two villages on opposite banks of the Congo River in an area where heavy rain and periodic flooding had reduced the iodine content of the soil. On one bank the village population was 80 percent goitrous; on the alluvial soil of the opposite bank the population was hardly goitrous at all. Iodine being leached by the heavy rain out of land upstream was being redeposited in the alluvial soil around the second vil-

lage, making the iodine concentration there just sufficient to prevent goiter.

The steady replenishment of iodine in terrestrial soils from atmospheric iodine tends in time to reverse the effects of glaciation. The degree of replenishment is complexly affected by the distance of an area from the ocean, the prevailing wind conditions and the amount of iodine in the precipitation. In addition some areas of the world have natural terrestrial iodine deposits that may also help to determine the iodine content of the local soil. In other words, the ecology of a human society as well as its principal staple diet is a major factor in the etiology of endemic goiter.

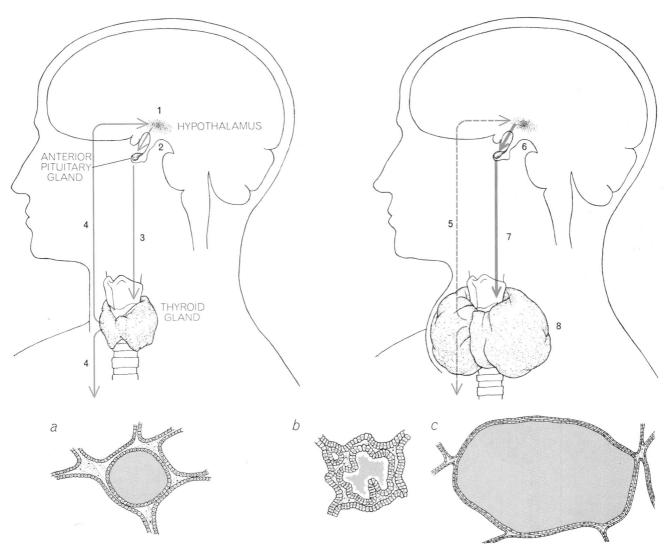

NEGATIVE-FEEDBACK SYSTEM controlling production of thyroid hormones begins with the neurosecretion from the hypothalamus (1) of thyrotropin-releasing factor (TRF), which goes directly to the pituitary (2) and causes it to release thyrotropin, or thyroid-stimulating hormone (TSH), into the bloodstream (3). In the thyroid gland TSH acts to bring about the synthesis and secretion into the circulation of the thyroid hormones thyroxine and tri-iodothyronine (4); the amount of thyroid hormones reaching the hypothalamus in turn controls the secretion of TSH, completing the negative-feedback loop. In the absence of iodine, an essential substrate for thyroid hormones, not enough hormone is produced (5) to "turn off" the system; excessive TRF (6) and TSH (7) are secreted, stimulating the iodine-depleted thyroid tissue to grow (8). A normal thyroid follicle, in which hormones are synthesized and stored, consists of an envelope of cells containing a colloid, thyroglobulin (a). In the absence of iodine TSH causes the cells to proliferate and become more columnar (b) and then to produce more colloid, so that the follicles become distended (c), forming a goiter.

Beginning in 1907 the extensive investigations of David Marine and O. P. Kimball of the Western Reserve University School of Medicine with laboratory animals provided the first direct experimental evidence that endemic thyroid hypertrophy is caused by iodine deficiency. These workers subsequently carried out the first large-scale program of goiter prophylaxis in Akron, Ohio. The study, completed in 1920, involved 4,500 schoolgirls between the fifth and the 12th grade. Half of them received two grams of iodized salt twice a year and the other half served as untreated controls. At the end of two and a half years 65.4 percent of the treated group showed regression of goiter and only five treated girls evinced thyroid enlargement. Meanwhile only 13.8 percent of the girls in the untreated group showed a regression of goiter and 495 untreated girls had developed thyroid hypertrophy. The study was a dramatic demonstration of the efficacy of iodine in the treatment and the prevention of simple goiter.

When these findings were published, many individuals and groups of health enthusiasts took to consuming iodine to the extent of a fetishism. Some people even hung around their neck little bottles of iodine from which they would occasionally take a swig. Iodine became the magic ingredient in the nostrums of certain charlatans. To everyone's surprise, rather than preventing goiter, iodine sometimes served to stimulate it. This apparently paradoxical effect of iodine on the etiology of goiter was later explained by Jan Wolff and Israel L. Chaikoff of the School of Medicine of the University of California at Berkeley, who found that very high iodine concentrations in the blood plasma inhibit the biosynthesis and secretion of thyroid hormone. This aspect of thyroid physiology, together with increasing reports of severe iodine toxicity and the fear that iodine might lead to toxic hyperthyroidism, elicited strenuous opposition to the iodization of table salt by many medical experts, lay people and politicians. The political and ethical controversy over the incorporation of iodine into table salt was even more intense than the present-day controversy over the fluoridation of water. It was not until the mid-1920's that iodine prophylaxis was generally accepted.

Although the idea that some positive agent in food or drink was responsible for goiter had antedated the discovery of iodine deficiency as a cause, it was not until 1941 that a goitrogenic substance was identified. Curt P. Rich-

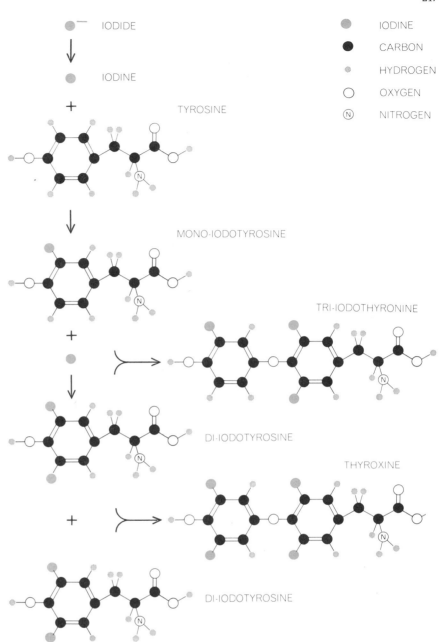

BIOSYNTHESIS of the thyroid hormones depends on the presence of ionic iodine, primarily as sodium iodide. The iodide is oxidized to elemental iodine and combines with the amino acid tyrosine to form mono-iodotyrosine and di-iodotyrosine. Two molecules of di-iodotyrosine may combine to form thyroxine, or mono- and di-iodotyrosine molecules may combine to form tri-iodothyronine. (Only hormone products are shown, not by-products.)

ter and Kathryn H. Clisby of the Johns Hopkins University School of Medicine were investigating the effects of certain rat poisons. When they fed laboratory rats the drug thiourea, they observed to their surprise that the rats survived but their thyroid began growing and soon became goitrous. At about the same time Julia B. and Cosmo G. MacKenzie, in another laboratory at Johns Hopkins, were studying the effect of a new sulfonamide drug on the bacterial flora of the rat intestine. They observed the same

phenomenon: the thyroid of their treated rats became hypertrophic, as if the animals had been maintained for several weeks on an iodine-deficient diet. The drugs were apparently preventing the proper utilization of iodine, which was present in normal concentrations in the animals' food and water. Since that time many additional antithyroid compounds have been discovered.

Theoretically these drugs could act by any of three different mechanisms. First, they could operate at the intestinal level to chelate, or sequester, iodine and so prevent its normal absorption into the bloodstream. Second, they could act at the surface of the thyroid epithelial cell to inhibit the selective absorption of iodine from the blood passing through the gland. (This trapping of iodine ions is an amazingly efficient process: the thyroid concentrates the ions to a level several hundred times higher than their concentration in the plasma.) Third, the goitrogenic compounds could gain admission to the cells of the thyroid and there in-

hibit the biosynthetic pathway at any of several crucial steps or prevent the release of thyroxine from its storage form in the follicles. It appears that the last two mechanisms are the significant ones. Thiocyanate and perchlorate inhibit the active transport processes of the iodide trap, thiouracil blocks the oxidation of iodide to iodine by certain peroxidase enzymes, and sulfonamides interfere with the incorporation of tyrosine [*see illustration below*].

Soon after the discovery of these goi-

trogenic compounds it was found that goiter endemic to some areas was a result of similar, naturally occurring compounds in local foods. Soybeans and members of the genus *Brassica*, which includes Brussels sprouts, cabbages, turnips and other vegetables, are among the foodstuffs containing significant amounts of goitrogenic compounds. In a nutritionally varied diet such foods do no harm, but they are a more serious matter in societies that survive on less varied diets.

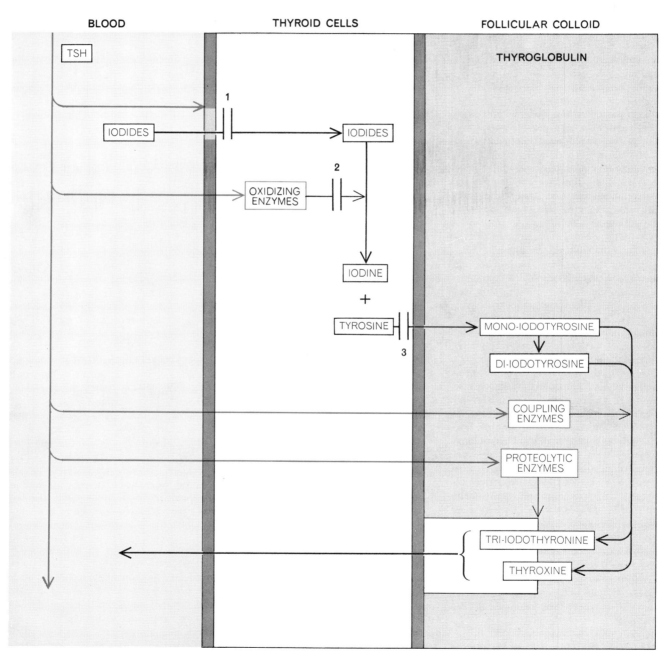

THYROID ACTIVITY is diagrammed schematically. Iodide trapped by thyroid-follicle cells is converted by oxidizing enzymes in the cells into iodine, which combines with tyrosine to form the thyroid hormones. The hormones are stored attached to thyroglobulin; on demand they are freed by proteolytic enzymes and pass in-to the blood. TSH stimulates hormone production by acting to abet iodide-trapping and the activity of three sets of enzymes. Goitrogenic substances interfere with hormone production. Thiocyanates and perchlorates block the iodide trap (*1*), thiouracil the oxidizing enzymes (*2*), sulfonamides the combination with tyrosine (*3*).

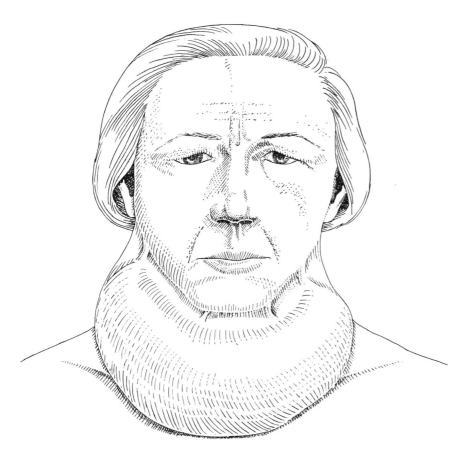

LARGE GOITER is seen frequently in regions where iodine-deficiency goiter is endemic. The drawing is based on a photograph made in the Alps near Innsbruck in Austria. Goiters have been reported that weighed four or five pounds, sometimes hanging below the chest.

The effect of the *Brassica* goitrogen was demonstrated not long ago in Tasmania, off the coast of southern Australia. The island was an area of endemic goiter, and so in 1949 a program was instituted to supply iodine-containing tablets to schoolchildren up to 16 years old. Five years later a survey revealed that the incidence of goiter in these children had not decreased; indeed, it had increased. The investigators verified their data and reevaluated their methods, and still they found that goiter had increased. F. W. A. Clements and J. W. Wishart, who had been instrumental in setting up the program, thereupon proposed that something other than iodine deficiency might be promoting goiter in these schoolchildren. As it happened, in 1950 the Australian government had begun a free-milk program in the schools. The increased demand for milk forced local dairies to keep their cows at pasture during seasons when grass was not available. As a consequence the cows were eating marrow-stem kale, which is more frost-resistant than grass and grows well all year. Marrow-stem kale is a member of the genus *Brassica* and contains a large amount of the goitrogenic compound. Further study revealed that this compound, present unaltered in the milk, was blocking utilization of the iodine being supplied in the tablets.

Clearly there are dangers inherent in administering to patients drug preparations that contain significant amounts of potentially goitrogenic compounds or elemental iodine. Although it is not common in this country, iatrogenic goiter—goiter caused by medical treatment—is becoming a more significant factor. Sulfonamides prescribed for urinary-tract infections, thiouracil drugs given routinely for the relief of hyperthyroidism and many iodine-containing compounds administered as expectorants in the treatment of asthma are potentially goitrogenic. The unborn infants of pregnant mothers who take these drugs have in some instances been killed *in utero* by goiters that develop when the drugs diffuse across the placenta and enter the fetal circulation. Because these drugs are concentrated in the lactating breast they may also induce goiter in a nursing infant. The most serious effect of these drugs in pregnancy is that they decrease the availability of maternal thyroxine to the early fetus, and thyroxine is of fundamental importance in the physical and mental development of the baby.

Several epidemiological surveys have indicated that goiter can arise spontaneously in a society, persist for a short time and then regress, all without any apparent change in the food or living habits of the people. The possibility of an infectious origin of goiter has been proposed to explain such epidemics, but no instance of this has been proved. It does seem possible that a strain of iodine-trapping bacteria could become resident among the normal flora of the intestine and decrease the availability of dietary iodine for absorption.

There is at least one documented case of goiter related to bacteria, although in a different way. While studying goitrous populations in the Himalayas in 1906, Robert McCarrison visited several neighboring villages in the valley of the Gilgit River. He was immediately impressed by the fact that whereas the village that was farthest upstream showed a low incidence of goiter (12 percent), as he moved downstream the incidence increased in each village, until in the lowest village more than 45 percent of the population had goiter. An isolated village that was near the river but whose residents did not drink river water did not have goiter. McCarrison undertook a controlled experiment with 30 volunteers divided into two groups. One group drank the muddy river water after boiling it and the other (including McCarrison himself) drank unboiled river water. Within a month most of the people in McCarrison's group began to develop goiter; those in the other group did not. He concluded from the experiment that bacteria were to blame for the goiter. Poor sanitation meant that the waste material from the villages went into the river, which became more contaminated as it flowed past each village, increasing the dose of bacteria in the drinking water of villagers in proportion to their distance downriver. It has since been shown that some strains of *Escherichia coli*, a bacterium normally found in fecal material, can produce thiouracil.

There is a vicious circle aspect to endemic goiter. Poor societies with an unvaried diet are likely to be the most susceptible to goiter and the most vulnerable to its biological, social and economic consequences. Where iodine-deficiency goiter is endemic in a human population domestic animals will probably be hypothyroid too. Goitrous sheep often produce less wool; goiter in cattle causes sterility, poor milk production and sickly calves; horses do less work;

hens with decreased thyroid activity produce eggs with insufficient calcium in the shell, leading to egg breakage and higher chick mortality. A poor society can scarcely afford to have these serious handicaps afflict the animals on which its survival may depend.

Long-standing endemic goiter has had particularly serious consequences in some remote communities, such as alpine valleys, where inbred populations have persisted for many generations in an iodine-deficient environment. Familial goitrous hypothyroidism can lead to a high incidence of individuals with the severe developmental defects of cretinism. Cretins manifest varying degrees of idiocy and are also physically dwarfed and often malformed. The mental retardation is believed to result from a deficiency of thyroxine during the first three months of pregnancy, when it must be supplied by the mother; the physical anomalies are probably due to a deficiency of the baby's own thyroxine during maturation.

The role of mountainous topography and isolation in cretinism is evident. There are many goitrous regions that do not show a high incidence of cretinism; the "goiter belt" in the Great Lakes region is an example. Presumably population mobility through this channel of westward migration supplied enough biological and social diversity so that cretinism did not develop.

The cretin is only the most extreme example of the consequences of decreased availability of thyroxine during the developmental stages of life. Because all the residents of a community affected by endemic goiter are potentially exposed to a suboptimal supply of thyroxine during their development, there may be serious but subtle effects on the quality of the society at large. Motivation, spontaneity, creativity and native intelligence may be diminished, and the resulting social stagnation may lead to further inbreeding.

Medical science and public health will eventually eliminate iodine-deficiency goiter as an endemic affliction. One must hope that this age-old and benign disorder will not be replaced by a different, nuclear-era thyroid dysfunction resulting from the ingestion of large amounts of radioactive iodine isotopes from nuclear fallout. The iodine is concentrated in the thyroid gland, where the radioactivity may damage cells irreversibly. The study of endemic goiter demonstrates the seriousness of this potential hazard and the effects it might have on the course of human evolution.

23

Atherosclerosis

australia

by David M. Spain
August 1966

The artery disease that is responsible for most heart attacks is on the rise in the U.S. Its prevalence seems to be related to diet, so there is hope that the epidemic can be controlled

The incidence of heart attacks among adult white males in relatively affluent occupations in the U.S. has reached epidemic proportions. From such attacks (coronary artery occlusions) the overall U.S. death rate is now 500,000 a year, and 200,000 more die from strokes. At least 5 percent of the adult males in the nation show signs of some form of heart disorder. The basic disease responsible for most of these disorders and deaths is atherosclerosis. There is every indication that the prevalence of atherosclerosis in the U.S. is steadily increasing.

It used to be thought that atherosclerosis was a disease of old age and that its rising incidence might be due simply to the lengthening of the average life-span by the control of infectious diseases. This idea has now been refuted by a number of studies. My colleagues and I have made a comparative examination in Westchester County, New York, of two samples of the population taken 20 years apart. The samples were comparable in that both groups covered the same age range (from 20 to 60), had records of good health before a fatal episode, had died of sudden causes not connected with heart disease and had been autopsied after death, so that the extent of atherosclerosis in their coronary arteries and aortas was known. The first sample consisted of people who had died of acute infections in the period between 1931 and 1935; the second was made up of people who had been killed in automobile or industrial accidents between 1951 and 1955. We found that the second group, representing a period 20 years later than the first, had a significantly greater amount of atherosclerosis. This was true for every age level: the young people in the second group had more atherosclero-

sis than the young ones in the first. A similar autopsy study in Sweden yielded the same finding; the degree of coronary atherosclerosis in a population sample in 1958 was greater than in a sample from 1934.

Laboratory studies of experimental animals and postmortem examinations of human infants have established that the development of atherosclerosis often begins shortly after birth. Fatty streaks signaling the beginning of atheromas have been found in many human aortas

as early as the age of three. In a group of U.S. soldiers killed in the Korean war whose average age was only 23, examination showed that most had extensive formations of atherosclerotic "plaques" in their arteries. In our study of accident victims in Westchester County we found that many 35-year-old males who had shown no indication of heart disease nevertheless had their coronary arteries so thickened by atherosclerosis that the channels were narrowed by 50 percent. It has become

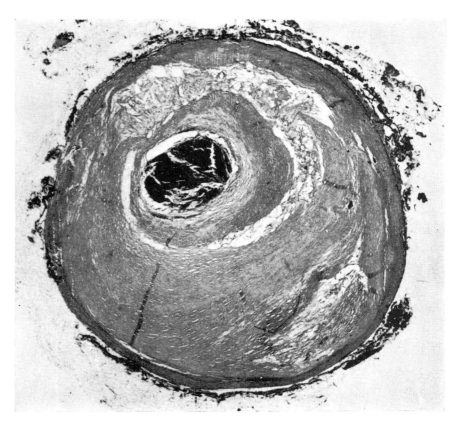

CRITICAL STAGE in the process under way in illustration at bottom of page 36 occurs when the atherosclerosis has advanced and blood clot almost fills the constricted channel.

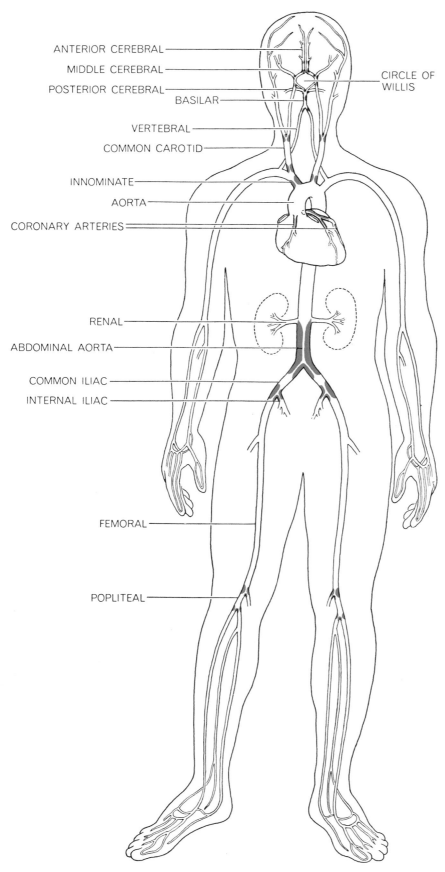

ANTERIOR CEREBRAL
MIDDLE CEREBRAL
POSTERIOR CEREBRAL
BASILAR
VERTEBRAL
COMMON CAROTID
INNOMINATE
AORTA
CORONARY ARTERIES
RENAL
ABDOMINAL AORTA
COMMON ILIAC
INTERNAL ILIAC
FEMORAL
POPLITEAL
CIRCLE OF WILLIS

FAVORED SITES of atherosclerosis are indicated in color in this diagram of the major arteries. There is a tendency for the disease to begin at points where an artery branches.

quite clear that atherosclerosis is a widespread disease of the young as well as the old.

The Nature of the Disease

Atherosclerosis appears to be at least as old as the civilization of mankind. The aortas of some Egyptian mummies that were entombed more than 3,500 years ago show the typical lesions of atherosclerosis. The modern name of the disease is derived from two Greek words: *athere,* meaning "porridge" or "mush," and *skleros,* meaning "hard." This apparently contradictory combination describes the fact that the lesion begins as a soft deposit and hardens as it ages. Materials that have been deposited from the bloodstream in the inner lining of the major arteries penetrate the arterial wall; they form plaques that gradually grow and thicken the wall, thus narrowing the blood channel. Eventually the thickening may close the channel entirely, or pieces of the plaques may break off and travel with the bloodstream until they are stopped in a smaller artery and thereby plug it. When the blockage occurs in the coronary artery, it produces a heart attack by cutting off the blood supply to the heart muscles; in the brain it produces a cerebral stroke; in the lower extremities it can lead to gangrene.

The circulatory system of the human body is a pipeline through which blood is pumped at a rate amounting to 4,300 gallons a day through 60,000 miles of pipe reaching every cell of the body. We might liken the atherosclerotic deposits in an artery to the rustlike encrustations that may form on the inner wall of a pipe. The living system, however, is vastly more complex than any ordinary pipeline. The fluid coursing through the arterial pipes contains living cells and a mixture of liquids that are continually changing in chemistry and physical characteristics. The flow is pulsatile, varying from moment to moment in velocity, volume and pressure. The living walls of the arteries themselves partake of the same changeability. They undergo a continual metabolism, conduct exchanges with the blood and the fluids bathing them externally and are subjected to various kinds of stress. In this dynamic system, subject to so many internal and external influences, unraveling the process that is responsible for atherosclerosis is akin to trying to solve a many-body problem in astronomy without knowing how many bodies are involved.

The atherosclerotic lesion is a complicated affair. When fully developed, it is composed of a considerable variety of structures and substances: blood and blood products, fibrous scar tissue, calcium deposits, complex carbohydrates, cholesterol (a fatlike, waxy substance normally present in the blood and body tissues), fatty acids and lipoproteins. Apparently the fatty acids and cholesterol are the crucial substances responsible for the development of the lesion, because they provoke inflammation and scarring of the arterial-wall tissue.

How does the process leading to atherosclerosis begin? Examination with electron and light microscopes shows that the first visible event is the invasion of the inner lining of the artery by fatty substances. These substances appear mainly in smooth muscle cells and foam cells found within the lining. In the spaces between the cells small amounts of cholesterol can be detected. Very fine fibers of a material that behaves like fibrin (a natural product of blood coagulation) also show up, both within the lining and on its surface. At this early stage the forerunner of the atherosclerotic lesion can be recognized in the form of fatty streaks, which when stained with a suitable dye are visible to the unaided eye as red streaks or spots on the lining surface.

Fats in the Arterial Wall

To solve the mystery of the origin of atherosclerosis one of the first questions we must answer is: How are the fatty materials deposited in the arterial wall? There are several current hypotheses. The one most widely accepted is that the fatty substances are transported into the wall by plasma, the blood fluid, and are trapped within the wall. It is believed that the plasma itself, under the force of the blood pressure, can leak all the way through the wall of the artery in small amounts, which then return to the bloodstream by way of the lymph-circulating system. The large lipoprotein molecules or complexes, on the other hand, cannot filter through the wall so easily; consequently they may tend to pile up within the wall, particularly if the plasma carries an excessive quantity of them.

The known structure of the walls of the major arteries gives support to this view. The wall of an artery consists essentially of three layers: outer, middle and inner. The outer layer and part of the middle one are nourished by a system of fine blood vessels (called vasa

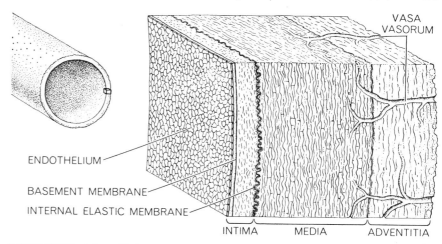

STRUCTURE of the wall of an "elastic" artery, the type usually involved in atherosclerosis, is shown in a somewhat schematic diagram. There is an inner lining of endothelial cells. The wall itself has three ill-defined layers of elastic tissue and muscle: the intima, media and adventitia. The vasa vasorum are small blood vessels that supply the artery wall.

vasorum) that come from the outer coat and go inward only as far as the middle layer. The nourishment of the inner portion of the arterial wall is taken care of by nutrients filtering into it from the bloodstream in the channel of the artery. Between the inner and the middle layer of the wall there is a curtain of elastic tissue. This tends to impede the flow of fluids through the wall. Hence it may act to trap substances that follow the gradient of flow, which in an artery is from inside to outside. Significantly, atherosclerosis rarely develops in veins, where the flow gradient is from outside to inside.

That lipids and other large molecules from the bloodstream can penetrate the arterial walls has been demonstrated conclusively by experiments with radioactively labeled cholesterol and other materials. These labeled materials usually turn up in highest concentration in areas in the walls that are already atherosclerotic. It has also been learned that in the early lesions of atherosclerosis the pattern of lipids present in the lesion is strikingly similar to the pattern in the blood.

Are there special conditions that favor the infiltration of lipids into the arterial wall? At least one interesting finding points in that direction. It was found that the administration of high doses of vitamin C to experimental animals inhibited the accumulation of lipids in the walls of their arteries. Conversely, when animals were fed a diet on which they developed a vitamin C deficiency, the inner lining of their arteries became more permeable: its cells were more widely spaced.

Abel Lazzarini-Robertson, Jr., of the Cleveland Clinic, who has studied the behavior of arterial-lining cells in tissue cultures, suggests that there may be a self-feeding process that generates expansion of an atherosclerotic lesion. Some of these cells, he says, respond to an excess of lipids by requiring more oxygen. When they fail to obtain enough oxygen to satisfy this increased need, the cell membranes become more permeable to lipids. Thus a vicious circle is set up: the more lipid enters the cells, the easier it is for additional lipid to invade them.

As I have mentioned, hypotheses other than the lipid-infiltration theory have been proposed to account for the

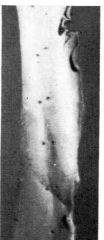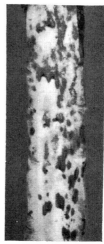

INNER SURFACES of the aortas of two rabbits were stained to visualize fatty material. Both animals had been fed cholesterol but one had also received estrogen, a female hormone. The aorta of that rabbit (left) was found to be almost free of atherosclerosis, whereas the other one was heavily affected.

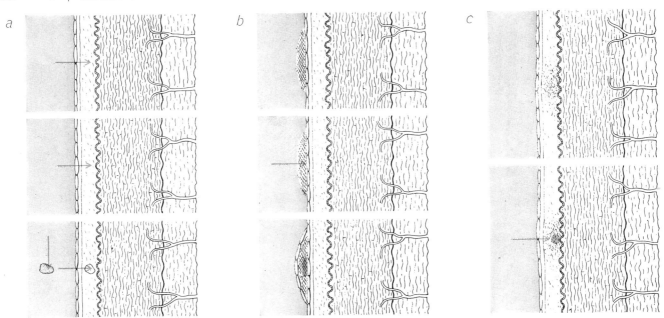

ENTRY OF FATTY MATERIAL into the arterial wall is the first sign of atherosclerosis. One theory holds that fat molecules infiltrate from the bloodstream (a) either by moving between endothelial cells or through them or by being carried between them by large cells called foam cells. Another theory is that the first event is the formation of a blood clot that is subsequently invaded by fats (b). A third idea is that an injury alters the wall's cementing substance so that fats can invade from the blood or be synthesized (c).

origin of atherosclerosis. One of these suggests that a disturbance of the blood-clotting mechanism, in combination with an injury to the inner wall of the artery, may result in the formation of a fibrin clot on the surface of the wall. Fatty substances from the bloodstream may then accumulate in the clot, particularly if there is a considerable amount of such substances in the blood, and this focus may generate the atherosclerotic lesion. Another hypothesis proposes that some alteration of the cementing substances (mucopolysaccharides) in the artery wall that occurs after an injury to the wall may open the way to local in-

vasions or synthesis of lipids. It may be, indeed, that there is some truth in all the hypotheses. There is reason to believe that atherosclerosis can originate in a number of different ways.

Once the process has started it develops a kind of life of its own. Enzymes within the artery wall break down the fatty complexes, liberating cholesterol and fatty acids. These act as noxious foreign agents and excite inflammation of the wall tissues. Scar tissue develops. Fragile capillaries growing into this tissue tend to rupture and thus lead to more inflammation. The artery lining may ulcerate, and blood

from the bloodstream clots around these breaks. Gradually the atherosclerotic lesion expands in size, and as the scar tissue and calcium deposits accumulate, the lesion stiffens and renders the arterial wall brittle and weak.

Atherosclerosis may occur simultaneously in many of the body's major arteries. There are, however, certain favored sites. Much depends on the shape and position of the vessel. For example, the coronary arteries, which receive the full impact of the pulsatile blood pressure against their walls during systole (the heart's pumping cycle), have a high tendency to develop atherosclerotic le-

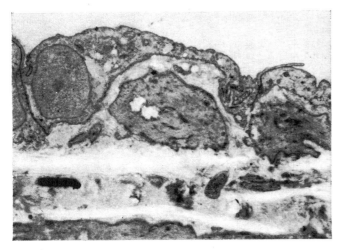

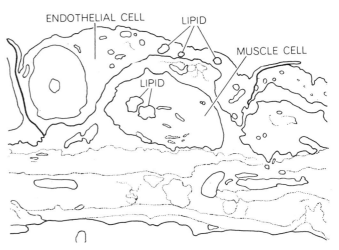

SECTION OF AORTA of a rabbit that had been fed cholesterol for two weeks is enlarged 5,000 diameters in an electron micrograph (left) made by Frank Parker and George F. Odland of the University of Washington School of Medicine. As the drawing (second from left) shows, an endothelial cell of the artery lining contains vacuoles filled with lipid, or fatty material. A single smooth-muscle

sions; on the other hand, the renal arteries, which branch from the aorta at right angles and have a low resistance to blood flow and therefore do not feel the pulsatile impact nearly as much, are relatively free of the disease. The vessels that are most often, and most critically, attacked are the coronary arteries, the aorta, the arteries in the neck and brain and the iliac and femoral arteries supplying blood to the lower extremities.

When thrombosis (formation of a blood clot) occurs in a narrowed coronary artery, the resulting partial or complete shutoff of blood supply to a portion of the heart muscle may have various effects: angina pectoris (pain in the chest), a myocardial infarct (destruction of part of the heart wall), irregularity or weakening of the heartbeat or sudden death due to complete failure of the heart. If the arteries to the brain become clogged, the result is a massive stroke causing paralysis or death. "Small" strokes, causing only slight or temporary paralysis of particular functions, may arise from fragments that break off from the atherosclerotic lesion and flow on to clog small vessels in the brain, thereby killing small areas of brain tissue. When atherosclerosis and clots clog a major artery to the legs, the result may be severe pain in these extremities and sometimes so much destruction of tissue that the gangrenous limb must be amputated.

In the aorta the lower section, passing through the abdomen, is particularly subject to atherosclerosis. The disease may so weaken the arterial wall that a portion of it balloons out, forming an aneurysm. Aneurysms of the aorta may press on the important organs in this area, interfering with their functions and causing pain. The rupture of one of these aneurysms usually produces massive hemorrhage and death.

One of the peculiarities of atherosclerosis is that even among the susceptible arteries it often selects particular ones for attack. For example, an individual may have severe atherosclerosis in his coronary arteries but very little of the disease in the cerebral arteries, or extensive lesions in the aorta with very little involvement of the coronary arteries. This form of selectivity is reflected in the disease rates of certain peoples. In Japan, for instance, strokes are common but heart attacks are relatively rare.

The Role of Diet

It is natural to suspect that diet has a great deal to do with atherosclerosis, and for more than a century the primary suspicion has focused on cholesterol. As early as 1847 a German anatomist, J. Vogel, reported that atherosclerotic arteries invariably contained cholesterol. In 1909 a Russian army medical officer, A. Ignatowski, observing that the army officers, who were of the meat-eating class, had many more heart attacks than the vegetarian peasants, undertook an experiment. He fed rabbits animal products and found that their aortas did indeed develop atherosclerotic lesions. A few years later a pair of Russian investigators, N. Anitschkow and S. Chalatow, followed up with a series of careful studies that became classic references in this field. When they fed rabbits fat and cholesterol, they observed that the cholesterol level in the animals' blood rose and atherosclerotic plaques appeared in their arteries. After cholesterol feedings were discontinued, lipids gradually disappeared from these plaques.

Cholesterol is indeed an inevitable suspect, because the formation of the atherosclerotic lesion is essentially an inflammatory response to this substance. The involvement of cholesterol in the disease has been demonstrated in many different ways. Experimenters have produced the disease by cholesterol feeding in many animals, including rabbits, rats, guinea pigs, chickens, dogs and monkeys. In almost every case in which the disease is induced experimentally the animals' serum shows a rise in cholesterol as a prelude to the atherosclerosis. In primates the disease exhibits all the features that occur in human beings. At the human level a cooperative study in Britain and the U.S. found that peptic ulcer patients who were treated with the Sippy diet (rich in milk and cream) had elevated levels of cholesterol in their serum and suffered twice as high a rate of heart attacks from coronary atherosclerosis as ulcer patients who did not use this diet. Conversely, patients with multiple myeloma, a malignant disease that tends to lower the serum-cholesterol level as one of its effects, have an unusually low rate of heart attacks. People who have died of so-called wasting diseases (essentially malnutrition) show a low lipid content in their arteries, which suggests that the loss of fat may have reduced their atherosclerotic lesions. On the other hand, people with diseases or conditions that are usually accompanied by a high cholesterol level (diabetes, nephrosis, hereditary elevation of lipids in the body) tend to develop atherosclerosis at

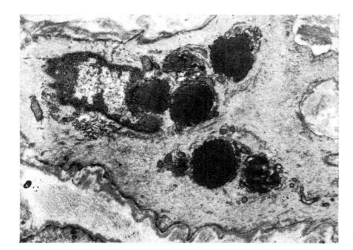
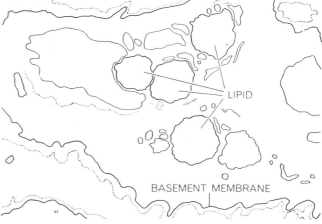

cell under the lining has two lipid vacuoles. In the other electron micrograph (third from left), made by Jack C. Geer and Marion A. Guidry of the Louisiana State University School of Medicine, a portion of a fatty streak from a human aorta has been enlarged 8,000 diameters. As indicated in the drawing (right), a smooth-muscle cell in the intima contains four lipid inclusions.

an earlier age and more extensively than usual.

Yet it has become increasingly clear that atherosclerosis cannot be explained simply in terms of cholesterol, or even a fatty diet. Certain species of pigeons spontaneously develop atherosclerotic lesions closely resembling those of human beings although these birds eat no animal fat. (Spontaneous atherosclerosis is also found in dogs, baboons, ostriches, pigs and whales.) Laboratory experiments have shown that exposure to cold, elevation of the blood pressure, antithyroid substances, high doses of vitamin D, lack of oxygen and other factors can contribute to the development of atherosclerosis. On the other hand, the disease process can be inhibited in animals by undernourishment, thyroid hormones, heparin (the anticlotting agent), fat-eliminating agents, unsaturated fats and sitosterol (a precursor of steroid hormones).

Epidemiology

Even the evidence of epidemiology is not entirely clear. It is true that populations whose diet contains a relatively small amount of saturated animal fats and cholesterol tend in general to have a low blood-cholesterol level and a low incidence of heart attacks. To illustrate with some often cited statistics: The South African Bantu, among whom death from coronary atherosclerosis is exceedingly rare, have a diet very low in fats (average: 17 percent of the total caloric intake) and a mean serum-cholesterol level of only 166. In Europe, where death from this disease is common, the average fat intake amounts to 35 percent of the diet and the serum-cholesterol level is 234. In the U.S., where the coronary death rate is very high, the average fat intake is between 40 and 45 percent and the serum-cholesterol level is about 250. Moreover, there is some evidence that people who migrate from a country with a low heart-disease death rate to one with a high death rate, and adopt the diet and cultural pattern of the latter country, tend to acquire a rise in the cholesterol level and an increase in the rate of heart attacks. This, at least, has been found to be true of Yemenite Jews and Japanese who have migrated to the U.S.

Nonetheless, it is not easy to determine exactly what factors separate the immune populations from the vulnerable ones, or the sheep from the goats. Among the peoples distinguished by exceptionally low rates of heart attack are the farmers of Guatemala, the Yemenite Jews, the South African Bantu, the Chinese, the Japanese and the Apache Indians living on reservations. Very high heart attack rates, on the other hand, are found among the adult white male inhabitants of New York, New Orleans, England, Sweden and parts of Finland. What do the latter populations have in common that differentiates them from the first group? This is one of the principal problems that today engages the attention of many investigators of the causes of atherosclerosis.

To narrow down the search for the significant environmental, biological or dietary factors, it would be very helpful if we could identify the individuals in each population who have atherosclerosis. Unfortunately this is difficult to do in a live population. Atherosclerosis has aptly been called an "iceberg" disease, because only five to 10 percent of those whose arteries are affected show any clinical sign of illness. Recently a method has been developed for examining the arteries in the body by X ray. In this method, called angiography, a radiopaque dye is injected into the bloodstream and the artery is then X-rayed to show whether or not the flow is normal. A narrowing or other abnormality of the channel is taken to indicate atherosclerosis. The technique is not, however, sufficiently simple, accurate or safe to be used as a screening procedure for the general population.

The cholesterol level in the blood is not itself a reliable index of the disease. In any population the level varies as a continuous spectrum, and one cannot find a dividing line that separates the atherosclerotic individuals from those with healthy arteries. Indeed, many people with low serum-cholesterol levels have heart attacks whereas many with high levels do not.

The investigation of atherosclerosis must therefore rely mainly on postmortem examinations and studies of people who clearly show signs of the disorder by their coronary disease or heart attacks. As everyone knows, there is now a very large accumulation of epidemiological studies that have sought to shed light on the factors associated with heart disease. These include the worldwide studies of Ancel Keys of the University of Minnesota and his associates, the famous mass studies in Framingham, Mass., Albany, N.Y., and Chicago and our own recently completed study of 10,000 males in Westchester County. All these studies have

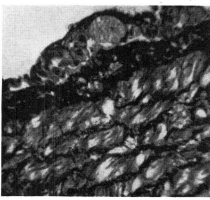

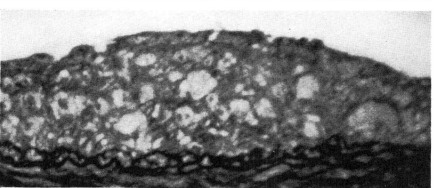

DEVELOPMENT of an atherosclerotic "plaque" in an arterial wall of a cholesterol-fed rabbit is traced in a sequence of photomicrographs made by the author. A normal section is shown at the upper left. A few foam cells penetrate the endothelium (*upper right.*) The bottom micrograph shows a larger accumulation of lipid—an early atherosclerotic plaque.

arrived at remarkably similar conclusions about the high-risk factors associated with coronary atherosclerosis. To sum them up in one profile, the most vulnerable person would be an adult male who has a high lipid content in his blood and high blood pressure, who engages in little physical activity and is markedly obese and who is a heavy smoker of cigarettes.

The difference between men and women in the rate of heart attacks from coronary atherosclerosis is striking. Our observations indicate that, in the age levels up to 55, deaths from such attacks are at least 10 times more common among men than among women. It seems that the factor protecting women is the female hormone estrogen. Women who have had their ovaries removed (thus reducing the estrogen output) tend to have more atherosclerosis than those with their ovaries intact. Injections of estrogens have been found to be capable of lowering the cholesterol level in the blood and of altering lipoproteins from the type associated with the development of atherosclerosis. At the Michael Reese Cardiovascular Research Institute in Chicago, Jeremiah Stamler and his colleagues demonstrated that the development of atherosclerosis in the coronary arteries of young male chickens that had been fed cholesterol could be stopped by injecting estradiol benzoate, a variant of the female hormone. On the strength of all the experimental evidence, estrogen injection has been tried as a treatment to inhibit atherosclerosis in men, but it is not promising for widespread use because of its feminizing effects.

High blood pressure is a serious contributor to atherosclerosis only when it is combined with a high cholesterol level in the blood, in which case the pressure forces cholesterol into the artery walls. The Apache Indians commonly have high blood pressure but seldom suffer heart attacks, probably because their blood content of cholesterol is low. Our studies of New York men indicated that the combination of high blood pressure and high cholesterol carries a high risk. In the age group between 36 and 50 men with this combination had a rate of atherosclerotic heart disease more than four times higher than that of men with normal blood pressure and lower serum cholesterol; the respective disease rates were 7.6 percent and 1.8 percent.

In the cases of the other risk factors revealed by the epidemiological studies —lack of physical activity, obesity, cigarette smoking—no direct tie to the athero-

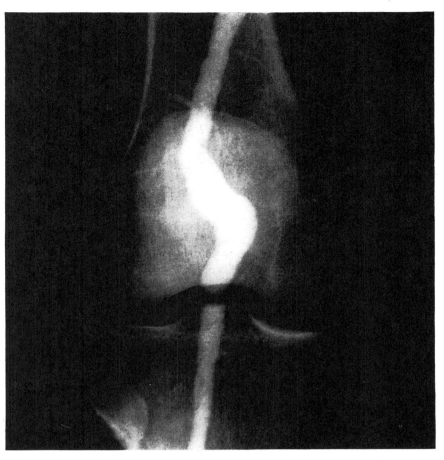

ANGIOGRAM, an X-ray photograph of a blood vessel injected with a radiopaque dye, can sometimes locate atherosclerotic damage. This one shows an aneurysm, or abnormally dilated segment, in a popliteal artery caused by atherosclerotic weakening of the arterial wall.

sclerotic process has been found. Just how these conditions contribute to heart disease remains to be determined.

Nondietary Factors

Many other elements that are suspected of contributing to atherosclerosis have been investigated. Undoubtedly heredity is an important factor. Atherosclerosis is frequently associated with diabetes and hypertension, diseases that are known to stem from genetic causes. Moreover, it seems likely that an individual's relative ability to metabolize and otherwise handle lipids plays a large part in his susceptibility to atherosclerosis. Studies have shown that identical twins tend to have about the same blood-cholesterol level, whereas twins who are not identical are much more likely to differ from each other in this respect. There have also been dramatic cases in which identical twins have had heart attacks at the same time in the prime of life.

Another factor that has had much attention is emotional stress, arising either from the individual's mode of life or his constitutional disposition. Unfortunately most of the studies of this factor have been so poorly conceived or executed that the conclusions are uncertain or questionable. There is no firm information so far to prove or disprove the hypothesis that emotional stress contributes to heart attacks.

We come back finally to the diet, which today holds the center of research attention as the factor most likely to be primarily responsible for the epidemic of atherosclerotic heart disease. There is no gainsaying the fact that this disease is a dominant feature of industrialized, affluent societies. If we look at metropolitan New York, where the disease has increased strikingly in the past 30 years, we can see that in the same period there has been a marked change toward a more luxurious and more passive manner of life, characterized by great increases in the use of the automobile, in automation of occupations and domestic tasks and in the animal-fat content of the average diet. The insurance companies have been compelled at frequent intervals (about 10 times in the past 30 years) to revise

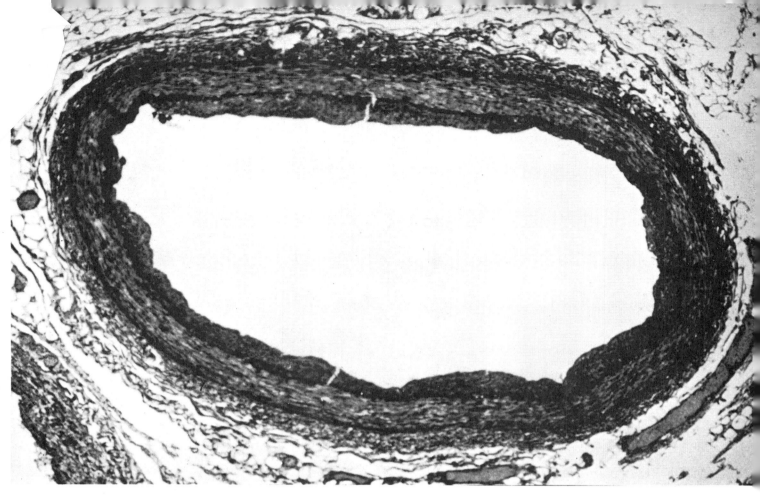

HUMAN CORONARY ARTERY is enlarged about 38 diameters in these photomicrographs made by the author. A normal artery is seen in cross section (*above*). In a diseased artery (*below*) the channel is partially occluded by atherosclerosis. Fibrous scar tissue, with fatty deposits (*clear areas*) in it, and other materials have thickened the arterial wall, reducing the blood-carrying capacity.

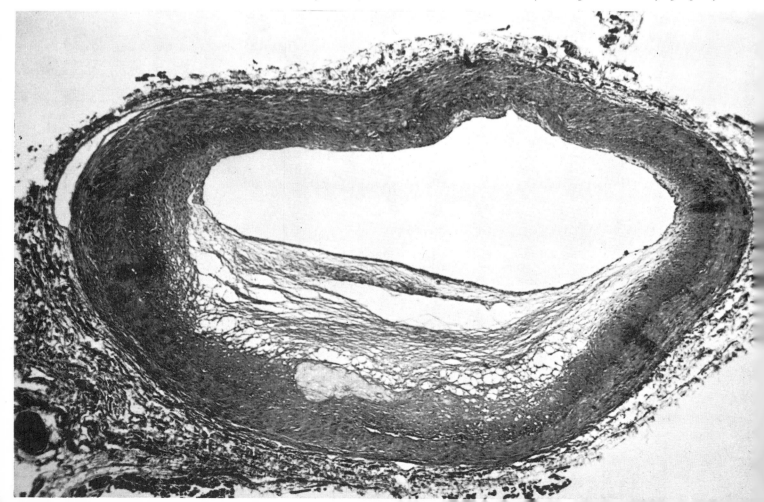

upward their statistical tables of average weights.

In a report to the White House Conference on Children and Youth, Stanley Marion Garn of the Fels Research Institute noted a disquieting trend in the eating habits of the younger generation in the U.S. today.

"If 35 percent of his calories comes from fats, is Junior being prepared, starting in nursery school, for a coronary occlusion?" asked Garn. "Reviewing the dietaries of some of our teen-agers, I am struck by the resemblance to the diet that Olaf Mickelsen uses to create obesity in rats. Frappes, fat-meat hamburgers, bacon-and-mayonnaise sandwiches, followed by ice cream, may be good for the farmer, good for the undertaker and bad for the population.... Through the stimulation of advertising, tap water is being replaced by sugared juices, milk and carbonated drinks. Snacks have become a ritualized part of the movies and are inseparably associated with television viewing."

To what extent can the animal-fat diet be specifically incriminated on the basis of the research done so far? The epidemiologist Ernest L. Wynder has suggested four criteria to determine whether or not a given factor can be regarded as a cause of a disease: (1) the incidence of the disease in a population must be proportional to the population's exposure to the factor; (2) the distribution of the disease—in geography, time, by sex and among various population groups—should be consistent with the distribution of the suspected factor; (3) the factor should produce the same disease, or one corresponding to it, in experimental animals in the laboratory, and (4) the removal of the factor or the reduction of exposure to it by the human population should reduce the incidence of the disease in the population.

The animal-fat diet has fulfilled the first three of these criteria for atherosclerosis in many tests. The fourth piece of incriminating evidence—reduction of the disease in man by reduction of the exposure—has not yet been established. It is currently being tested, however, in a massive dietary study, expected to involve ultimately 100,000 men, that is being conducted at five major centers under the auspices of the National Institutes of Health. If this and similar studies demonstrate that the fatty diet is indeed a major cause of atherosclerosis, there may be hope that the epidemic increase of the disease can be halted and reversed.

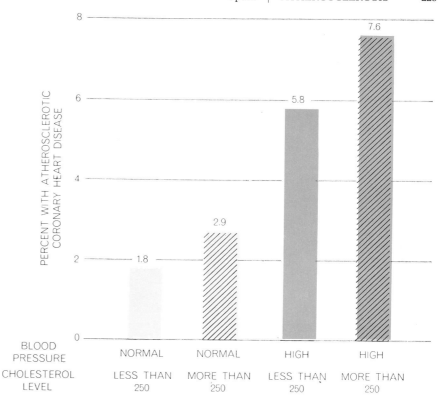

STUDY by the author of some 6,000 men showed that blood pressure and cholesterol level are correlated with the incidence of atherosclerosis. A diastolic blood pressure of 90 or less was called "normal"; that figure and the cholesterol count of 250 are necessarily arbitrary.

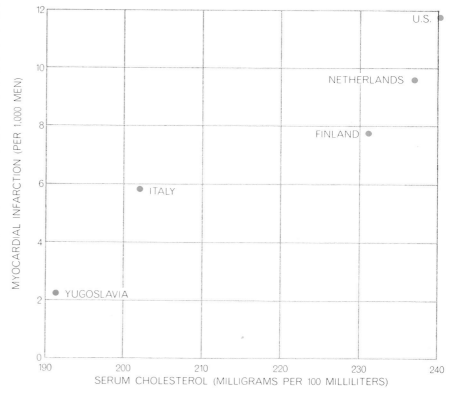

STATISTICS collected by Ancel Keys's group at the University of Minnesota indicate a correlation between the average cholesterol level in male populations and the amount of myocardial infarction, or heart-muscle damage. Cholesterol count may in turn be related to diet.

VI

THE GLOBAL PROBLEM OF NUTRITION

VI THE GLOBAL PROBLEM OF NUTRITION

INTRODUCTION

Man's history is replete with examples of groups of people who have suffered from lack of food. Inadequate nutrition or malnutrition takes several forms. A simple lack of calories is the most common. This can be sporadic, as when the vagaries of the hunt or the seasons occasionally leave primitive hunting and gathering societies without food. In societies dependent on agriculture, failure of a crop caused by weather, pests or war can lead to famine and widespread starvation. Populations that depend on a single food to meet the greater part of their dietary needs are especially vulnerable to crop failure. For example, the dependence of the Irish on potatoes (see "The Social Influence of the Potato" in Section III) caused mass starvation in 1845–1846 when the potato crop was devastated by a fungus infection. Such crisis situations, which never lasted more than a few years, are well-documented because they are out of the ordinary. But there have also always been groups suffering chronic undernutrition, i.e., seldom if ever having enough to eat. While this condition in the past was not sufficiently dramatic to warrant special historic documentation, we can now appreciate the profound consequences these events have on subsequent physical and mental development.

A second form of malnutrition, the specific deficiency of one or more essential nutrients, more commonly occurs when a people's way of living and traditional food patterns undergo change. Beri beri spread through the Far East in the wake of efficient milling machines as white, highly milled rice replaced brown rice and its thiamine-containing coat. Rickets became common in Britain during the Industrial Revolution when people moved from the open countryside to the smoke-filled cities. The change to more refined foods and the abandonment of simple ironware for food preparation has led to an increased incidence of iron deficiency anemia, the only widespread specific nutritional deficiency in the United States today.

The fortunate of the world not only have been able to avoid traditional types of malnutrition, they commonly eat beyond their daily needs and indulge in excessive amounts of certain foods. It is only now, with our appreciation of the role of overeating in the development of a variety of degenerative diseases, that we recognize this behavior as leading to malnutrition. In "The Dimensions of Human Hunger" Jean Mayer estimates the current incidence of the several types of malnutrition. Though the relative amount of malnutrition in the world may be no different than in years past, the increased population in the developing world and the increased wealth of industrialized countries have intensified the problem.

While the economic, cultural, and political factors involved in specific instances of undernutrition have been documented, overall the problem is a reflection of the ecological imperative that a species increase its population to the limits of available resources. Thomas Malthus, a British economist (d. 1834), postulated that while the growth of the human population could be exponential, the expansion of food resources is arithmetical, so that population eventually becomes limited by a shortage of food, if not sooner by moral actions, that is, birth control. Malthus's views created quite a stir when first made public but were never widely accepted. By mid-twentieth century the pervasive view was that man could so thoroughly manipulate nature that he would always be able to provide abundant food. This euphoria was a product of the spectacular successes in feeding countries devastated by World War II, the large grain and food surpluses of the United States, the successful development of disease-resistant, high-yield wheat and corn, and the promise of unlimited nuclear power.

Then came the first realization that in some parts of the world, especially among the developing poorer nations, increases in food supplies barely kept pace with increases in population. During the 1950s an appreciation of the consequences of an exponential growth became more widespread, and some countries initiated policies aimed at restricting rather than encouraging the birth rate. Those who considered the problem at that time could be divided into two groups. The optimists felt that advancing technology would solve the problems of increasing food supplies and that improved living standards would lead to a lowered birth rate and stabilized population; the pessimists saw no end to the increasing population, predicted widespread famine, and advocated drastic policies. In "The Human Population" Edward Deevey, Jr. looks at the history of population growth and suggests that food supply has probably not been the limiting factor in determining birth rate. In evaluating some of the consequences of an increasing population, he is cautiously optimistic about the ability to support 2 to 3 times the current population but stresses the impossibility of dealing with a tenfold increase in population. In 1960, when this article was first published, the rate of population growth was still accelerating; but since then policies restricting this growth in the Western world have begun to take effect. Although demographic predictions are notoriously risky, it appears that the world population will come to a new equilibrium of 6 to 8 billion within about two generations. The major increases in population will take place in those countries least able to feed themselves now and least able to take advantage of the advanced agricultural techniques of industrialized countries. In "Orthodox and Unorthodox Methods of Meeting World Food Needs" N. W. Pirie explores food sources that have yet to be exploited or have not been exploited to their full potential. It has become apparent in the 10 years since the first appearance of this article that the increasing demand for grain as animal feed in the industrialized countries, the decreasing availability and increased costs of energy, and the susceptibility of the new high-yield grains to drought make it impossible for the less-developed countries to fulfill food requirements from conventional sources. Consequently, hitherto neglected food resources are now the subject of active investigation.

24

The Dimensions of Human Hunger

by Jean Mayer
September 1976

The number of people who are poorly nourished or undernourished can only be roughly estimated, but they probably represent an eighth of the human population. Most of them are found in Asia and Africa

Famine, fearsome and devastating though it is, can at least be attacked straightforwardly. A famine occurs in a definable area and has a finite duration; as long as food is available somewhere, relief agencies can undertake to deal with the crisis. Malnutrition, on the other hand, afflicts a far larger proportion of mankind than any famine but is harder to define and attack. Only someone professionally familiar with nutritional disease can accurately diagnose malnutrition and assess its severity. Malnutrition is a chronic condition that seems to many observers to be getting worse in certain areas. In one form or another it affects human populations all over the world, and its treatment involves not mobilization to combat a crisis but long-term actions taken to prevent a crisis—actions that affect economic and social policies as well as nutritional and agricultural ones. In the background always is the concern that too rapid an increase in population, combined with failure to keep pace in food production, will give rise to massive famines that cannot be combated.

The statistics with which the public is bombarded are of little help. What is the layman to make of statements that a billion people suffered from hunger and malnutrition last year, that 10 million children the world over are so seriously malnourished that their lives are at risk, that 400 million people live on the edge of starvation, that 12,000 people die of hunger each day and that in India alone one million children die each year from malnutrition? If the world's food problem is to be brought under control, and I believe it can be, we must first draw conceptual boundaries around it and place it in a time frame as we would a famine.

First, then, just what is the chronic hunger of malnutrition and how widespread is it? The first part of the question can be answered with assurance; the second, in spite of the statistics cited in the preceding paragraph, is really a matter of informed guesswork.

Malnutrition may come about in one of four ways. A person may simply not get enough food, which is undernutrition. His diet may lack one essential nutrient or more, which gives rise to deficiency diseases such as pellagra, scurvy, rickets and the anemia of pregnancy due to a deficiency of folic acid. He may have a condition or an illness, either genetic or environmental in origin, that prevents him from digesting his food properly or from absorbing some of its constituents, which is secondary malnutrition. Finally, he may be taking in too many calories or consuming an excess of one component or more of a reasonable diet; this condition is overnutrition. Malnutrition in this sense is a disease of affluent people in both the rich and the poor nations. In countries such as the U.S. diets high in calories, saturated fats, salt and sugar, low in fruits and vegetables and distorted toward heavily processed foods contribute to the high incidence of obesity, diabetes, hypertension and atherosclerotic disease and to marginal deficiencies of certain minerals and B vitamins. Bizarre reducing diets, which exclude entire categories of useful foods, are self-inflicted examples of the first two causes of malnutrition. The nutritional diseases of the affluent are not, however, the subject of this article. In areas where the food supply is limited the first three causes of malnutrition are often found in some combination.

In children a chronic deficiency of calories causes listlessness, muscle wastage and failure to grow. In adults it leads to a loss of weight and a reduced inclination toward and capacity for activity. Undernourished people of all ages are more vulnerable to infection and other illness and recover more slowly and with much greater difficulty. Children with a chronic protein deficiency grow more slowly and are small for their age; in severe deficiency growth stops altogether and the child shows characteristic symptoms: a skin rash and discoloration, edema and a change in hair color to an orange-reddish tinge that is particularly striking in children whose hair would normally be dark. The spectrum of protein-calorie malnutrition (PCM, as it is known to workers in the field) varies from a diet that is relatively high in calories and deficient in protein (manifested in the syndrome known as kwashiorkor) to one that is low in both calories and protein (manifested in marasmus).

Although protein-calorie malnutrition is the most prevalent form of undernourishment, diseases caused by deficiencies of specific vitamins or minerals are also widespread. It is true that the prevalence of certain classic deficiency diseases has decreased drastically since World War II. Beriberi is now rare and pellagra has been essentially eradicated, at least in its acute form; rickets is seen mostly in its adult form (osteomalacia) in Moslem women whose secluded way of life keeps them out of the sun, and scurvy is unlikely to be seen except in prisoners who are not provided with enough vitamin C. In contrast, blindness caused by the lack of vitamin A occurs with particular frequency in India, Indonesia, Bangladesh, Vietnam, the Philippines, Central America, the northeast of Brazil and parts of Africa. In remote inland areas (central Africa, the mountainous regions of South America and

POOR ALABAMA FARM FAMILY OF 1936 was photographed by Walker Evans for the Farm Security Administration of the Department of Agriculture. The farmer was Bud Fields, who lived in Hale County, in the west-central part of the state. In the intervening 40 years much of the poverty in the area has been eliminated by development programs such as the Tennessee Valley Authority. Here, as in areas of developing countries where hunger is endemic today, effects of malnutrition were severest among pregnant women and growing children.

the Himalayas) goiter, the enlargement of the thyroid resulting from a deficiency of iodine, is common. The World Health Organization estimates that up to 5 percent of such populations are afflicted with cretinism, the irreversible condition caused by iodine deficiency in the mother before or during pregnancy. From 5 to 17 percent of the men and from 10 to 50 percent of the women in countries of South America, Africa and Asia have been estimated to have iron-deficiency anemia.

The human beings most vulnerable to the ravages of malnutrition are infants, children up to the age of five or six and pregnant and lactating women. For the infant protein in particular is necessary during fetal development for the generation and growth of bones, muscles and organs. The child of a malnourished mother is more likely to be born prematurely or small and is at greater risk of death or of permanent neurological and mental dysfunction. Brain development begins *in utero* and is complete at an

early age (under two). Malnutrition during this period when neurons and neuronal connections are being formed may be the cause of mental retardation that cannot be remedied by later corrective measures. The long-term consequences, not only for the individual but also for the society and the economy, need no elaboration.

Growing children, pound for pound, require more nutrients than adults do. A malnourished child is more susceptible to the common childhood diseases, and illness in turn makes extra demands on nutritional reserves. In addition many societies, still believing the old adage about starving a fever, withdraw nourishing foods from the child just when he needs them most, thus often pushing him over the borderline into severe malnutrition. So common is the cycle of malnutrition, infection, severe malnutrition, recurrent infection and eventual death at an early age that the death rate for children up to four years old in general, and the infant mortality rate in par-

ticular, serve as one index of the nutritional status of a population as a whole. For infants less than a year old the death rate is about 250 per 1,000 births in Zambia and Bolivia, 140 in India and Pakistan and 95 in Brazil (for all its soaring gross national product). The rate in Sweden is 12 per 1,000 births; in the U.S. the average is 19, but in the country's affluent suburbs the rate equals Sweden's, whereas it rises to about 25 in the poor areas of the inner cities and as high as 60 for the most poverty-stricken and neglected members of the society: the migrant farm workers.

How reliable the figures for the developing nations are, however, is another matter. In most instances statistical reporting is as underdeveloped as the rest of the economy. Deaths, particularly of one-day-old infants, often go unreported. In all probability the rates are higher than the ones I have cited.

More precise nutritional assessments

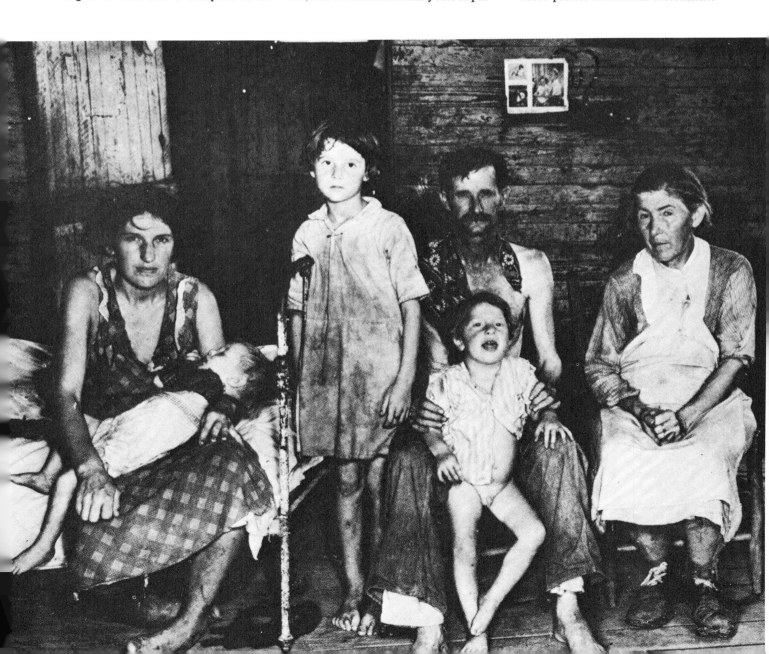

are attempted in two ways. One is to construct a "food balance sheet," which puts agricultural output, stocks and purchases on the supply side and balances them against the food used for seed for the next year's crop, animal feed and wastage and hence derives an estimate of the food that is left for human consumption. That amount can then be matched against the United Nations Food and Agriculture Organization's tables of nutritional requirements to obtain an estimate of the adequacy of the national diet.

This method has a number of drawbacks. For several reasons it tends to result in underestimates. One is that it is difficult to estimate the agricultural production in developing countries with any degree of accuracy. Farmers have every incentive to underestimate their

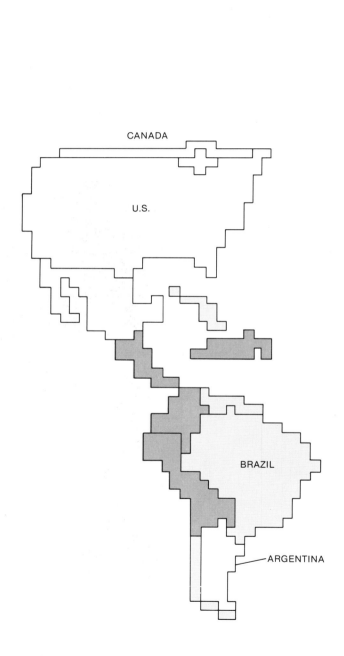

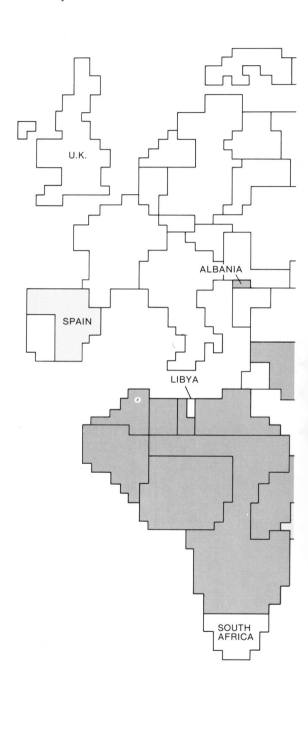

LEVEL OF ENERGY obtained from food is portrayed on a map where the area of each nation is proportional to its population. Canada, for example, occupies a large area but has a relatively small population, whereas Japan has a large population in a relatively small area. The level of energy intake is indicated by the presence or absence of color. In the countries shown in dark color the average calo-

crop: they may be able to reduce taxes and the obligatory payment of crops (often as much as 60 percent of the harvest) in rent to the landlord. Second, the foods included in the balance sheet tend to be the items that figure prominently in channels of trade: grain, soybeans and

large livestock. Other farm products—eggs, small animals, fruits and vegetables—vital to a good diet but grown for family consumption or sold locally are almost impossible to count and so are ignored.

On the other hand, the balance-sheet

method has certain tendencies toward overestimates. For example, it is extremely difficult to estimate the postharvest loss of crops to insects, rodents and microorganisms. The loss is known to be close to 10 percent for the U.S. wheat crop and is probably higher for other

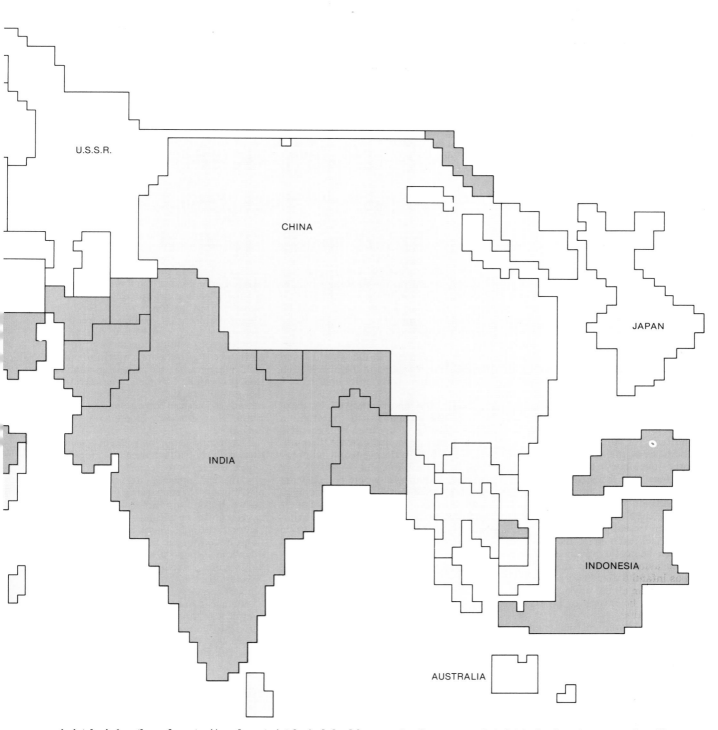

rie intake is less than adequate. (An adequate intake is defined by United Nations agencies as being about 3,000 calories per day for a man and 2,200 for a woman.) In the countries indicated by the light color the average calorie intake is adequate or as much as 10 percent above adequate, and in the countries represented in white the average calorie level is higher than adequate by at least 10 percent.

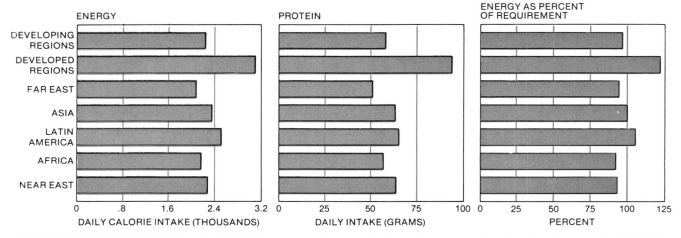

AVAILABILITY OF CALORIES AND PROTEIN is portrayed for the developed and developing regions and for several specific developing regions. The figures reflect the average daily diet per person in the various regions and are based on data assembled by the International Task Force on Child Nutrition for the UN Children's Fund. The figures for Asia refer to the centrally planned economies.

crops, even with the advanced technology available. In some tropical countries the loss can run as high as 40 percent. For all these reasons figures on food production do not provide a particularly accurate index of the amount of food actually available for consumption or the types of food actually consumed, and they make no attempt to differentiate patterns of consumption within a population. They do, however, provide rough estimates of the state of nutrition by regions [see illustration on preceding two pages].

The second way of estimating the degree of malnutrition within an area is to extrapolate from data compiled from hospital records and cross-sectional surveys. Statistics on illness, however, tend to be as unreliable as mortality statistics. The criteria for admission to a hospital on the basis of malnutrition vary from country to country; the records from rural areas may be sparse; the poor, among whom malnutrition and its related conditions are most likely to be found, are the least likely segment of the population to seek medical help, and if they do seek such help, the condition may then be so far advanced that the diseases associated with malnutrition, such as infantile diarrhea and pneumonia, may claim all the physician's attention, so that he misses or ignores the underlying cause.

Projections based on the results of 77 studies of nutritional status made among more than 200,000 preschool children in 45 countries of Asia, Africa and Latin America place the total number of children suffering from some degree of protein-calorie malnutrition at 98.4 million. Percentages ranged from 5 to 37 in Latin America, from 7 to 73 in Africa and from 15 to 80 in Asia (excluding China). These surveys, however, did not employ standardized proce-

dures. In some of them clinical assessments were made and in others the children were measured against international weight tables. Thus, although the general indications of such studies are useful, figures derived from them are rough at best. In order to assign reliable figures to the degree of hunger and malnutrition in the world today we would need large-scale surveys that included both clinical examinations based on an established definition of malnutrition and individual consumption surveys that determine the amount and types of food eaten and the distribution of food within each family unit.

Even if the figures derived by these methods are doubtful, the situation they reflect is clear. In my judgment it would seem reasonable to set the number of people suffering from malnutrition at 500 million and to add to that another billion who would benefit from a more varied diet. The largest concentration of such people is in Asia, Southeast Asia and sub-Saharan Africa. Clinical surveys and hospital records indicate that malnutrition wherever it exists is severest among infants, preschool children and pregnant and lactating women; that it is most prevalent in depressed rural areas and the slums of great cities; that the problem is lack of calories as much as lack of protein; that (except in areas where the people subsist largely on manioc or bananas) where calories are adequate protein tends to be adequate too, and that although a lack of food is the ultimate factor in malnutrition, that lack results from a number of causes, operating alone or in combination. A nation may lack both self-sufficiency in food production and the money to buy food or to provide the farm inputs necessary to increase production; the poorer members of the population

may lack income to buy the food that is available, and regional factors, such as customs in child-feeding and restrictions on the movement of supplies, may prevent the food from getting to the people who need it most.

On the basis of these findings one can divide the nations of the world into five groups. The first group consists of the industrialized nations, where food is plentiful but pockets of poverty persist. Here governments are able to deal with problems of malnutrition through food assistance to the poor, nutrition and health programs and nutrition-education programs. The chief members of the group are the U.S., Canada, the nations of Western Europe, Japan, Australia, New Zealand, Hong Kong and Singapore.

The second group consists of the nations with centrally planned economies, where whatever the economic philosophy the egalitarian pattern of income distribution together with government control of food supplies and distribution have seemed in the past few years to insure the populations against malnutrition due to hunger. In this category are mainland China, Taiwan, North Korea, South Korea, North Vietnam and South Vietnam. In the third group are the nations of the Organization of Petroleum Exporting Countries (OPEC), whose overall wealth is undeniable but whose pattern of income distribution does not ensure that this wealth will benefit the poor. Fourth is a group of countries in Asia, the Near East, Central America and South America that are already self-sufficient or almost self-sufficient in food production at their present level of demand. The demand, however, is impeded by an uneven distribution of income that is reflected in malnutrition in large segments of the population. Brazil, for example, has the highest economic growth rate in the world, but malnutrition is rampant in the northeast and widespread in the shantytowns surrounding the large cities.

The fifth group includes the nations the UN designates as "least developed." They have too few economic resources to provide for the people in the lowest income groups. Many of the countries are exposed to recurring droughts, floods or cyclones; some are ravaged by war. All 25 of the least developed nations are poor in natural resources and investment capital.

Looking back today, it seems incredible that in 1972 it appeared the world might soon, for the first time, be assured of an abundant food supply. The new wheat varieties of the "green revolution" had taken hold in Mexico and northwestern India, and the new varieties of rice developed in the Philippines promised a high-yield staple crop for the peoples of Southeast Asia. The harvest from the seas was still rising spectacularly (from 21 million metric tons in 1950 to 70 million in 1970—a steady increase of about 5 percent per year, outstripping the world's annual population increase of 2 percent). The worldwide production of grain was rising by an average of 2.8 percent per year, and there were substantial reserves in the form of carry-over stocks held by the principal exporting countries and of cropland held idle in the U.S. under the soil-bank program. The prospect was so rosy that the FAO suggested in 1969 that the food problems of the future might be those of surplus rather than shortage.

Although two sudden and short-term simultaneous crop failures in a number of areas and the sharp rise in oil prices were the immediate cause of the food crisis of 1972–1974, it has since become clear that four long-term factors that had been building up quietly for a long time were in any case about to alter the hopeful situation permanently. (The first short-term reversal, a reduction of crops in several parts of the world because of unfavorable weather in 1972, gave rise to a second: the massive purchases of grain by the U.S.S.R. that eliminated American reserves and caused the international prices of wheat, corn and rice to rise sharply. Moreover, the increase in oil prices effectively put the green revolution out of the reach of such countries as India, Pakistan and Bangladesh, which are poor in petroleum and other resources and have gone about as far as they can in increasing yields with traditional methods of farming. The increase in oil prices also dislocated the economies of the wealthy nations, reducing their contributions to international aid.)

Even though the situation is less serious now than it was in 1974, it is more

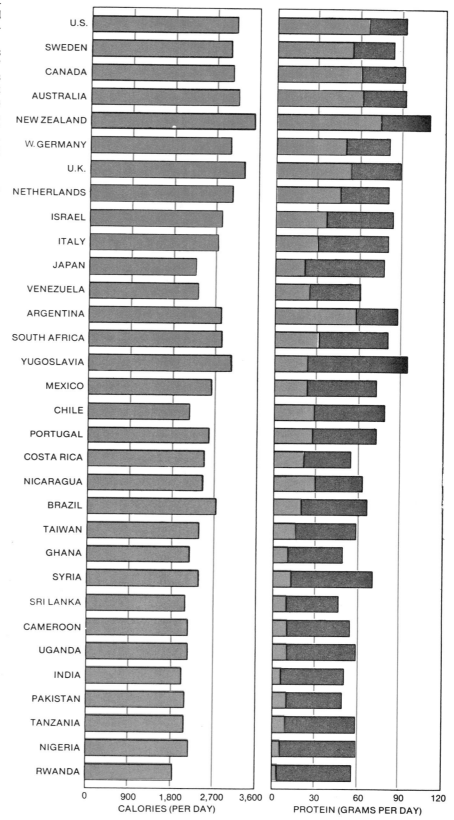

NUTRITION AND NATIONAL ECONOMY are compared in a chart that lists countries according to their gross national product as apportioned on a per capita basis. The bars at the left show the average daily calorie intake of the people in each country. In the bars at the right the full length of the bar represents the average daily protein intake of each person in grams per day, and the colored portion of the bar indicates how much of that intake is animal protein.

precarious as a result of the long-term factors. The primary long-term factor is the growth of the human population: 80 million people per year, the equivalent of the population of the U.S. every 30 months. Moreover, the population is growing most rapidly in the areas that are experiencing the greatest nutritional difficulties.

In considering the effects of population growth, however, one must bear in mind the phenomenon known as the demographic transition. It is the process whereby societies move from a stage of high birth and death rates to one of low birth and death rates. Usually the decline in death rates precedes the decline in birth rates by from one generation to three generations. On both sides of the transition the result is a stable level of population. The developed countries have made the transition or are well along in it; the developing countries are now making the transition but have traveled varying distances through it.

Alongside the inequality in population growth as a long-term factor affecting the food supply is an even greater inequality in the patterns of producing and utilizing food. It appears to be historically inevitable that as people or societies become wealthier their consumption of animal products increases. This means that more of their basic foodstuffs (grains, legumes and even fish) that could feed human beings directly are instead fed to domesticated animals such as cattle and chickens. The efficiency of the conversion of plant food into

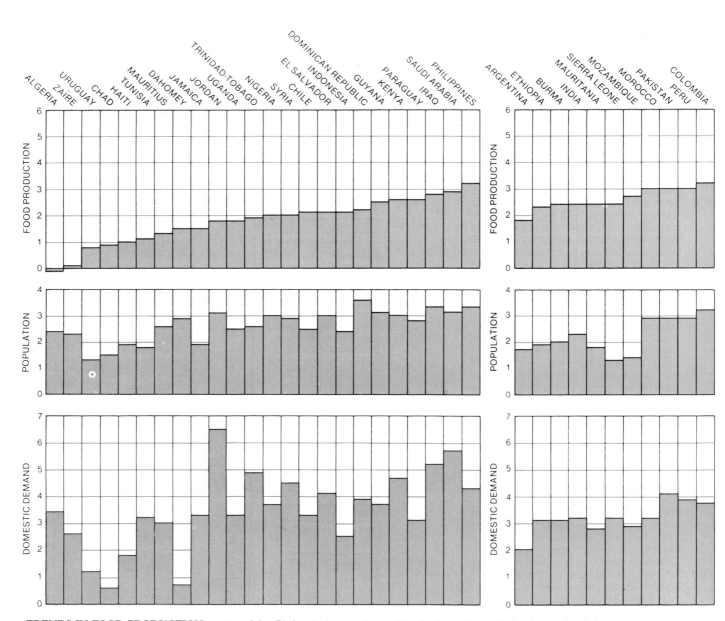

PRODUCTION FAILED TO EQUAL
POPULATION GROWTH

PRODUCTION GROWTH FAILED TO
EQUAL GROWTH OF DOMESTIC DEMAND

TRENDS IN FOOD PRODUCTION are traced for 71 developing countries on the basis of how each country's average annual change in food production (an increase for every country except Algeria) compares with the country's change in population and in domestic demand for food, a category that reflects not only increases in population but also the economic status of the people and their changes in preferences for food, as in a tendency to eat more meat. Each bar reflects an average annual percentage change for the period from 1953

animal food varies with the animal product but is in no case higher than the level of about 25 percent attained in milk and eggs.

The net effect of this trend is that rich countries consume far more food per capita than poor ones. For example, it has been estimated that in China each person is adequately fed on 450 pounds of grain per year; 350 pounds are consumed directly as cereal or cereal products and 100 pounds are fed to domesticated animals. In the U.S. the average

individual consumes more than 2,000 pounds of grains per year; 150 pounds are eaten directly (as bread, pasta, breakfast cereal and the like) and the rest, more than 90 percent of the total, is fed to animals.

The third source of pressure on the world's food supply has been the diminishing effectiveness of the fishing industry, an important source of protein for many poor nations. In 1970 and 1971 the total catch remained steady at

about 70 million tons. It dropped abruptly in 1972 to less than 55 million tons. The reasons for the decline are overfishing and pollution.

Finally, it has become apparent that the "miracle" of the green revolution requires more time, more work and more capital than was thought in the first flush of enthusiasm. I shall not elaborate on this point, since the green revolution is discussed in other articles in this issue. In sum, the situation as it exists today is precarious but manageable, barring

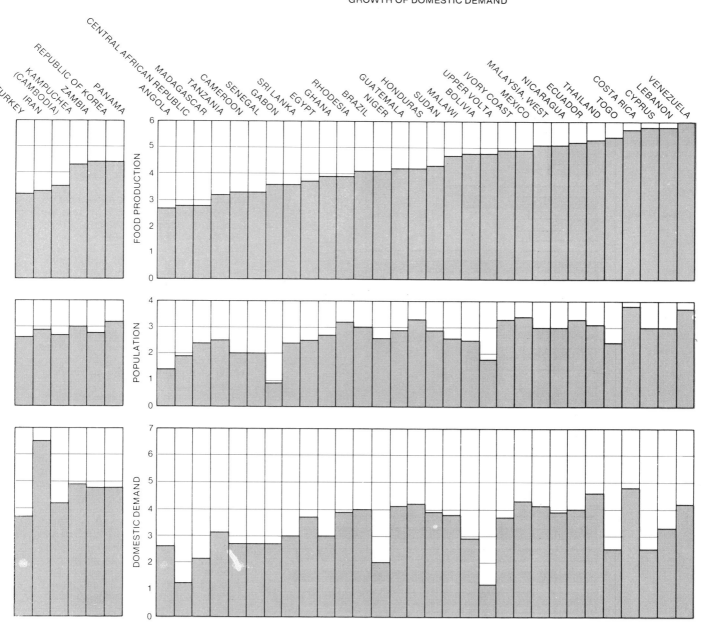

PRODUCTION GROWTH EQUALED OR EXCEEDED
GROWTH OF DOMESTIC DEMAND

through 1971. In the group of 24 nations beginning with Algeria and ending with the Philippines the rise in food production failed to keep pace with the growth of population. In the next 17 nations (Argentina through Panama) the growth of food production exceeded the population growth but fell short of the change in domestic demand. In the final group of 30 nations (from Angola through Venezuela) the rise in food production exceeded population growth and rise in domestic demand. Data are from UN Economic and Social Council.

some catastrophe such as a massive crop failure in the U.S., which is currently the granary of the world.

What of the future? Let us first consider three advances that could be made in dealing with famine. Their common aim is to sight and attack incipient famines in an early stage of development.

The first requirement is an early-warning system. It would employ weather satellites, economic indexes (such as the movement and amounts of food in a region) and clinical indicators. One of the most sensitive clinical indicators is provided by the charted weight and growth curves for children in the most vulnerable socioeconomic sectors of a society.

The second requirement is a permanent small international organization that would keep track of such information for every region and monitor it for any sign of an impending emergency. The agency would maintain manuals on how to proceed against disaster and famine, would hold periodic training sessions for key people from each nation, would draft contingency plans (listing likely requirements and sources of food, medicine, transportation and personnel) and would explore such matters as stockpiling essential supplies and setting up alternative systems of distribution. In an emergency the organization would stand ready to assist a national relief director.

The third requirement is an adequate grain reserve, distributed strategically around the world. It would serve as a standby supply for nearby countries while grain shipments intended for them were diverted to the stricken area. This arrangement might not avert a famine, but it would prevent one from becoming a major disaster.

Several things can also be done to deal with malnutrition. For the next few years it will be necessary to continue to provide food relief where it is needed. The least developed countries may require special assistance in the form of food distribution and feeding programs for some years to come. Those nations should also be helped to develop methods to increase their ability to store food and to distribute it to vulnerable areas in times of emergency.

Simple and inexpensive programs are available to eradicate certain diseases of malnutrition, and they should be instituted. The blindness resulting from a deficiency of vitamin A can be prevented with two injections per year of 100,000 units of the vitamin, at a cost of a few cents per person. Goiter can be prevented by the iodization of salt, also at infinitesimal cost.

In the intermediate term (the next 15 years or so) the goal must be to make the developing nations independent in their food supply. The fish catch appears to have stabilized at the 1970° level. The production of animal foods that compete with human beings for grain should be reduced. (Grazing animals, which utilize land that cannot be cultivated and crops that cannot be eaten by human beings, are another matter.) The development of new foods is still in the future. The only sure resource is the green revolution, which still has the potential of doubling or tripling yields in some areas.

Therefore it is important to begin immediately the construction of fertilizer plants, preferably right at the source of supply (the flare gas around the Persian Gulf and in Nigeria, for example) or in the needy countries. The task should be furthered by international assistance and by oil sold by the OPEC nations at concessional prices.

Another step, which entails something that Americans do well, is to help the food-deficit nations set up agricultural research and extension services, with the aim of adapting the green revolution to a tropical, labor-intensive agriculture and of assisting the small farmer to obtain an increased yield while maintaining a varied production of small animals, fruits and vegetables so that he is not dependent on large tonnages of one crop for an adequate income. Such countries can also be helped to develop ways of protecting a crop once it is har-

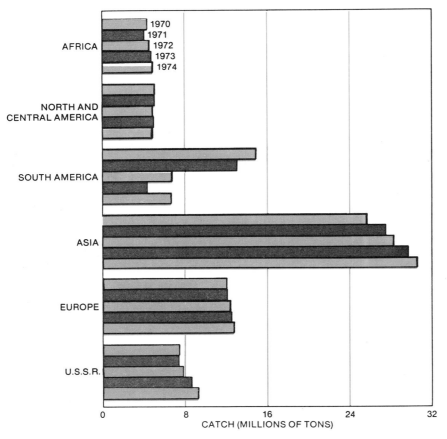

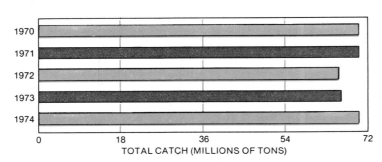

WORLD FISH CATCH appears to have stabilized at about the level of 1970 after declines in 1972 and 1973 that resulted mainly from drops in the South American catch. In most other regions catch has increased slightly. Data are from UN Food and Agriculture Organization.

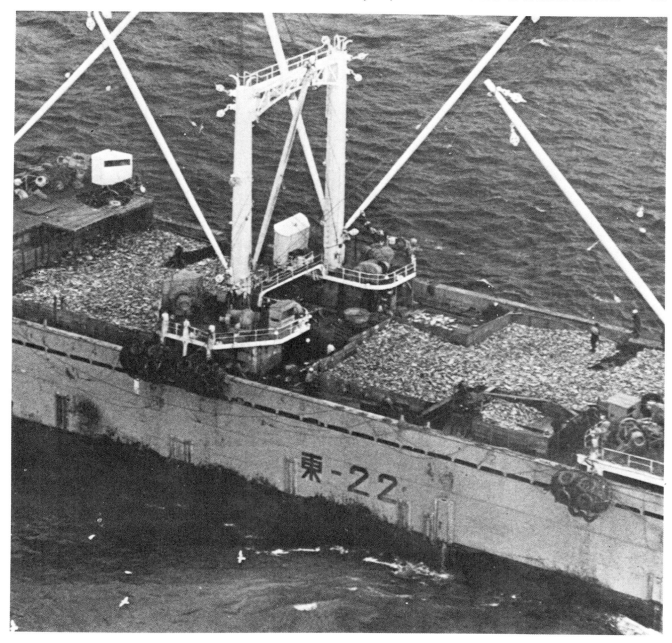

MODERN FISHING METHODS are exemplified by large factory ships such as this Japanese vessel, the *Soyo Maru*. It is a mother ship for several trawlers, processing their catch while at sea. The fish visible in this photograph of the ship are mainly sole and halibut.

vested and of establishing an indigenous food industry that can package and distribute the food. A system of international credit that favors the small farmer and the small businessman and promotes a more equitable distribution of income and opportunity should be established. Finally, an international system of weather forecasting should be activated so that future crop failures will not come as a surprise.

These actions will buy time for the next 25 years. If the population of the world is then between six and seven billion, as seems likely, new sources of food will have to be at hand—on the dinner table, not in the development stage. Unfortunately the nations that will need the new foods the most desperately have neither the financial resources nor the technological skill to do the necessary research, and the nations that do have these things have so far felt no urgency about doing it. The objectives of the research should include the intensive development of aquaculture, the establishment through genetic techniques of new species of animals (such as the beefalo) and of grazing animals that can utilize forage more efficiently, the domestication of some wild animals, the development of one-cell microorganisms as food and the direct synthesis of food from oil. Work on all these objectives should now be under way.

To sum up, we know who is hungry, if not precisely how many people are affected. We also know why. Economists often say that expanded food production will solve the problem. Social reformers maintain that the need is for more equitable distribution. The evidence shows that we must and can have both.

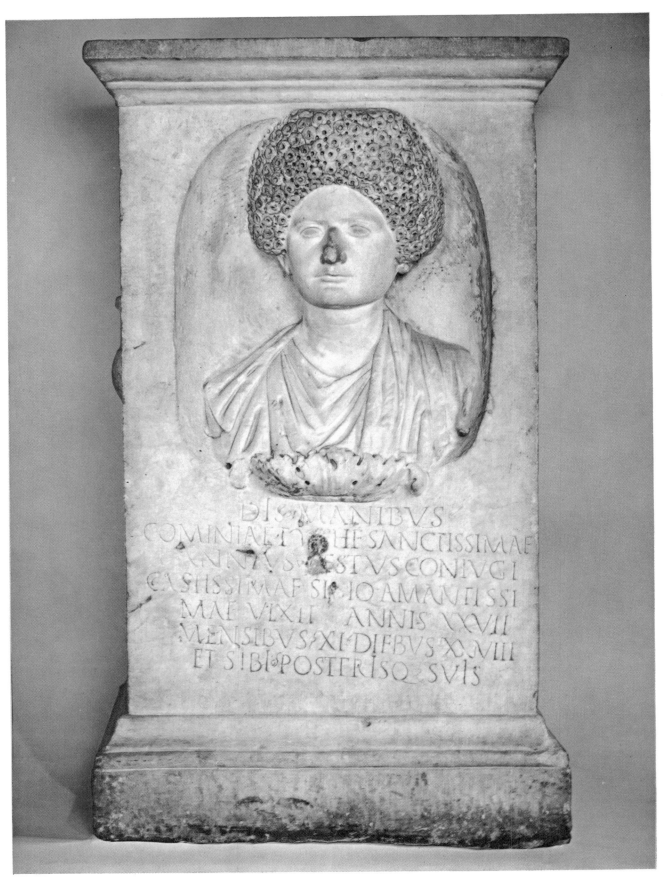

ROMAN TOMBSTONE from the first century A.D. records the death of Cominia Tyche, aged 27 years, 11 months, 28 days. Tombstones are a source of information on life expectancy in the ancient world. Stone is in the Metropolitan Museum of Art in New York.

The Human Population

25

Edward S. Deevey, Jr.
September 1960

In the short span of his existence man has come to consume more food than all other land animals put together. This raises the question of how many men the earth can support

Almost until the present turn in human affairs an expanding population has been equated with progress. "Increase and multiply" is the Scriptural injunction. The number of surviving offspring is the measure of fitness in natural selection. If number is the criterion, the human species is making great progress. The population, now passing 2.7 billion, is doubling itself every 50 years or so. To some horrified observers, however, the population increase has become a "population explosion." The present rate of increase, they point out, is itself increasing. At 1 per cent per year it is double that of the past few centuries. By A.D. 2000, even according to the "medium" estimate of the careful demographers of the United Nations, the rate of increase will have accelerated to 3 per cent per year, and the total population will have reached 6.267 billion. If Thomas Malthus's assumption of a uniform rate of doubling is naive, because it so quickly leads to impossible numbers, how long can an accelerating annual increase, say from 1 to 3 per cent in 40 years, be maintained? The demographers confronted with this question lower their eyes: "It would be absurd," they say, "to carry detailed calculations forward into a more remote future. It is most debatable whether the trends in mortality and fertility can continue much longer. Other factors may eventually bring population growth to a halt."

So they may, and must. It comes to this: Explosions are not made by force alone, but by force that exceeds restraint. Before accepting the implications of the population explosion, it is well to set the present in the context of the record of earlier human populations. As will be seen, the population curve has moved upward stepwise in response to the three major revolutions that have marked the evolution of culture [*see bottom illustration on page 248*]. The tool-using and toolmaking revolution that started the growth of the human stem from the primate line gave the food-gatherer and hunter access to the widest range of environments. Nowhere was the population large, but over the earth as a whole it reached the not insignificant total of five million, an average of .04 person per square kilometer (.1 person per square mile) of land. With the agricultural revolution the population moved up two orders of magnitude to a new plateau, multiplying 100 times in the short span of 8,000 years, to an average of one person per square kilometer. The increase over the last 300 years, a multiplication by five, plainly reflects the first repercussions of the scientific-industrial revolution. There are now 16.4 persons per square kilometer of the earth's land area. It is thus the release of restraint that the curve portrays at three epochal points in cultural history.

But the evolution of the population size also indicates the approach to equilibrium in the two interrevolutionary periods of the past. At what level will the present surge of numbers reach equilibrium? That is again a question of restraint, whether it is to be imposed by the limitations of man's new command over his environment or by his command over his own nature.

The human generative force is neither new nor metabiological, nor is it especially strong in man as compared to other animals. Under conditions of maximal increase in a suitable environment empty of competitors, with births at maximum and deaths negligible, rats can multiply their numbers 25 times in an average generation-time of 31 weeks. For the water flea *Daphnia*, beloved by ecologists for the speedy answers it gives, the figures are 221 times in a generation of 6.8 days. Mankind's best efforts seem puny by contrast: multiplication by about 1.4 times in a generation of 28 years. Yet neither in human nor in experimental populations do such rates continue unchecked. Sooner or later the births slow down and the deaths increase, until—in experiments, at any rate—the growth tapers off, and the population effectively saturates its space. Ecologists define this state (of zero rate of change) as equilibrium, without denying the possibility of oscillations that average out to zero, and without forgetting the continuous input of energy (food, for instance) that is needed to maintain the system.

Two kinds of check, then, operate to limit the size of a population, or of any living thing that grows. Obviously the environment (amount of space, food or other needed resources) sets the upper limit; sometimes this is manipulable, even by the population itself, as when it exploits a new kind of food in the same old space, and reaches a new, higher limit. More subtly, populations can be said to limit their own rates of increase. As the numbers rise, female fruit-flies, for example, lay fewer eggs when jostled by their sisters; some microorganisms battle each other with antibiotics; flour beetles accidentally eat their own defenseless eggs and pupae; infectious diseases spread faster, or become more virulent, as their hosts become more numerous. For human populations pestilence and warfare, Malthus's "natural restraints," belong among these devices for self-limitation. So, too, does his "moral restraint," or voluntary birth control. Nowadays a good deal of attention is being given, not only to voluntary methods,

YEARS AGO	CULTURAL STAGE	AREA POPULATED	ASSUMED DENSITY PER SQUARE KILOMETER	TOTAL POPULATION (MILLIONS)
1,000,000	LOWER PALEOLITHIC		.00425	.125
300,000	MIDDLE PALEOLITHIC		.012	1
25,000	UPPER PALEOLITHIC		.04	3.34
10,000	MESOLITHIC		.04	5.32
6,000	VILLAGE FARMING AND EARLY URBAN		1.0 .04	86.5
2,000	VILLAGE FARMING AND URBAN		1.0	133
310	FARMING AND INDUSTRIAL		3.7	545
210	FARMING AND INDUSTRIAL		4.9	728
160	FARMING AND INDUSTRIAL		6.2	906
60	FARMING AND INDUSTRIAL		11.0	1,610
10	FARMING AND INDUSTRIAL		16.4	2,400
A.D. 2000	FARMING AND INDUSTRIAL		46.0	6,270

but also to a fascinating new possibility: mental stress.

Population control by means of personality derangement is probably a vertebrate patent; at least it seems a luxury beyond the reach of a water flea. The general idea, as current among students of small mammals, is that of hormonal imbalance (or stress, as defined by Hans Selye of the University of Montreal); psychic tension, resulting from overcrowding, disturbs the pituitary-adrenal system and diverts or suppresses the hormones governing sexuality and parental care. Most of the evidence comes from somewhat artificial experiments with caged rodents. It is possible, though the case is far from proved, that the lemming's famous mechanism for restoring equilibrium is the product of stress; in experimental populations of rats and mice, at least, anxiety has been observed to increase the death rate through fighting or merely from shock.

From this viewpoint there emerges an interesting distinction between crowding and overcrowding among vertebrates; overcrowding is what is perceived as such by members of the population. Since the human rate of increase is holding its own and even accelerating, however, it is plain that the mass of men, although increasingly afflicted with mental discomfort, do not yet see themselves as overcrowded. What will happen in the future brings other questions. For the present it may be noted that some kind of check has always operated, up to now, to prevent populations from ex-

POPULATION GROWTH, from inception of the hominid line one million years ago through the different stages of cultural evolution to A.D. 2000, is shown in the chart on the opposite page. In Lower Paleolithic stage, population was restricted to Africa (*colored area on world map in third column*), with a density of only .00425 person per square kilometer (*fourth column*) and a total population of only 125,000 (*column at right*). By the Mesolithic stage, 10,000 years ago, hunting and food gathering techniques had spread the population over most of the earth and brought the total to 5,320,-000. In the village farming and early urban stage, population increased to a total of 86,500,000 and a density of one person per square kilometer in the Old World and .04 per square kilometer in the New World. Today the population density exceeds 16 persons per square kilometer, and pioneering of the antarctic continent has begun.

ceeding the space that contains them. Of course space may be non-Euclidean, and man may be exempt from this law.

The commonly accepted picture of the growth of the population out of the long past takes the form of the top graph on the next page. Two things are wrong with this picture. In the first place the basis of estimates, back of about A.D. 1650, is rarely stated. One suspects that writers have been copying each other's guesses. The second defect is that the scales of the graph have been chosen so as to make the first defect seem unimportant. The missile has left the pad and is heading out of sight—so it is said; who cares whether there were a million or a hundred million people around when Babylon was founded? The difference is nearly lost in the thickness of the draftsman's line.

I cannot think it unimportant that (as I calculate) there were 36 billion Paleolithic hunters and gatherers, including the first tool-using hominids. One begins to see why stone tools are among the commonest Pleistocene fossils. Another 30 billion may have walked the earth before the invention of agriculture. A cumulative total of about 110 billion individuals seem to have passed their days, and left their bones, if not their marks, on this crowded planet. Neither for our understanding of culture nor in terms of man's impact upon the land is it a negligible consideration that the patch of ground allotted to every person now alive may have been the lifetime habitat of 40 predecessors.

These calculations exaggerate the truth in a different way: by condensing into single sums the enormous length of prehistoric time. To arrive at the total of 36 billion Paleolithic hunters and gatherers I have assumed mean standing populations of half a million for the Lower Paleolithic, and two million for the Middle and Upper Paleolithic to 25,000 years ago. For Paleolithic times there are no archeological records worth considering in such calculations. I have used some figures for modern hunting tribes, quoted by Robert J. Braidwood and Charles A. Reed, though they are not guilty of my extrapolations. The assumed densities per square kilometer range from a tenth to a third of those estimated for eastern North America before Columbus came, when an observer would hardly have described the woods as full of Indians. (Of course I have excluded any New World population from my estimates prior to the Mesolithic climax of the food-gathering and hunting phase of cultural evolution.) It is only

because average generations of 25 years succeeded each other 39,000 times that the total looms so large.

For my estimates as of the opening of the agricultural revolution, I have also depended upon Braidwood and Reed. In their work in Mesopotamia they have counted the number of rooms in buried houses, allowing for the areas of town sites and of cultivated land, and have compared the populations so computed with modern counterparts. For early village-farmers, like those at Jarmo, and for the urban citizens of Sumer, about 2500 B.C., their estimates (9.7 and 15.4 persons per square kilometer) are probably fairly close. They are intended to apply to large tracts of inhabited country, not to pavement-bound clusters of artisans and priests. Nevertheless, in extending these estimates to continent-wide areas, I have divided the lower figure by 10, making it one per square kilometer. So much of Asia is unirrigated and nonurban even today that the figure may still be too high. But the Maya, at about the same level of culture (3,000 or 4,000 years later), provide a useful standard of comparison. The present population of their classic homeland averages .6 per square kilometer, but the land can support a population about a hundred times as large, and probably did at the time of the classic climax. The rest of the New World, outside Middle America, was (and is) more thinly settled, but a world-wide average of one per square kilometer seems reasonable for agricultural, pre-industrial society.

For modern populations, from A.D. 1650 on, I have taken the estimates of economic historians, given in such books as the treatise *World Population and Production*, by Wladimir S. and Emma S. Woytinsky. All these estimates are included in the bottom graph on the next page. Logarithmic scales are used in order to compress so many people and millennia onto a single page. Foreshortening time in this way is convenient, if not particularly logical, and back of 50,000 years ago the time-scale is pretty arbitrary anyway. No attempt is made to show the oscillations that probably occurred, in glacial and interglacial ages, for example.

The stepwise evolution of population size, entirely concealed in graphs with arithmetic scales, is the most noticeable feature of this diagram. For most of the million-year period the number of hominids, including man, was about what would be expected of any large Pleistocene mammal—scarcer than horses, say, but commoner than elephants. Intellectual superiority was simply a successful adaptation, like longer legs; essential to stay in the running, of course, but making man at best the first among equals. Then the food-gatherers and hunters became plowmen and herdsmen, and the population was boosted by about 16 times, between 10,-000 and 6,000 years ago. The scientific-industrial revolution, beginning some 300 years ago, has spread its effects much faster, but it has not yet taken the number as far above the earlier base line.

The long-term population equilibrium implied by such base lines suggests

something else. Some kind of restraint kept the number fairly stable. "Food supply" offers a quick answer, but not, I think, the correct one. At any rate, a forest is full of game for an expert mouse-hunter, and a Paleolithic man who stuck to business should have found enough food on two square kilometers, instead of 20 or 200. Social forces were probably more powerful than mere starvation in causing men to huddle in small bands. Besides, the number was presumably adjusted to conditions in the poorest years, and not to average environments.

The main point is that there were ad-

justments. They can only have come about because the average female bore two children who survived to reproduce. If the average life span is 25 years, the "number of children ever born" is about four (because about 50 per cent die before breeding), whereas a population that is really trying can average close to eight. Looking back on former times, then, from our modern point of view, we might say that about two births out of four were surplus, though they were needed to counterbalance the juvenile death toll. But what about the other four, which evidently did not occur? Unless the life expectancy was very much less

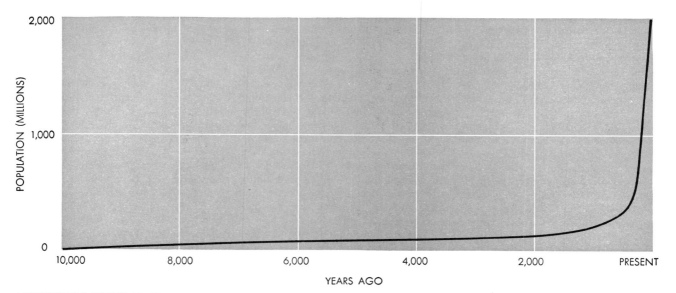

ARITHMETIC POPULATION CURVE plots the growth of human population from 10,000 years ago to the present. Such a curve suggests that the population figure remained close to the base line for an indefinite period from the remote past to about 500 years ago, and that it has surged abruptly during the last 500 years as a result of the scientific-industrial revolution.

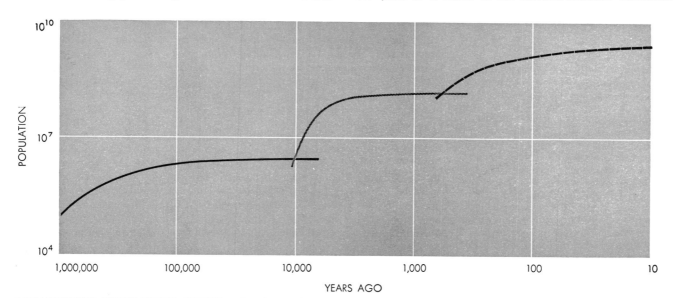

LOGARITHMIC POPULATION CURVE makes it possible to plot, in a small space, the growth of population over a longer period of time and over a wider range (from 10^4, or 10,000, to 10^{10}, or 10 billion, persons). Curve, based on assumptions concerning relationship of technology and population as shown in chart on page 4, reveals three population surges reflecting toolmaking or cultural revolution (solid line), agricultural revolution (gray line) and scientific-industrial revolution (broken line).

than I have assumed (and will presently justify), some degree of voluntary birth control has always prevailed.

Our 40 predecessors on earth make an impressive total, but somehow it sounds different to say that nearly 3 per cent of the people who have ever lived are still around. When we realize that they are living twice as long as their parents did, we are less inclined to discount the revolution in which we are living. One of its effects has just begun to be felt: The mean age of the population is increasing all over the world. Among the more forgivable results of Western culture, when introduced into simpler societies, is a steep drop in the death rate. Public-health authorities are fond of citing Ceylon in this connection. In a period of a year during 1946 and 1947 a campaign against malaria reduced the death rate there from 20 to 14 per 1,000. Eventually the birth rate falls too, but not so fast, nor has it yet fallen so far as a bare replacement value. The natural outcome of this imbalance is that acceleration of annual increase which so bemuses demographers. In the long run it must prove to be temporary, unless the birth rate accelerates, for the deaths that are being systematically prevented are premature ones. That is, the infants who now survive diphtheria and measles are certain to die of something else later on, and while the mean lifespan is approaching the maximum, for the first time in history, there is no reason to think that the maximum itself has been stretched. Meanwhile the expectation of life at birth is rising daily in most countries, so that it has already surpassed 70 years in some, including the U. S., and probably averages between 40 and 50.

It is hard to be certain of any such world-wide figure. The countries where mortality is heaviest are those with the least accurate records. In principle, however, mean age at death is easier to find out than the number of children born, the frequency or mean age at marriage, or any other component of a birth rate. The dead bones, the court and parish records and the tombstones that archeology deals with have something to say about death, of populations as well as of people. Their testimony confirms the impression that threescore years and ten, if taken as an average and not as a maximum lifetime, is something decidedly new. Of course the possibilities of bias in such evidence are almost endless. For instance, military cemeteries tend to be full of young adult males. The hardest bias to allow for is the deficiency of in-

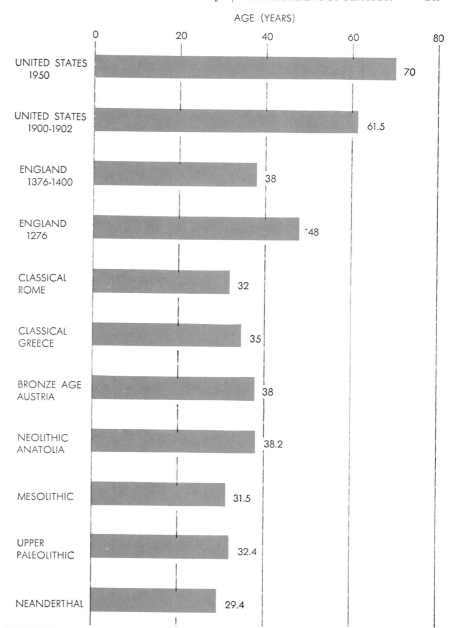

LONGEVITY in ancient and modern times is charted. From time of Neanderthal man to 14th century A.D., life span appears to have hovered around 35 years. An exception is 13th-century England. Increase in longevity partly responsible for current population increase has come in modern era. In U.S. longevity increased about 10 years in last half-century.

fants and children; juvenile bones are less durable than those of adults, and are often treated less respectfully. Probably we shall never know the true expectation of life at birth for any ancient people. Bypassing this difficulty, we can look at the mean age at death among the fraction surviving to adolescence.

The "nasty, brutish and short" lives of Neanderthal people have been rather elaborately guessed at 29.4 years. The record, beyond them, is not one of steady improvement. For example, Neolithic farmers in Anatolia and Bronze Age Austrians averaged 38 years, and even the

Mesolithic savages managed more than 30. But in the golden ages of Greece and Rome the life span was 35 years or less. During the Middle Ages the chances of long life were probably no better. The important thing about these averages is not the differences among them, but their similarity. Remembering the crudeness of the estimates, and the fact that juvenile mortality is omitted, it is fair to guess that human life-expectancy at birth has never been far from 25 years— 25 plus or minus five, say—from Neanderthal times up to the present century. It follows, as I have said, that about half

250

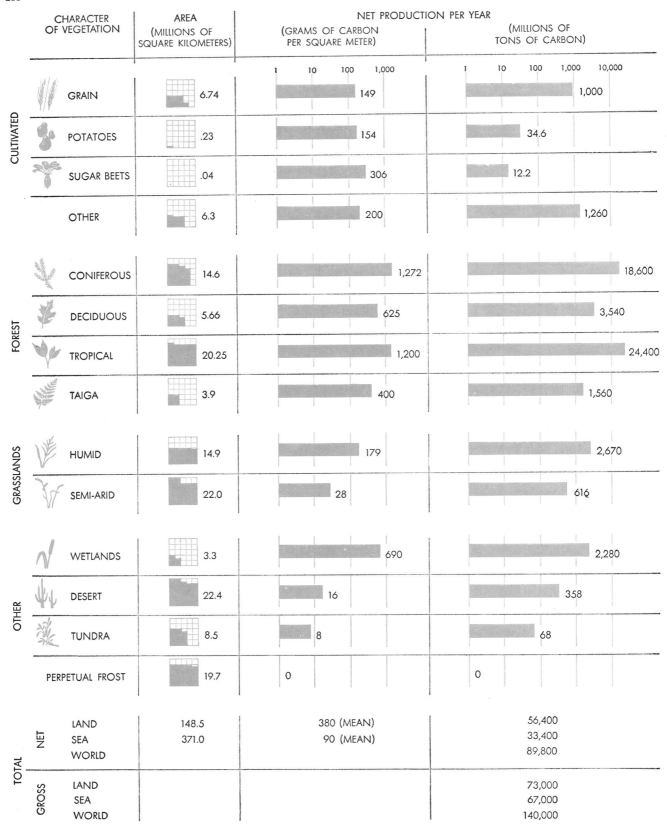

CHARACTER OF VEGETATION		AREA (MILLIONS OF SQUARE KILOMETERS)	NET PRODUCTION PER YEAR	
			(GRAMS OF CARBON PER SQUARE METER)	(MILLIONS OF TONS OF CARBON)
CULTIVATED	GRAIN	6.74	149	1,000
	POTATOES	.23	154	34.6
	SUGAR BEETS	.04	306	12.2
	OTHER	6.3	200	1,260
FOREST	CONIFEROUS	14.6	1,272	18,600
	DECIDUOUS	5.66	625	3,540
	TROPICAL	20.25	1,200	24,400
	TAIGA	3.9	400	1,560
GRASSLANDS	HUMID	14.9	179	2,670
	SEMI-ARID	22.0	28	616
OTHER	WETLANDS	3.3	690	2,280
	DESERT	22.4	16	358
	TUNDRA	8.5	8	68
	PERPETUAL FROST	19.7	0	0
TOTAL NET	LAND	148.5	380 (MEAN)	56,400
	SEA	371.0	90 (MEAN)	33,400
	WORLD			89,800
TOTAL GROSS	LAND			73,000
	SEA			67,000
	WORLD			140,000

PRODUCTION OF ORGANIC MATTER per year by the land vegetation of the world—and thus its ultimate food-producing capacity—is charted in terms of the amount of carbon incorporated in organic compounds. Cultivated vegetation (*top left*) is less efficient than forest and wetlands vegetation, as indicated by the uptake of carbon per square meter (*third column*), and it yields a smaller over-all output than forest, humid grasslands and wetlands vegetation (*fourth column*). The scales at top of third and fourth columns are logarithmic. Land vegetation leads sea vegetation in efficiency and in net and gross tonnage (*bottom*). The difference between the net production and gross production is accounted for by the consumption of carbon in plant respiration.

the children ever born have lived to become sexually mature. It is not hard to see why an average family size of four or more, or twice the minimum replacement rate, has come to seem part of a God-given scheme of things.

The 25-fold upsurge in the number of men between 10,000 and 2,000 years ago was sparked by a genuine increase in the means of subsistence. A shift from animal to plant food, even without agricultural labor and ingenuity, would practically guarantee a 10-fold increase, for a given area can usually produce about 10 times as much plant as animal substance. The scientific-industrial revolution has increased the efficiency of growing these foods, but hardly, as yet, beyond the point needed to support another 10 times as many people, fewer of whom are farmers. At the present rate of multiplication, without acceleration, another 10-fold rise is due within 230 years. Disregarding the fact that developed societies spend 30 to 60 times as much energy for other purposes as they need for food, one is made a little nervous by the thought of so many hungry mouths. Can the increase of efficiency keep pace? Can some of the apparently ample energy be converted to food as needed, perhaps at the cost of reducing the size of Sunday newspapers? Or is man now pressing so hard on his food supply that another 10-fold increase of numbers is impossible?

The answers to these questions are not easy to find, and students with different viewpoints disagree about them. Richard L. Meier of the University of Michigan estimates that a total of 50 billion people (a 20-fold increase, that is) can be supported on earth, and the geochemist Harrison Brown of the California Institute of Technology will allow (reluctantly) twice or four times as many. Some economists are even more optimistic; Arnold C. Harberger of the University of Chicago presents the interesting notion that a larger crop of people will contain more geniuses, whose intellects will find a solution to the problem of feeding *still* more people. And the British economist Colin Clark points out that competition for resources will sharpen everyone's wits, as it always has, even if the level of innate intelligence is not raised.

An ecologist's answer is bound to be cast in terms of solar energy, chlorophyll and the amount of land on which the two can interact to produce organic carbon. Sources of energy other than the sun are either too expensive, or nonrenewable or both. Land areas will continue for a very long time to be the places where food is grown, for the sea is not so productive as the land, on the average. One reason, sometimes forgotten, is that the plants of the sea are microscopic algae, which, being smaller than land plants, respire away a larger fraction of the carbon they fix. The culture of the fresh-water alga *Chlorella* has undeniable promise as a source of human food. But the high efficiencies quoted for its photosynthesis, as compared with agricultural plants, are not sustained outdoors under field conditions. Even if Chlorella (or another exceptionally efficient producer, such as the water hyacinth) is the food plant of the future, flat areas exposed to sunlight will be needed. The 148.5 million square kilometers of land will have to be used with thoughtful care if the human population is to increase 20-fold. With a population of 400 per square kilometer (50 billion total) it would seem that men's bodies, if not their artifacts, will stand in the way of vital sunshine.

Plants capture the solar energy impinging on a given area with an efficiency of about .1 per cent. (Higher values often quoted are based on some fraction of the total radiation, such as visible light.) Herbivores capture about a 10th of the plants' energy, and carnivores convert about 10 per cent of the energy captured by herbivores (or other carnivores). This means, of course, that carnivores, feeding on plants at second hand, can scarcely do so with better than 1 per cent efficiency ($1/10 \times 1/10$ equals $1/100$). Eugene I. Rabinowitch of the University of Illinois has calculated that the current crop of men represents an ultimate conversion of about 1 per cent of the energy trapped by land vegetation. Recently, however, I have re-examined the base figure—the efficiency of the land-plant production—and believe it should be raised by a factor of three or four. The old value came from estimates made in 1919 and in 1937. A good deal has been learned since those days. The biggest surprise is the high productivity of forests, especially the forests of the Temperate Zone.

If my new figures are correct, the population could theoretically increase by 30 or 40 times. But man would have to displace all other herbivores and utilize all the vegetation with the 10 per cent efficiency established by the ecological rule of tithes. No land that now supports greenery could be spared for nonagricultural purposes; the populace would have to reside in the polar regions, or on artificial "green isles in the sea, love"—scummed over, of course, by 10 inches of Chlorella culture.

The picture is doubtless overdrawn. There is plenty of room for improvement in present farming practice. More land could be brought under cultivation if a better distribution of water could be arranged. More efficient basic crops can be grown and used less wastefully. Other sources of energy, notably atomic energy, can be fed back into food production to supplement the sun's rays. None of these measures is more than palliative, however; none promises so much as a 10-fold increase in efficiency; worse, none is likely to be achieved at a pace equivalent to the present rate of doubling of the world's population. A 10-fold, even a 20-fold, increase can be tolerated, perhaps, but the standard of living seems certain to be lower than today's. What happens then, when men perceive themselves to be overcrowded?

The idea of population equilibrium will take some getting used to. A population that is kept stable by emigration, like that of the Western Islands of Scotland, is widely regarded as sick—a shining example of a self-fulfilling diagnosis. Since the fall of the death rate is temporary, it is those two or more extra births per female that demand attention. The experiments with crowded rodents point to one way they might be corrected, through the effect of anxiety in suppressing ovulation and spermatogenesis and inducing fetal resorption. Some of the most dramatic results are delayed until after birth: litters are carelessly nursed, deserted or even eaten. Since fetuses, too, have endocrine glands, the specter of maternal transmission of anxiety now looms: W. R. Thompson of Wesleyan University has shown that the offspring of frustrated mother mice are more "emotional" throughout their own lives, and my student Kim Keeley has confirmed this.

Considered abstractly, these devices for self-regulation compel admiration for their elegance. But there is a neater device that men can use: rational, voluntary control over numbers. In mentioning the dire effects of psychic stress I am not implying that the population explosion will be contained by cannibalism or fetal resorption, or any power so naked. I simply suggest that vertebrates have that power, whether they want it or not, as part of the benefit—and the price—of being vertebrates. And if the human method of adjusting numbers to resources fails to work in the next 1,000 years as it has in the last million, subhuman methods are ready to take over.

26

Orthodox and Unorthodox Methods of Meeting World Food Needs

N. W. Pirie
February 1967

*The orthodox methods must be pressed, but it seems
they cannot solve the problem without the aid of the
unorthodox ones. And the adoption of unorthodox
methods calls for basic changes in cultural attitudes*

The world has been familiar with famine throughout recorded history. Until the present century some people have been hungry all the time and all the people have been hungry some of the time. Now a few industrialized countries have managed, by a mixture of luck, skill and cunning, to break loose from the traditional pattern and establish systems in which most of the population can expect to go through life without knowing hunger. Instead their food problems are overnutrition (about which much is now being written) and malnutrition. Malnutrition appears when the food eaten is supplying enough energy, or even too much, but is deficient in some components of a satisfactory diet. Its presence continually and on a large scale is a technical triumph of which primitive man was incapable because he lacked the skill to process the food he gathered in a manner that would remove some of the essential components but leave it palatable and pleasing in appearance. Furthermore, until the development of agriculture few foods contained the excess carbohydrate that characterizes much of the world's food today. The right policy in technically skilled countries, however, is not to try to "go back to nature" and eat crude foods. Processing does good as well as harm. What we now need is widespread knowledge of the principles of nutrition and enough good sense to use our technical skill prudently.

It is salutary to remember how recently this pattern was established. There was some hunger in Britain 50 years ago and much hunger 50 years before that. Still earlier many settlements in now well-fed regions of Australia and the U.S. had to be abandoned because of starvation. It is said that scurvy killed about 10,000 "forty-niners," and California was the scene of some of the classic descriptions of the disease. One has to learn how to live and farm in each new region; it cannot be assumed that methods that are successful in one country will work elsewhere. It is therefore probable that methods will be found for making the currently ill-fed regions productive and self-sufficient. The search for them should be started immediately and should be conducted without too much regard for traditional methods and preconceptions.

The problem can be simply stated: How can human affairs be managed so that the whole world can enjoy the degree of freedom from hunger that the industrialized countries now have?

It is well known that in many parts of the world not only is there a food shortage but also the population is increasing rapidly. Some of the reasons for this situation are fairly easy to establish. When the conditions of life change slowly, compensating changes can keep pace with them. In Europe during the 16th century half of the children probably never reached the age of five. There are no general statistics for this period, but in the 17th century 22 out of the 32 British royal children (from James I to Anne) died before they were 21, and it is unlikely that the poor fared better than royalty. The establishment of our present standards of infant mortality had little to do with medical knowledge. Until this century the farther away one could keep from doctors, except for the treatment of physical injury, the better. It was increasing technical skill in bringing in clean water and getting rid of sewage that made communities healthy, and this skill was applied by people who had never heard of germs or, like Florence Nightingale, disbelieved what they were told. But the change came slowly enough for families to adjust the birthrate to suit the new conditions. Moreover, there was incompletely filled land to be used. What René Dubos calls the "population avalanche" is on us because it is now possible to undertake public health measures on a larger scale and finish them quicker than heretofore.

254

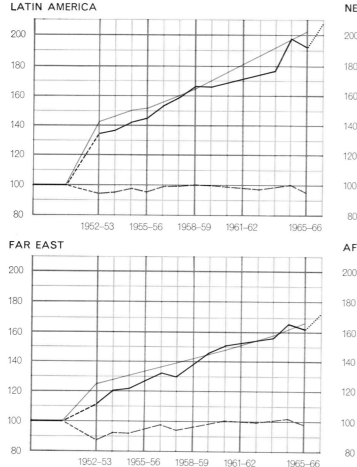

LATIN AMERICA

NEAR EAST

FAR EAST

AFRICA

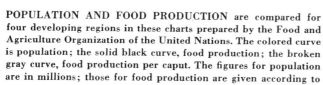

POPULATION AND FOOD PRODUCTION are compared for four developing regions in these charts prepared by the Food and Agriculture Organization of the United Nations. The colored curve is population; the solid black curve, food production; the broken gray curve, food production per caput. The figures for population are in millions; those for food production are given according to an index of 100 for the prewar average. The food production figures for 1965–1966 (July 15, 1965, to July 15, 1966) show the effects of adverse weather in many parts of the world. In that period world food production per caput fell 2 percent. The dots at end of food production curve show increase required to regain per caput level of 1964–1965. Mainland China is not represented in Far East figures.

Once the principles are understood the hygiene of an area can be improved quickly by a few people, and the population as a whole gets the advantage of improved health without having to take any very active steps to achieve it. Even where methods for improving conventional agriculture are known their application is of necessity slower, because it depends on a change in the outlook of most of the people in a farming community rather than in the outlook of the few who control water and sewage. Furthermore, fecundity is potentially unlimited but food production is not. Clearly, therefore, the "avalanche" will have to be stopped. It is important to remember, however, that it cannot be stopped in any noncoercive way without the cooperation of the people; that means more education, which means more hygiene and so, at least for a time, a still greater increase in the population. The

first result of an effective campaign for contraception will be an increase in population rather than a diminution. More effort should be put into the encouragement of contraception. And more research is needed on improved methods, leading to the ideal: that people should have to do something positive to reverse a normal state of infertility, so that no conception would be inadvertent. This, however, is a complement to, and not a substitute for, work on the production of more food. Strained as existing supplies are, it seems inevitable that they will be strained still further during the next half-century. After that the entire world may have established the population equilibrium that now exists in some industrialized countries.

The normal humane reaction in the presence of misery is pity, and this reaction is followed, where appropriate,

by charity. Hence the immense effort that is now being put into shipping the food surpluses, accumulated in some parts of the world, to areas of need. This is commendable and spiritually satisfying to the donor, but for two reasons it has little effect on the real problem. The amount of surplus food is not large enough to make much of a dent in the world's present need. The surplus could be increased, but the logistic problem of shipping still greater quantities of food would be formidable. The more serious objection to charity, except during temporary periods of crisis, is that it discourages the recipient. A century ago the philanthropist Edward Denison remarked: "Every shilling I give away does fourpence worth of good by keeping the recipients' miserable bodies alive and eightpence worth of harm by helping to destroy their miserable souls." Nearly 1,000 years ago Maimonides categorized the forms of charity and concluded that the most commendable form was to act in such a way that charity would become unnecessary.

Trade is the obvious alternative to charity. Unfortunately the developing countries are in a poor bargaining position. Since 1957 the prices paid for their primary products declined so much that the industrialized countries made a saving of $7,000 million and an extra profit of $3,000 million because of the increased cost of manufactured goods. The developing countries thus lost $10,000 million—about the same as the total "aid" they received from commercial, private and international sources. (The figures are from the *Financial Times* of London for July 19, 1965.) With the market rigged against them in this way it is not likely that they will soon be able to buy their food as countries such as Britain do. At present the industrialized countries are exporting about 30 million tons of grain a year, largely against credit. It is unlikely that this state of affairs can last; half of the world cannot permanently feed the other half.

The idea that the developing parts of the world should be fed by either charity or trade depends on the assumption that they are in some way unsuited for adequate food production. This idea is baseless. Once the methods have been devised, food can be produced in most places where there is sunlight and water; for political stability food must be produced where the mouths are. Any country dependent on imports for its main foodstuffs is to some extent controlled by others.

The problem can be more narrowly stated: How to produce enough food in the more populous parts of the world?

Food production can and will be increased in many orthodox ways. There is still some uncultivated but cultivable land, irrigation and drainage can be improved and extended, fertilizers can be used on a much greater scale and the general level of farming technique can be improved. If all the farmers in a region were as skilled as the best 10 percent of them, there would probably be enough food for everyone today. These improvements could be achieved by vigorous government action and without further research.

In the Temperate Zone plant breeders have greatly increased cereal yields during the past 20 years, and these improved varieties could be used more widely. There have been no comparable developments with food crops in the Tropical Zone, but there is no reason

to think that progress there could not be equally spectacular. This research should not be limited to cereals. In many parts of the wet Tropics yams (*Dioscoria* and *Colocasia*) are staple foods but the varieties used contain little protein. There is, however, some evidence that the protein content of yams varies; a New Guinea variety called Wundunggul contains 2.5 percent nitrogen. If this nitrogen is all in protein, the yam contains 15 percent protein and is worthy of serious study.

It is generally agreed that pests and

diseases rob us of as much as a third of our crops. When the improvements outlined above have been made, the proportional loss as well as the absolute one could become greater, since wellnourished crops, growing uniformly in large fields, are particularly susceptible. The cost of treatment may be only a tenth of the value of the crop saved; the methods are well publicized by firms making pesticides. There is no need to labor this aspect of the problem here. More attention should, however, be given to losses during storage; the need for

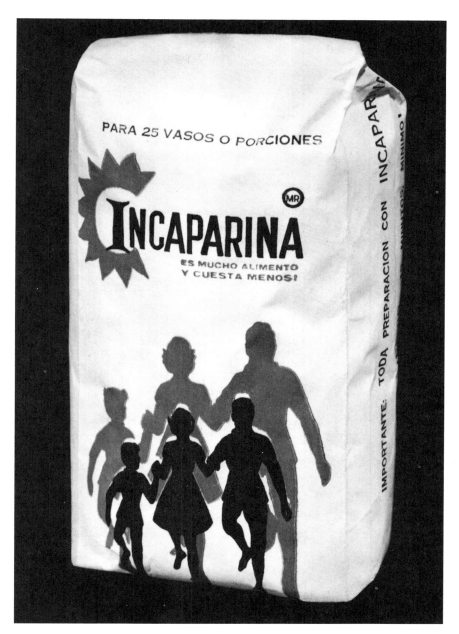

SYNTHETIC FOOD is represented by Incaparina, made of maize, sorghum and cottonseed by the Quaker Oats Company. The product has been skillfully promoted by Quaker Oats in Central America. The Spanish words at the top of this 500-gram package mean: "For 25 glasses or portions." Those below "Incaparina" mean: "It is very nourishing and costs little."

satisfactory storage techniques for use in primitive conditions is especially acute. So much mystical nonsense has been written by believers in the merits of "natural" foods that most scientists show understandable impatience at the idea that pesticide residues may be harmful to the ultimate consumer of the protected crop. Furthermore, a food shortage may well do more harm to a community than sensibly applied pesticides can do. There is, nevertheless, great scope here for research on improved techniques.

There are such good prospects that productivity can be increased by each, or even all, of these methods if they are assiduously developed that it seems to many experts that there is no immediate need for any more radical approach to the problem of world feeding. This is the attitude of the United Nations Food and Agriculture Organization (F.A.O.). One cannot praise too highly its work in compiling statistics and persistently calling attention to the need for agricultural improvements. On the other hand, while recognizing that the F.A.O. is not a research organization, one can deplore its equally persistent tendency to denigrate every unorthodox approach to the problem. History may partly excuse this attitude. Ever since the time of Malthus prophets have been making our flesh creep with warnings of impending famine. Conditions have remained much the same—or have improved. These prophecies remain unfulfilled because 400 years of explora-

tion enabled new land to be cultivated, 200 years of biological research laid the foundation for scientific agriculture, and 50 years of rational chemistry made it possible to produce fertilizers by fixing the nitrogen of the air. The cautious prophet should therefore not say that hunger is inevitable but that it is probable unless the relevant research is done on an adequate scale. The time to do it is now, before the need has become more acute.

The main product of agriculture is carbohydrate. The foods that make up the world's diet—the cereals, potatoes, yams, cassava and so on—are from 1 to 12 percent protein on the basis of dry weight. An adult man needs 14 percent protein in his food; children and pregnant or lactating women need from 16 to 20 percent. However great an increase there may be in the consumption of conventional bulk foods, there will be a protein deficit. Moreover, it will be exacerbated if food is made palatable by the addition of fats and sugar, which give energy but contain no protein. Too much stress cannot be laid on the fact that the percentage of protein in a diet is the vital thing; increased consumption of low-protein food makes the consumer fat but as malnourished as before.

Recognition of the importance of protein sources, and their deficiency in most of the world's diet, has come slowly. It is nonetheless gathering momentum. Fifteen years ago little attention was paid to protein sources by international agencies and gatherings such as the International Nutrition Congress. Now protein

is one of the main themes. Audiences at these gatherings are a step ahead of the management. At the International Congress of Food Science and Technology last year, for example, the session "Novel Protein Sources" proved more popular than those who had allocated the rooms had foreseen; that session was more uncomfortably overcrowded than any other. The remainder of this article will be exclusively concerned with protein. All the components of a diet are needed, but the need for protein will be the most difficult to meet.

Animal products—meat, milk, cheese, eggs, fish—are widely esteemed and are used as protein concentrates to improve diets that are otherwise mainly carbohydrate. About a third of the world's cattle population is in Africa and India; most of these animals are relatively unproductive and are maintained largely for reasons of prestige and religion. It is easy to sidestep the main problem and argue that the protein shortage in these countries could be ameliorated, even if it could not be abolished, if herds were culled and the remainder made fully productive. The more thoughtful Africans and Indians realize this, and the situation will doubtless change. But every community tends to devote an amount of effort to nonproductive activity that seems to outsiders unreasonable. In the Middle Ages cathedrals were built by people who lived in hovels, and we now spend more on space research than on research in agriculture and medicine. Change is inevitable, and contemporary forms of religious observance and prestige are certain to be modified; the transition will not be hastened by nagging from outside.

According to most forecasters, the need to grow crops on land now used to maintain animals will lead to a decline in meat consumption in industrial countries, and the essential disappearance of meat is sometimes predicted. Although the decline is probable, the disappearance is not. There is much land that is suitable for grazing but not for tillage. Furthermore, there will always be a great deal of plant residue that (perhaps after supplementation with urea) can be more conveniently used as animal feed than in any other way. It is by no means certain, however, that we will always use the ideal herbivore. There is good reason to think that several species of now wild herbivore, running together, give a greater return of human food in many areas of tropical bush or savanna than domesticated species [see "Wildlife Hus-

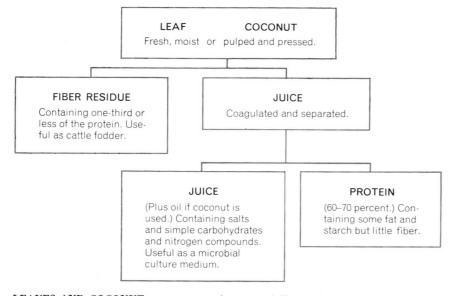

LEAVES AND COCONUT are a source of protein if fiber and juice are removed from them. This chart shows the steps of the process and also indicates the uses of by-products.

bandry in Africa," by F. Fraser Darling; SCIENTIFIC AMERICAN, November, 1960]. In addition, wild herbivores generally yield more protein per pound "on the hoof" than domestic species. These are matters that are being investigated by the International Biological Program. Even better results may be achieved after a few years of skilled breeding. Ruminants such as the antelope and the water buffalo are not the only species worthy of attention, and land is not the only site available for grazing. The capybara, a large rodent, is well adapted to South America and is palatable. Water weeds, and plants growing in swamps and on lake margins, contribute hardly anything to human nutrition. They could be collected and fed to land animals, but it would seem to be more efficient to domesticate the *Sirenia* (the freshwater manatee and the marine dugong) and use them as sources of meat. These herbivores are wholly aquatic and so, unlike semiaquatic species such as tapirs and hippopotamuses, do not compete for food with more familiar animals.

It is usual in articles such as this one to stress the importance of fish. This is admirable, but stress should not be allowed to drift into obsession. The more cautious forecasters estimate that the fish catch could be increased only two- or threefold without depleting stocks. Moreover, much of the world's population lives far from large bodies of water, and since fishing has an accident rate twice as high as coal mining it is likely to remain a relatively unattractive occupation. In the past decade the wet weight of fish caught annually increased from 29 million tons to 52 million, but the proportion used as human food decreased from 83 percent to 63. The remainder was used as fodder, mainly in the already well-fed countries. When still more fish are caught, the temptation to use a still larger proportion as fodder will be greater because much of the extra catch will consist of unfamiliar species. By grinding and solvent extraction these unfamiliar fishes can be turned into an edible product containing 80 percent protein. This process has suffered from every form of misfortune: the use of unsuitable solvents, commercial overstatement, excessive hygienic caution and political intrigue. It is nevertheless sound in principle and will do much to increase the amount of food protein made on an industrial scale and distributed through international channels.

One also hears of "fish farming." Activity that could properly be given this

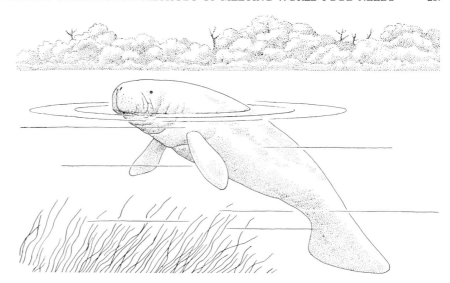

MANATEE, an aquatic mammal, is an example of an unorthodox source of meat. It can also control aquatic weeds, which it eats. An adult manatee is between nine and 15 feet long.

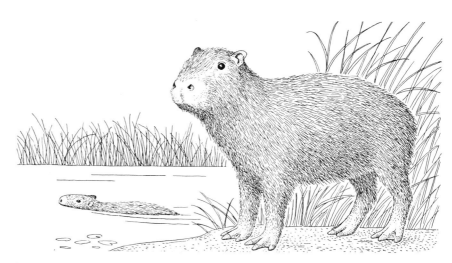

CAPYBARA, a large rodent that lives in South America, has also been suggested as a source of meat. Like the manatee, it feeds on aquatic weeds. An adult is about four feet long.

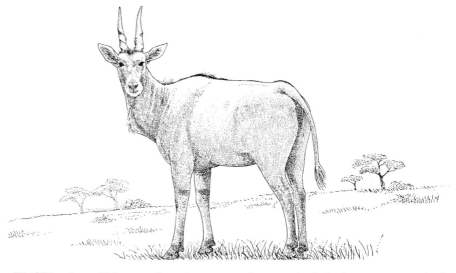

ELAND, a large African antelope, is an accepted meat animal. Its importance as a food source is that it is adapted to grazing on marginal lands that are not suited to agriculture.

title is possible in lagoons but unlikely in the oceans because fish move too freely, and fertilizer, intended to encourage the growth of their food, spreads too easily into the useless unlit depths. With mollusks and crustaceans, farming becomes much more promising and deserves more scientific attention than it gets. Food for such marine invertebrates does not seem to be the limiting factor; many of them can use the world's largest biological resource, the million million tons of organic matter in suspension in the sea. Sedentary mollusks are limited by predators and attachment sites. The predators could be controlled and the sites, with modern materials, could be increased.

Animals that live on something that we could not use as food—forage growing in rough country, straws and other residues, phytoplankton and other forms of marine organic matter—cannot properly be said to have a "conversion efficiency." We either use an animal converter or these materials are wasted. Efficiency has a real meaning when we consider animals that live either on crops that people could eat or on crops grown on land that could have grown food. The inefficiency of animal conversion, expressed as pounds of protein the animal must eat to make a pound of protein in the animal product that people eat, is much greater than is generally realized. This unawareness probably arises from the tendency among animal feeders to present their results as the ratio of the dry food eaten to the wet weight (including all inedible parts) of the carcass produced. Furthermore, the figures generally relate only to one phase of the animal's life, without allowance for unproductive periods. It is unlikely that the true efficiency of protein conversion is often greater than one pound of food protein for every seven pounds of fodder protein; it is generally less. Although animal products are highly esteemed in most countries, their production is an extravagance when it depends on land or fodder that could have been used to feed people. The extravagance may be tolerated in well-fed countries but not in those that are short of food.

As I have indicated, the world's main food crops need to be supplemented with protein. Peas and beans, which are 25 to 40 percent protein, are traditionally used. Green vegetables and immature flowers are gaining recognition. They can yield 400 pounds of edible protein per acre in a three-to-four-month growing period, but because they contain fiber and other indigestible components a person cannot get more than two or three grams of protein from them in a day. This amount, however, is much more than is normally consumed, and such plants offer a rewarding field for research. The varieties cultivated in industrialized countries are often ill-adapted to other climatic conditions. The work of vegetable improvement that was done in Europe in the 18th and 19th centuries should now be replicated in the wet Tropics. Biochemical control would be needed to ensure that what is being produced is not only nontoxic but also nutritionally valuable. This would be an excellent project for the International Biological Program; the raw materials have worldwide distribution and the need is also worldwide.

The residue that is left when oil is expressed from soya, groundnut, cottonseed and sunflower is now for the most part used as animal feed or fertilizer or is simply discarded. It contains about 20 million tons of protein, that is, twice the world's present estimated deficit. Because its potential value is not yet widely realized, most of this material is at present so contaminated, or damaged by overheating during the expressing of the oil, that it is useless as a source of human food. But methods are being devised, notably in the Indian state of Mysore and in Guatemala, for processing the oilseeds more carefully in order to produce an acceptable food containing 40 to 50 percent protein. The avoidance of damage during processing is not the only problem that arises with oilseeds; each species contains, or may contain, harmful components, for example gossypol in cottonseed, enzyme inhibitors in soya and aflatoxin in peanuts. Gossypol can be extracted or low-gossypol strains of cotton can be used (it is said, however, that these are particularly attractive to insect pests); enzyme inhibitors can be destroyed, and the infestation that produces aflatoxin can be prevented by proper harvesting and storage. The alternative of extracting a purified protein concentrate from the residues is often advocated. This approach seems mistaken; it increases the cost of the protein fivefold. In addition, the process is in the main simply the removal of starch or some other digestible carbohydrate, and carbohydrate has to be added to the protein concentrate again during cooking.

The residue left after expressing oil from an oilseed can be used because it contains little fiber. Coconuts and the leaves from many species of plants are also potential protein sources, but they contain so much fiber that it is essential to separate the protein if more than two or three grams is being eaten each day. The process of separation, although simple, is still in its infancy, and many improvements remain to be made. Units for effecting it are working in Mysore, at the Rothamsted Experimental Station and elsewhere. In wet tropical regions the conventional seed-bearing plants often do not ripen, but coconuts thrive and leaves grow exuberantly. It is in these

TANKS ARE FILLED WITH LITTLE FISH from a truck (*left*) at a fish meal plant in the Peruvian port of Callao. The fish are anchovetas, a variety of anchovy. By grinding and solvent extraction they are converted into a product that contains 80 percent protein.

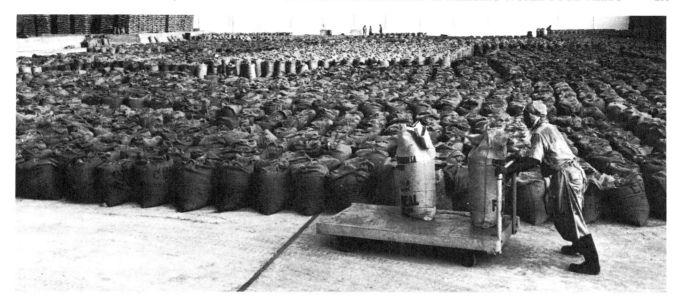

BAGS OF FISH MEAL are piled in the yard of the same plant. Fish meal is currently used primarily as a supplement to feed for domestic animals. In 1965 Peru harvested 7.46 million metric tons of fish, a catch that makes it the world's leading fishing nation.

regions that protein separation has its greatest potentiality.

The protein sources discussed in the last two paragraphs would be opened up by handling conventional agricultural products in unusual ways. Attention is also being given to completely novel forms of production based on photosynthesis by unicellular algae and other microorganisms. The early work was uncritical and, considering the small increases in the rate of fixation of carbon dioxide given by these methods compared with conventional agriculture, the necessary expenditure on equipment was out of proportion. It is an illusion to think that algae have any special photosynthetic capacity. Their merit is that it is much easier to spread an algal suspension, rather than a set of slowly expanding seedlings, uniformly over a sunlit surface so as to make optimal use of the light. Recently more realistic methods, using open tanks and the roofs of greenhouses in which other plants can be grown during the winter, have been tried in Japan and Czechoslovakia. The product resembles leaf protein in many ways but contains more indigestible matter because the algal cell walls are not removed; it may prove possible either to separate the protein from the cell walls or to digest the walls with enzymes.

All the processes discussed so far depend on what might be called current photosynthesis. Microorganisms that do not themselves photosynthesize can produce foodstuffs from the products of photosynthesis in the immediate past (straw, sawdust or the by-product liquor from leaf-protein production) or in the remote past (petroleum, coal or methane). The former substrates would have to be collected over a wide area, whereas the latter are concentrated in a few places and so lend themselves to convenient large-scale industrial processing. At first sight this seems advantageous, and in fact it would be so were we merely concerned with increasing the amount of food in the world. That will be the problem later; now the important thing is, as I have said, to make food where the mouths are, and elaborate and sophisticated techniques are not well adapted to this end. The most valuable aspect of the research now being done in many countries on microbial growth on fossil substrates such as petroleum is that it will familiarize people with the idea of microbial food and so will hasten its acceptance when it is produced from local materials.

Finally, there is synthetic food. Plants make fats and carbohydrates so economically that it is unlikely synthesis could be cheaper. Many of the abundant plant proteins do not have an amino acid composition ideally suited to human needs. These proteins are sometimes complementary, so that the deficiencies of each can be made good by judicious mixing. When this is not possible, the deficient amino acids can be synthesized or made by fermentation and then added to the food. Production of amino acids for this purpose will probably be possible only in industrialized countries; their use may therefore seem to violate the principle that food must be where the mouths are. The quantities needed, however, are small. It is obviously better to upgrade an abundant local protein by adding .5 percent of methionine to it rather than import a whole protein to make up this one deficiency.

The food that is now needed or that will soon be needed in the underprivileged parts of the world might be supplied by charity, by the extension of existing methods of agriculture or by novel processes. I have argued that the first cannot be satisfactory and that it would be dangerous to assume that the second will suffice. Without wishing in any way to minimize the importance of what is being done in these two directions, it seems necessary to take novelties seriously. By definition a novelty is novel. That is to say, it may have an unfamiliar appearance, texture or flavor. In commenting on any of the proposals made— the use of strange animals, oilseed residues or leaf and microbial protein—it is irrelevant to say that they are unfamiliar. If the world is to be properly fed, products such as these will probably have to be used. Our problem is to make them acceptable.

Socrates, when one of his companions said he had learned little by foreign travel, replied: "That is not surprising. You were accompanied by yourself." Similarly, food technologists, accustomed to the dietary prejudices of Europe and the U.S., are apt to project their prejudices onto other communities. They have two opposite obsessions: to fabricate a "chewy" texture in their product and to produce a bland stable powder with an indefinite shelf life. Neither quality is universal in the familiar foods of most of the world. The former may have merits, although these probably do not outweigh the extra difficulties involved. It is odd that, at a time when people in industrialized countries are beginning to revolt against uniform and prepacked foods, we should be bent on foisting the latter quality off on others. Instead, novelties should be introduced into regions where they will most smoothly conform with local culinary habits. Novel forms of fish and mollusks are probably well adapted to Southeast Asia, where fermented fish is popular. Leaf, oilseed or microbial protein would fit smoothly into a culture accustomed to porridge, gruel and curry. It is important to remember the irrational diversity of our tastes. Even in Europe and the U.S. a flavor and appearance unacceptable in an egg is acceptable in cheese, a smell unacceptable in chicken is acceptable in pheasant or partridge, and a flavor unacceptable in wine is acceptable in grapefruit juice. These things are a matter of habit, and habits, although they will not change in a day or even a month, can readily be changed by suitable example and persuasion. The essential first step is to find out what is meant by the word "suitable."

Enough experience is now accumulating for us to define the parameters of success. The four most important are:

First, research on the novelty should be done privately and completely, so that when popularization starts there can be no rationally based doubts about the merits of the product.

Second, the novelty should manifestly be eaten by the innovators themselves. It is folly to ask people to practice what we only preach—we must practice it ourselves.

Third, example is the main factor leading to a change in habits; it is therefore essential to get the support of influential local people—from film stars to political leaders. Care should be taken that the first users are not underprivileged groups (prisoners, refugees and so on), because the stigma will not easily be removed.

Last, an adequate and regular supply of the product should be assured before there is any publicity, because it is hard to reawaken interest that has waned because the product is not obtainable.

All these proposals, except that of the simplest form of agricultural extension, call for research. It is worth considering who should do it and what form opposition is likely to take. Opposition to innovation is an interesting and underinvestigated part of psychopathology. It takes three main forms: total, quasi-logical and "instant."

Total opposition is the denial of the problem. Even today there are those who, in the course of condemning some specific proposal, sometimes deny that a protein shortage exists or is impending. This is a point that should be settled at the very beginning: "Do we have a problem or not?" Fortunately for research, and for humanity, the international agencies are in agreement that we do.

Quasi-logical opposition comes from economists. They may accept the problem but argue that some proposed solutions will be too expensive. There are two relevant questions: "Compared with what?" and "How do you know when it has not been tried?" When there are several equally feasible methods for getting the extra food that is needed in a region, a comparison of their probable costs is obviously worthwhile. But when all costs are, for various reasons, unknown, the exercise becomes futile because assumptions play a larger part in it than rigid economic argument, and scientists are better qualified than economists to make the assumptions; they know more of the facts, are aware of more possibilities and are less subject to romantic illusion.

"Instant opposition" arises because innovators are apt to irritate right-minded people, and enthusiasm invites skepticism. The innovator must therefore expect to run into trouble. When someone made the old comment that genius was an infinite capacity for taking trouble,

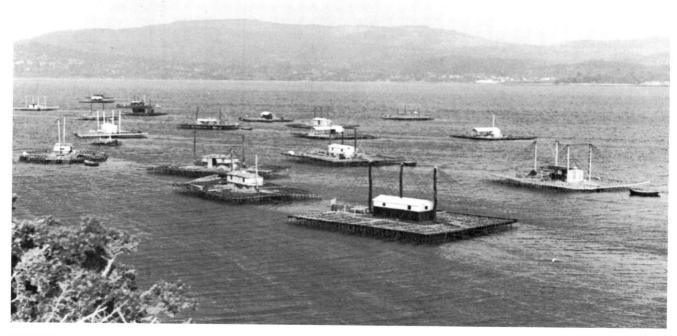

MUSSELS ARE GROWN in this floating "park" in Vigo Bay on the northwestern coast of Spain. Suspended from each of the large anchored raftlike structures are ropes on which the mussels are seeded and grow to maturity (see photograph on opposite page).

Samuel Butler replied: "It isn't. It is an infinite capacity for getting into trouble and for staying in trouble for as long as the genius lasts." In an attenuated form the principle applies even when genius is not involved. There are many different ways of getting into trouble, and it is as naïve and illogical to assume that an idea must be correct because it is meeting opposition as it is to take "instant opposition" seriously.

The governments of countries with a food shortage know that, for a decade at least, more people will be better fed if money is spent on importing food rather than on setting up a research project on means to make more food from local products for local consumption. The more farsighted statesmen realize that ultimately the research will have to be done, but it is hard to resist political pressure, and resistance is hampered by the high cost of primitive agriculture. In a market in New Guinea local sweet potatoes cost three times as much per calorie as imported wheat, and fresh fish cost twice as much per gram of protein as canned fish. So poor countries are hardly likely to mount research projects.

At the other extreme are the giants of private enterprise. They already do very well selling soft drinks and patent foods in underdeveloped countries, and their skill in creating a market, regardless of the real merits of their product, is unrivaled. Thus baby foods, which few experts regard as superior to mother's milk, were used in Uganda by 42 percent of the families in 1959, whereas only 14 percent had used them in 1950. Undoubtedly there are efficient firms that operate with strict integrity, and a few of them have ventured into the production of low-cost protein-rich foods. After the necessary research and preliminary publicity had been done with money from international sources, the Quaker Oats Company has done a masterly job in making, distributing and popularizing Incaparina (maize, sorghum and cottonseed) in Central America. And skilled advertising increased the sales of Pronutro (soya, peanuts and fish) tenfold in two years. Other attempts have failed because the possible profit, when one is selling to poor people without misleading them with meretricious advertising, is too small to cover the costs of the preliminary educational campaign. That, as I have suggested, can be managed only with the cooperation of governments and the local leaders of opinion.

Large-scale private enterprise will probably not find this activity lucrative, and from some points of view the methods of production that would be used may not be desirable. Already more than a third of the world's city population (12 percent of the total population) live in shantytowns on the fringes of cities, and rural depopulation is accelerating. This, together with transport difficulties, makes it at least arguable that research attention should be focused on simple techniques adapted for use in a large village or small town, rather than on fully industrialized techniques. The latter have their place, but they should not become our exclusive concern.

If neither the governments of needy countries nor private enterprise is likely to undertake the necessary research and development, it remains for the governments of industrialized countries, the international agencies and the foundations. So far these groups have been reluctant to admit that any radical changes in research policy will be needed, but times are changing. The novelties are now at least mentioned by the F.A.O. even if only to be gently damned with a few misstatements. On the Barnum principle, "I don't care what people say about me so long as they talk about me," this is a step forward. The governments of wealthy countries supply most of the support for the international agencies, they support other forms of aid, and much knowledge that is of use in poorer countries is an international by-product of their more parochial research. They may feel that they are already doing their share. Our best hope must therefore lie with the foundations. Several institutes of food technology are needed to undertake fundamental and applied research on the production of food from local products for local consumption. At least one of the institutes should be in the wet Tropics and all should give particular attention to protein sources. Using locally available material, each institute should study all the types of raw material discussed here. This will ensure that similar criteria are applied to all of them and that the assessment of their merits is made objectively and is not colored by interinstitutional rivalry. These institutes should also be responsible for work on the presentation and popularization of the products made. It may be that an extension of normal agriculture will meet the world's food needs for a few more years, but ultimately more radical research will be needed. It would be prudent to start it before the need is even more pressing than it is at present.

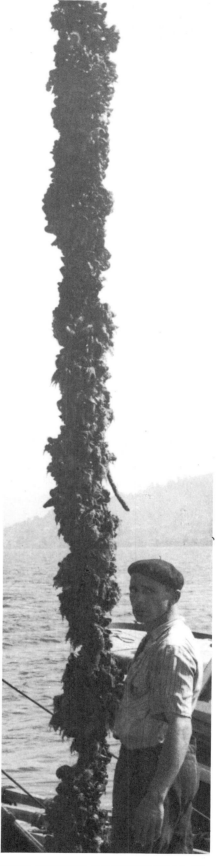

ROPE COVERED WITH MUSSELS is lifted from the water after mussels are mature.

EPILOGUE

The eventual aim of human nutrition is for every person in the world to eat a diet that contributes maximally to health and well-being. As is evident from the articles in this volume, we are still a long way from achieving that aim. Possibly no person now eats a diet that contributes maximally to health. There is, however, an increasing awareness both among individuals and among governments that something must be done to improve nutrition. Fad diets and the current high sales of popular books on nutrition, particularly those advocating exotic diets as a means to improving health, attest to the concern of individuals. Presidential commissions and White House Conferences on Nutrition, and the establishment in 1968 of a U.S. Senate Select Committee on Nutrition and Human Needs, are evidence of increasing public activity in this area. Within the past few years a number of less-developed countries, previously interested primarily in industrial development, have belatedly realized the importance of good nutrition in achieving their aims and have begun to formulate national nutrition policies.

Two complementary areas of nutritional activity must be pursued. One is continued research into man's utilization of and reactions to food and nutrients. The other is development of the technology for making available appropriate diets as well as educational techniques for assuring that people will utilize these diets.

In light of the tragedies of malnutrition throughout the world, many observers believe that simply making sufficient food available is the answer to proper nutrition. In fact, however, there are major economic, political, and cultural barriers to overcome, although it is clear that increased knowledge and appropriate technologic advances will facilitate the process. Certain topics of research have been designated by the National Research Council Study on World Food and Nutrition as having high priority because they are directly applicable to the problem of world hunger. These areas include (1) photosynthesis, (2) biological nitrogen fixation, (3) plant breeding and genetic manipulation, (4) pest control, (5) prevention of post-harvest losses, (6) sources of fertilizer, (7) use of tropical soils, (8) prediction and modification of weather and climate, (9) use of water, (10) use of ruminants, and (11) aquatic food sources. In addition to these areas of research, which rely primarily on science or technology, the Council has established several priority areas for social and political research. These include (1) policies affecting nutrition, (2) market expansion, (3) trade policy, (4) food reserves, and (5) information systems We would add a sixth: sociocultural needs. By now it is universally accepted that any long-term solution to the world food problem, as well as many other global problems, depends on our ability to limit population growth. Research on all aspects of population and reproduction, and especially on how to deal with the burgeoning urban population, should receive highest priority.

Current Knowledge of Human Nutritional Requirements

	Infants			Children			Adults			
	Pre-mature	0-6 months	6-23 months	Pre-school	School Age	Adoles-cent	Young	Aged	Preg-nant	Lacta-ting
Total Energy	O	O	O	O	●	●	●	O	O	O
Carbohydrates:										
Starch										
Sugars	O	O	O	O	O	O	●			
Fibers						O	O			
Total Fat		●								
Essential Fatty Acids		O					O	O		
Protein	●	O	O	O	O	O	●	O	●	O
Amino Acids:										
Arginine		●		O			●			
Histidine	O	●		O			●			
Isoleucine	O	●		O			●			
Leucine	O	●		O			●			
Lysine		●		O			●	O		
Methionine		●		O			●	O		
Phenylalanine		●		O			●			
Threonine		●		O			●	O		
Tryptophan		●		O			●	O		
Valine	O	●		O			●			
Minerals:										
Calcium	●	●	●	O	O	O	●	O	O	O
Magnesium				O	O	O	O			
Iron	●	●	●	●	●	O	●	●	●	●
Phosphorus				O	O				O	O
Sulfur				O	O				O	O
Sodium				O	O		O	O		
Potassium	O	O	O	O	O		O	O		
Copper	O	O		O	O		O			
Molybdenum										
Manganese				O						
Zinc	O	O	O	O	O	O	O		O	O
Chromium				O						
Selenium							O			
Nickel										
Vanadium										
Chlorine										
Fluorine				O	●	O		O		
Iodine				O	O	O	O			
Vitamins:										
Vitamin A	●	●		O	O		●			
Vitamin D	●	●	O	O	O	O				
Vitamin E	O						O			
Vitamin K	O	O						O		
Thiamin	O	O		O	O	O	●	O	O	O
Riboflavin	O	O		O	O	O	●	O	O	O
Niacin							O	O	O	O
Pyridoxine		O					O	O		
Pantothenate							O			
Cobalamin		O					O			
Folic Acid	O	O					O	O	O	
Biotin										
Choline										
Ascorbic Acid	●	●		O	O	O	●	O	O	O

☐ LITTLE OR NO DATA O FRAGMENTARY DATA ● SUBSTANTIAL PROGRESS MADE 1976 DATA

Knowledge of human nutritional requirements as of 1976. (Prepared by the Nutrition Institute, Agricultural Research Service, U.S. Department of Agriculture; courtesy of Dr. J. M. Iacono.)

Contrary to the common view that knowledge in the field of nutritional science was essentially completed with the discovery of the last vitamin or trace element, precise knowledge of human nutrition has many gaps (see the chart on the next page). Successful research in these areas should have as profound an impact on man's health as did the discovery of the essential nutrients. Indeed, we know more about the nutrient requirements for pigs, cattle, and chickens than for man.

The nutritional status of individuals or communities is often used as a basis for making medical or political decisions; yet present techniques for evaluating types of malnutrition other than the obvious case of undernutrition are extremely imprecise. Development of new methodologies for detecting subtle nutritional deficiencies is urgently needed. The long-term effects of modest deficiencies and imbalances or excesses of nutrients need exploration. The role of nonnutrient components of foods, such as fiber content, spices, or additives, should be scientifically documented and not based on anecdotal experience. The specific role of diet in the prevention and therapy of diseases must be better established. With the increased use of potent drugs as therapeutic agents, it has become apparent that some pharmacological agents increase the requirement of specific nutrients while others inhibit metabolism of certain foods. The interaction of drugs and diet is now a promising area of research.

While much of the necessary background knowledge in the above areas can be acquired through the use of experimental animals, the eventual application to man must inevitably involve the use of humans for testing. Until a few years ago the responsibility for using humans as subjects in experiments was left to the individual scientist. In some notorious instances investigators have been overzealous in obtaining scientific results, without giving adequate consideration to possible damage to the individual. Today the decision of whether or not humans may be used in a given study is generally made by committees that include nonscientists and other members of a community. (For a discussion of this problem see "The Ethics of Experimentation with Human Subjects" by B. Barbour, *Scientific American*, February 1976.) There is no question but that concern with the rights of our fellow man as expressed in new regulations dealing with the use of human subjects is highly laudable. However, it may mean that we shall always have to base certain nutritional knowledge, especially that applicable to the fetus and young children, on extrapolation from results obtained in other age groups and with experimental animals.

SUGGESTED GENERAL READINGS

Abelson, Philip H. "Food." *Science*, Vol. 183, No. 4188, (May 9, 1975).

Biosphere. Reprint of *Scientific American*, September 1970. W. H. Freeman, 1970.

Davidson, Stanley, R. Passmore, and J. F. Brock. *Human Nutrition and Dietetics*, 5th ed. Williams and Wilkins, 1972.

Galdston, Iago. *Human Nutrition: Historic and Scientific*. International Universities Press, 1960.

Heiser, Charles B. *Seed to Civilization: The Story of Man's Food*. W. H. Freeman, 1973.

Kallen, David J. *Nutrition, Development and Social Behavior*. U.S. Department of Health, Education, and Welfare Publication No. (NIH) 73-274.

Lehninger, Albert. *Biochemistry*. Worth, 1975.

Mayer, Jean. *Human Nutrition: Its Physiological, Medical, and Social Aspects*. Charles C. Thomas, 1972.

Mayer, Jean. *U.S. Nutrition Policies in the Seventies*. W. H. Freeman, 1973.

Recommended Dietary Allowances, 8th ed. Food and Nutrition Board, National Research Council, National Academy of Sciences, 1974.

Robson, John R. K. *Malnutrition: Its Causation and Control*, 2 vols. Gordon and Breach, 1972.

Sauer, Carl. O. *Seeds, Spades, Hearths, and Herds: The Domestication of Animals and Foodstuffs*. MIT Press, 1969.

Siu, R. G. H. *et al.* "Evaluation of Health Aspects of GRAS Food Ingredients: Lessons Learned and Questions Unanswered." *Federation Proceedings*, 36:2519–2561, 1977.

World Food and Nutrition Study. Steering Committee, Study on World Food and Nutrition of the Commission on International Relations, National Research Council, National Academy of Sciences, 1977.

BIBLIOGRAPHIES

I NUTRITION AND THE FLOW OF ENERGY AND MATTER

1. How Cells Transform Energy

ENERGY RECEPTION AND TRANSFER. Melvin Calvin. In *Biophysical Science—A Study Program*, edited by J. L. Oncley *et al.*, pages 147–156. Wiley, 1959.

FREE ENERGY AND THE BIOSYNTHESIS OF PHOSPHATES. M. R. Atkinson and R. K. Morton, In *Comparative Biochemistry*, edited by Marcel Florkin and Howard S, Mason, Vol II, pages 1–95. Academic Press, 1960.

RESPIRATORY-ENERGY TRANSFORMATION. Albert L. Legninger. In *Biophysical Science—A Study Program*, edited by J. L. Oncley *et al.*, pages 136–146. Wiley, 1959.

2. Biological Nitrogen Fixation

THE BIOLOGY OF NITROGEN FIXATION. Edited by A. Quispel. North Holland, 1974.

SURVEY OF NITROGENASE AND ITS EPR PROPERTIES: A COMPREHENSIVE TREATISE. R. H. Burris, and W. H. Orme-Johnson. In *Microbial Iron Metabolism*, edited by J. B. Neilands. Academic Press, 1974.

NITROGEN FIXATION IN BACTERIA AND HIGHER PLANTS. R. C Burns and R. W. F. Hardy. Springer-Verlag, 1975.

REGULATION AND GENETICS OF BACTERIAL NITROGEN FIXATION. Winston J. Brill. In *Annual Review of Microbiology*, Vol. 29, 1975, pages 109–129.

3. From Cave to Village

REPORT OF ROBERT J. BRAIDWOOD ON WORK IN NORTHERN IRAQ. *American Journal of Archaeology*, Vol. 56, No. 1 (January 1952), pages 47–49.

4. The Cycles of Plant and Animal Nutrition

THE NATURE AND PROPERTIES OF SOILS. Harry O. Buckman and Nyle C. Brady. Macmillan, 1960.

ENERGY EXCHANGE IN THE BIOSPHERE. David M. Gates. Harper & Row, 1962.

ANIMAL NUTRITION. Leonard A. Maynard and John K. Loosli. McGraw-Hill, 1969.

NUTRIENT REQUIREMENTS OF DOMESTIC ANIMALS: NUTRIENT REQUIREMENTS OF BEEF CATTLE (1970), DAIRY CATTLE (1971), POULTRY (1971), SWINE (1973), SHEEP (1975). National Academy of Sciences.

AGRICULTURAL PRODUCTION AND ENERGY RESOURCES. G. H. Heichel. In *American Scientist*, Vol. 64 No. 1 (January–February, 1976), pages 64–72.

5. Human Food Production as a Process in the Biosphere

MALNUTRITION AND NATIONAL DEVELOPMENT. Alan D. Berg. In *Foreign Affairs*, Vol. 46, No. 1 (October, 1967), pages 126–136.

ON THE SHRED OF A CLOUD. Rolf Edberg. Translated by Sven Ahmån. University of Alabama Press, 1969.

POLITICS AND ENVIRONMENT: A READER IN ECOLOGICAL CRISIS. Edited by Walt Anderson. Goodyear, 1970.

POPULATION, RESOURCES, ENVIRONMENT: ISSUES IN HUMAN ECOLOGY. Paul R. Ehrlich and Anne H. Erlich. W. H. Freeman, 1970.

SEEDS OF CHANGE: THE GREEN REVOLUTION AND DEVELOPMENT IN THE 1970's. Lester R. Brown. Praeger, 1970.

II MAN'S FOOD

6. The Plants and Animals That Nourish Man

THE DOMESTICATION AND EXPLOITATION OF PLANTS AND ANIMALS. Edited by P. J. Ucko and D. W. Dimbleby. Aldine, 1969.

PALAEOETHNOBOTANY: THE PREHISTORIC FOOD PLANTS OF THE NEAR EAST AND EUROPE. Jane M. Renfrew. Columbia University Press, 1973.

CROPS AND MAN. Jack R. Harlan. American Society of Agronomy, 1975.

7. Wheat

THE ORIGIN, VARIATION, IMMUNITY AND BREEDING OF CULTIVATED PLANTS. Nikolai I. Vavilov. Chronica Botanica, 1951.

THE WHEAT PLANT. John Percival. Duckworth, 1921.

8. Cattle

BREEDING LIVESTOCK ADAPTED TO UNFAVORABLE ENVIRONMENTS. Ralph W. Phillips. FAO Agricultural Studies No. 1, 1948.

THE CATTLE OF INDIA. Ralph W. Phillips in *Journal of Heredity*, Vol. 35, No. 9 (September, 1944), pages 273–288.

FLAYING AND CURING OF HIDES AND SKINS AS A RURAL INDUSTRY. A. Aten, R. Faraday Innes and E. Knew. FAO Agricultural Development Paper No. 49, 1955.

YEARBOOK OF FOOD AND AGRICULTURAL STATISTICS, 1955. Vol. 9, PART 1: PRODUCTION. Food and Agriculture Organization of the United Nations, 1956.

YEARBOOK OF FOOD AND AGRICULTURAL STATISTICS, 1955. Vol. 10, PART 1: PRODUCTION. Food and Agriculture Organization of the United Nations, 1957.

9. Milk

PRINCIPLES OF DAIRY CHEMISTRY. Robert Jenness and Stuart Patton. Wiley, 1959.

MILK: THE MAMMARY GLAND AND ITS SECRETION. Edited by S. K. Kon and A. T. Cowie. Academic Press, 1961.

MILK PROTEINS. H. A. Mc Kenzie, In *Advance in Protein Chemistry*, Vol. 22, edited by C. B. Anfinsen, Jr., M. L. Anson, John T. Edsall and Frederic M. Richards, 1967, pages 55–234.

THE ROLE OF THE PLASMA MEMBRANE IN THE SECRETION OF MILK FAT. Stuart Patton and Frederick M. Fowkes in *Journal of Theoretical Biology*, Vol. 15, No. 3 (June, 1967), pages 274–281.

10. Captain Bligh and the Breadfruit

A VOYAGE TO THE SOUTH SEAS. William Bligh. Published by permission of the Lords Commissioners of the Admiralty. Printed for George Nicol, Bookseller to His Majesty, Pall-Mall, 1792.

III SELECTION OF FOOD AND ITS INFLUENCE UPON HUMAN BEHAVIOR

11. Food Additives

FOOD STANDARDS COMMITTEE REPORTS. Great Britain Ministry of Agriculture, Fisheries and Food. Her Majesty's Stationery Offie London.

REPORTS OF THE CODEX COMMITTEE ON FOOD ADDITIVES. Food and Agriculture Organization of the United Nations, Rome.

REPORTS OF THE JOINT FAO/IAEA/WHO EXPERT COMMITTEE ON FOOD IRRADIATION. Food and Agriculture Organization of the United Nations, Rome.

REPORTS OF THE JOINT FAO/WHO EXPERT COMMITTEE ON FOOD ADDITIVES. Food and Agriculture Organization of the United Nations, Rome.

HANDBOOK OF FOOD ADDITIVES. Edited by Thomas E. Furia. The Chemical Rubber Co., 1968.

12. The Social Influence of the Potato

THE HISTORY AND SOCIAL INFLUENCE OF THE POTATO. Redcliffe N. Salaman. Cambridge University Press, 1949.

13. The Social Influence of Salt

CAUSES AND CONSEQUENCES OF SALT CONSUMPTION. Hans Kaunitz in *Nature*, Vol. 178, No. 4543 (November 24, 1956), pages 1141–1144.

SALT AND THE SALT INDUSTRY. Albert F. Calvert. Pitman & Sons, 1919.

SODIUM CHLORIDE: THE PRODUCTION AND PROPERTIES OF SALT AND BRINE. Edited by Dale W. Kaufmann. Reinhold, 1960.

14. Lactose and Lactase

A RACIAL DIFFERENCE IN INCIDENCE OF LACTASE DEFICIENCY. Theodore M. Bayless and Norton S. Rosensweig in *The Journal of the American Medical Association*, Vol. 197, No. 12 (September 19, 1966), pages 968–972.

MILK. Stuart Patton. In *Scientific American*, Vol. 221, No. 1 (July, 1969), pages 58–68.

PRIMARY ADULT LACTOSE INTOLERANCE AND THE MILKING HABIT: A PROBLEM IN BIOLOGIC AND CULTURAL INTERRELATIONS. II: A CULTURAL HISTORICAL HYPOTHESIS. Frederick J. Simoons. In *The American Journal of Digestive Diseases*, Vol. 15, No. 8 (August, 1970), pages 695–710.

LACTASE DEFICIENCY: AN EXAMPLE OF DIETARY EVOLUTION. R. D. McCracken in *Current Anthropology*, Vol. 12, No. 4–5 (October–December, 1971), pages 479–517.

MEMORIAL LECTURE: LACTOSE AND LACTASE—A HISTORICAL PERSPECTIVE. Norman Kretchmer. In *Gastroenterology*, Vol. 61, No. 6 (December, 1971), pages 805–813.

IV NUTRIENTS REQUIRED BY MAN AND THEIR UTILIZATION

15. Biotin

BIOTIN AND BACTERIAL GROWTH. I: RELATION TO ASPARTATE, OLEATE AND CARBON DIOXIDE. Harry P. Broquist and Esmond E. Snell. In *The Journal of Biological Chemistry*, Vol. 188, No. 1, (January, 1951), pages 431–444.

THE CHEMISTRY OF BIOTIN. Donald B. Melville. In *Vitamins and Hormones* Vol. 2 (1944), pages 29–69.

EVIDENCE FOR THE PARTICIPATION OF BIOTIN IN THE ENZYMIC SYNTHESIS OF FATTY ACIDS. Salih J. Wakil, Edward B. Titchener and David M. Gibson. In *Biochimica et Biophysica Acta*, Vol. 29, No. 1 (July, 1958), pages 225–226.

POSSIBLE BIOCHEMICAL IMPLICATIONS OF THE CRYSTAL STRUCTURE OF BIOTIN. W. Traub. In *Science*, Vol. 129, No. 3343 (January 23, 1959), page 210.

16. The Chemical Elements of Life

TRACE ELEMENTS IN BIOCHEMISTRY. H. J. M. Bowen. Academic Press, 1966.

CONTROL OF *Environmental* CONDITIONS IN TRACE ELEMENT RESEARCH: AN EXPERIMENTAL APPROACH TO UNRECOGNIZED TRACE ELEMENT REQUIREMENTS. Klaus Schwarz, In *Trace Element Metabolism in Animals*, edited by C. F. Mills. E & S. Livingstone, 1970.

THE PROTEINS: METALLOPROTEINS, VOL V. Edited by Bert L. Vallee and Warren E. C. Wacker. Academic Press, 1970.

CERULOPLASMIN: A LINK BETWEEN COPPER AND IRON METABOLISM. Earl Frieden. In *Bioinorganic Chemistry*, Advances in Chemistry Series 100. American Chemical Society, 1971.

TRACE ELEMENTS IN HUMAN AND ANIMAL NUTRITION. E. J. Underwood, Academic Press, 1971.

17. The Requirements of Human Nutrition

RECOMMENDED DIETARY ALLOWANCES. Food and Nutrition Board, National Research Council. National Academy of Sciences, 1974.

DIETARY STANDARDS. D. Mark Hegsted. In *Journal of the American Dietetic Association*, Vol. 66, No. 1 (January, 1976), pages 13–21.

SHATTUCK LECTURE—STRENGTHS AND WEAKNESSES OF THE COMMITTEE APPROACH: AN ANALYSIS OF PAST AND PRESENT RECOMMENDED DIETARY ALLOWANCES FOR PROTEIN IN HEALTH AND DISEASE. Nevin S. Scrimshaw. In *The New England Journal of Medicine*, Vol. 294, No. 3 (January 15, 1976), pages 136–142; No. 4 (January 22, 1976), pages 198–203.

18. Total Intravenous Feeding

GROWTH OF PUPPIES RECEIVING ALL NUTRITIONAL REQUIREMENTS BY VEIN. Stanley J. Dudrick, Harry M. Vars and Jonathan E. Rhoads. In *Fortschritte der parenteralen Ernährung*. Symposium of the International Society of Parenteral Nutrition, 1966; West Germany, 1967.

GROWTH AND DEVELOPMENT OF AN INFANT RECEIVING ALL NUTRIENTS EXCLUSIVELY BY VEIN. Douglas W. Wilmore and Stanley J. Dudrick. In *Journal of the American Medical Association*, Vol. 203, No. 10 (March 4, 1968), pages 860–864.

LONG TERM TOTAL PARENTERAL NUTRITION WITH GROWTH, DEVELOPMENT, AND POSITIVE NITROGEN BALANCE. Stanley J. Dudrick, Douglas W. Wilmore, Harry M. Vars, and Jonathan E. Rhoads. In *Surgery*, Vol. 64, No. 1 (July, 1968), pages 134–142.

CONTINUOUS LONG-TERM INTRAVENOUS INFUSION IN UNRESTRAINED ANIMALS. S. J. Dudrick, E. Steiger D. W. Wilmore and H. M. Vars. In *Laboratory Animal Care*, Vol. 20 (1970), pages 521–529.

INTRAVENOUS HYPERALIMENTATION. Stanley J. Dudrick and Jonathan E. Rhoads. In *Critical Surgical Illness*, edited by James D. Hardy. Saunders, 1971.

19. Prostaglandins

NOBEL SYMPOSIUM 2: PROSTAGLANDINS. Edited by Sune Bergström and Bengt Samuelsson. Wiley, 1967.

PROSTAGLANDINS: A REPORT ON EARLY CLINICAL STUDIES. J. W. Hinman. In *Postgraduate Medical Journal*, Vol. 46, No. 539 (September, 1970), pages 562–575.

NON-STEROIDAL ANTIFERTILITY AGENTS IN THE FEMALE N. Wiqvist, M. Bygdeman and K. T. Kirton. In *Nobel Symposium 15: Control of Human Fertility*, edited by Egon Diczfalusy and Ulf Borell. Wiley, 1971.

PROSTAGLANDINS. Edited by Peter W. Ramwell and Jane E. Shaw. In *Annals of the New York Academy of Sciences*, Vol. 180 (April 30, 1971).

V IMPACT OF DIET ON HUMAN HEALTH AND DISEASE

20. Rickets

THE ETIOLOGY OF RICKETS. Edwards A. Park. In *Physiological Reviews*, Vol. 3, No. 1 (January, 1923), pages 106–163.

RICKETS INCLUDING OSTEOMALACIA AND TETANY. Alfred F. Hess. Lea & Febiger, 1929.

INVESTIGATIONS ON THE ETIOLOGY OF RICKETS VITAMIN D. Elmer Verner McCollum. In *A History of Nutrition: The Sequence of Ideas in Nutritional Investigations*. Houghton Mifflin, 1957.

SKIN-PIGMENT REGULATION OF VITAMIN-D BIOSYNTHESIS IN MAN. W. Farnsworth Loomis. In *Science* Vol. 157, No. 3788 (August 4, 1967), pages 501–506.

21. Night Blindness

THE BIOLOGICAL FUNCTION OF VITAMIN A ACID. John E. Dowling and George Wald. In *Proceedings of the National Academy of Sciences*, Vol. 46, No. 5 (May 15, 1960), pages 587–616.

INHERITED RETINAL DYSTROPHY IN THE RAT. John E. Dowling and Richard L. Sidman. In *The Journal of Cell Biology*, Vol. 14, No. 1 (July, 1962), pages 73–109.

VITAMIN A. Thomas Moore. Elsevier, 1957.

22. Endemic Goiter

ETIOLOGY AND PREVENTION OF SIMPLE GOITER. David Marine in *Medicine*, Vol. 3, No. 4 (November, 1924), pages 453–479.

THYROXINE. Edward C. Kendall. Chemical Catalog Company, Inc., 1929.

ENDEMIC GOITRE. World Health Organization Monograph Series No. 44. World Health Organization, 1960.

THE THYROID GLAND. Rulon W. Rawson in *Clinical Symposia, Ciba Pharmaceutical Company*, Vol. 17, No. 2 (April–May–June, 1965), pages 35–63.

23. Atherosclerosis

ATHEROMA LESIONS. *Cardiovascular Pathology; Vol 1.* Reginald E. B. Hudson. Williams and Wilkins, 1965.

EPIDEMIOLOGY OF CARDIOVASCULAR DISEASES: METHODOLOGY. Edited by Herbert Pollack and Dean E. Krueger. Supplement to *American Journal of Public Health and the Nation's Health*, Vol. 50, No. 10 (October, 1960).

THE ETIOLOGY OF MYOCARDIAL INFARCTION. Edited by Thomas N. James and John W. Keyes. Henry Ford Hospital International Symposium. Little, Brown, 1963.

METABOLISM AND STRUCTURE OF THE ARTERIAL WALL IN ATHEROSCLEROSIS. Abel L. Robertson, Jr., in *Cleveland Clinic Quarterly*, Vol. 32, No. 3 (July, 1965), pages 99–117.

PROBLEMS IN THE STUDY OF CORONARY ATHEROSCLEROSIS IN POPULATION GROUPS. David M. Spain. In *Annals of the New York Academy of Sciences*, Vol. 84, Article 17 (December 8, 1960), pages 816–834.

VI THE GLOBAL PROBLEM OF HUMAN NUTRITION

24. The Dimensions of Human Hunger

FOOD AND POPULATION: THE WRONG PROBLEM? Jean Mayer in *Daedalus,* Vol. 93, No. 3 (Summer, 1964), pages 830–844.

THE NUTRITION FACTOR: ITS ROLE IN DEVELOPMENT. Alan Berg. Brookings Institution. 1973.

NUTRITION. *Science,* Vol. 188, No. 4188 (May 9, 1975), pages 557–577.

THE WORLD FOOD PROSPECT. Lester R. Brown in *Science,* Vol. 190, No. 4219 (December 12, 1975), pages 1053–1059.

25. The Human Population

THE NEXT HUNDRED YEARS: MAN'S NATURAL AND TECHNICAL RESOURCES. Harrison Brown, James Bonner, and John Weir. Viking, 1957.

POPULATION AHEAD. Roy Gustaf Francis. University of Minnesota Press, 1958.

SCIENCE AND ECONOMIC DEVELOPMENT: NEW PATTERNS OF LIVING. Richard L. Meier. Wiley 1956.

WORLD POPULATION AND PRODUCTION: TRENDS AND OUTLOOK. W. S. Woytinsky and E. S. Woytinsky. Twentieth Century Fund, 1953.

26. Orthodox and Unorthodox Methods Of Meeting World Food Needs

THE STATE OF FOOD AND AGRICULTURE 1966. Food and Agriculture Organization of the United Nations. Rome, 1966.

INDEX